An Introduction to Clinical Research for Health and Social Care Professionals

Ario Santini, **Kenneth** A Eaton

authorHOUSE°

AuthorHouse™ UK
1663 Liberty Drive
Bloomington, IN 47403 USA
www.authorhouse.co.uk
Phone: UK TFN: 0800 0148641 (Toll Free inside the UK)
*   UK Local: (02) 0369 56322 (+44 20 3695 6322 from outside the UK)*

Published by AuthorHouse   05/20/2022

ISBN: 978-1-6655-9751-7 (sc)
ISBN: 978-1-6655-9750-0 (e)

Principal Authors

Ario Santini Doc (hc), BDS, DDS (Univ. Edin), PhD; FDS RCPS Glasgow.; FDS RCS Eng.; DipFMed, (Univ Glasg) DGDP, DipFFGDP, FCGDent, FADM. Professor Postgraduate Studies, George Emil Palade University of Medicine and Pharmacy Science and Technology of Targu Mures, Romania; former director of biomaterial research and senior lecturer, the University of Edinburgh; Honorary Fellow, The University of Edinburgh.

Kenneth A. Eaton BDS, MSc, PhD, MGDS RCS (Eng.), FFGDP (UK) (hon), FCGDent, FFPH, FHEA, FICD, FNCUP, DHC. Visiting Professor University College London, Honorary Professor University of Kent. Chair, British Dental Editors and Writers Forum.

Contributing Authors

I Blum DDS, PhD, Dr Med Dent, MSc, MFDS RCs (Eng.), MFDS RCS (Edin), FDS (REST Dent) RCS (Eng.), FFGDP(UK), PGCHE, FCGDent, FHEA, LLM. Consultant and Specialist in Restorative Dentistry, King's College Hospital, Reader in Primary Dental Care & Advanced General Dental Practice, Faculty of Dentistry, Oral & Craniofacial Sciences, King's College, London.

Roger Farbey OBE Immediate Past Head Librarian British Dental Association.

Mark-Steven Howe BDS DGDP (UK) MGDS RCS (Eng.) MSc(Oxon) FFGDP(UK) General Dental Practitioner, Doctoral Researcher, Peninsula Dental School, University of Plymouth.

Nicola R. Palmer BA, MA, PGCert, Research Ethics and Governance Manager, University of Kent.

Debbie Reed Ed (D) MSc, PGCHE, BA(Hons) Cert Ed FHEA, Chartered MCIPD, GCGI, ANCUP. Department of Digital and Lifelong Learning, University of Kent.

Derek Richards BDS, MSc, DDPH RCS, FDSRCPS, FDS(DPH)RCPS. Director, Centre for Evidence-based Dentistry and Senior Lecturer, School of Dentistry, University of Dundee, UK.

Jeanie Suvan DipDH, MSc, CRA, FHEA, PhD, Clinical Research Coordinator, Associate Professor and Programme Director DH MSc, UCL Eastman Dental Institute, Unit of Periodontology, 21 University Street, London WC1E 6DE,

Laura Wiles BA (Hons), Scientific Manuscript Editor, Basel, Switzerland.

Acknowledgements

The principal authors thank the contributing authors for their work and support in the production of this book. Without them, it would have been difficult to write. They also thank Yann Maidment and Ian Mills for reviewing the first draft and for their comments and advice. Paul Batchelor and Vishal Aggarwal are also thanked for reviewing the next draft and for their helpful comments.

Contents

Chapter 1. The Need for Practice-Based Research

EATON K.A., SANTINI A.

1.1. Overview

This chapter explains the need for practice-based research and describes how this publication aims to explain the principles and practices of research to first-time or early researchers. It then considers the need to critically appraise literature before carrying out a research project and introduces readers to the different stages of research, which are then described. It also stresses the need for patient and public involvement (PPI) and recognises that other potential stakeholders, including commissioners, governmental organizations, and education providers. such the Health Education England, corporate bodies, and others are also important when planning and funding research.

1.2. The need for practice-based research

In the United Kingdom, the importance of evidence-informed professional practice is well established. Such evidence comes from research. If the research is clinical or work-based, instead of laboratory-based, it should ideally be carried out at work, where the care or services is provided. Translation of research from one setting to another can be justified but may dilute the strength of the evidence and lead to errors of judgement. For example, because more than 90 per cent of oral healthcare is provided in a primary dental-care setting, it is logical that much research should take place in dental practices to reflect the setting, the environment, and the circumstances in which care is likely to be delivered. The vast majority of research has hitherto taken place in universities, research institutes, medical and dental schools, secondary-care facilities and laboratories. and the inherent weakness in this situation has been acknowledged.[1]

A survey of general dental practitioners (GDPs) in 2005[2] found that, although they appreciated the importance of research for providing evidence to improve patients' care, only a small percentage had been involved in research. Nevertheless, the majority were interested in taking part, and just under half thought that research in primary care should be performed by those working in this area.

A survey of Irish primary care clinicians found that "Despite awareness of the importance of R&D in primary care and investment therein, primary healthcare professionals remain largely unengaged with the R&D process. This study highlights the issues that need to be addressed in order to encourage a shift towards a culture of R&D in primary care: lack of research training particularly in basic research skills and increased opportunities for research involvement."[3]

In 2007, to help oral healthcare professionals acquire a basic understanding of the different aspects of research, the Faculty of General Dental Practice (UK) (FGDP [UK]) commissioned the production of a series of research leaflets. Between 2010 and 2012, the content of these leaflets was expanded, and the resulting nine papers were published in *Primary Dental Care* in London.

The series provided an overview of the different stages in a research project and the relevance to primary dental care. It introduced readers to the basic principles of research methodology but did not provide an in-depth review of all aspects of research. This new publication aims to address this task and to provide a source of information for all healthcare and social-care professionals, not just dental ones. Thus, although some of the examples in this publication relate to oral healthcare, it provides an introduction to workplace/professional practice-based research for any healthcare or social-care professional who is undertaking research for the first time or is an early researcher.

1.3. Evidence-based practice and critical appraisal of the literature

Understanding the principles of evidence-based practice and skills in critically appraising literature is key before embarking on research. This topic is therefore covered in chapter 2.

1.4. The stages of a research project

After Chapter 2, the following chapters cover the ten stages of a research project, which are:

1. The initial idea (asking a research question);
2. Searching the literature;
3. Refining the research question
4. Designing the study;
5. Writing a protocol;
6. Obtaining ethics approval and funding;
7. Piloting the methodology and project management;
8. Collecting data;
9. Analysing the data; and
10. Writing and disseminating the results.

The first three stages are covered in Chapter 3. Stage 4 has many aspects and is covered in eight chapters (4,5,6,7,8,9,10,11). Apart from obtaining ethics approval and funding, which are split into two chapters (13 and 14), the other stages are each covered in one chapter. At the end of the publication, appendices on guidelines and checklists, a glossary of terms and further details of the apprenticeship scheme provide further information to complement the 18 chapters. Chapters are written to be read, in the main, without the need to turn to other chapters. This inevitably produces minor duplication of material. Readers should also note that the content of the chapters is presented in several different ways, which their authors felt to be appropriate, some with multiple tables and others in a more narrative style. It should be stressed that this publication is an introduction to research and, as such, does not seek to go into the different facets of research in-depth. However, each chapter signposts readers to other publications, both in hard copy and online, to enable them to find further information.

References

1   R&D in Primary Care—National Working Group Report. UK Department of Health, Leeds, November 1997. Catalogue no. 97CC0138.

2   Palmer N.O.A and Grieveson B. "An Investigation into Merseyside general dental practitioners' interest in primary care research, their views on research and their training needs," *Primary Dental Care*, 2005 Oct;12(4):145–149.

3   Glynn, L., O'Riordan, C., MacFarlane A. et al. "Research activity and capacity in primary healthcare: the REACH study: a survey," *BMC Family Practice* 2009, 10:33

Chapter 2. Evidence-Based Practice and Critical Appraisal of Literature

SANTINI A., HOWE M-S.

2.1. Overview

Before taking part in any research, it is essential to understand the principles of evidence-based practice (EBP) and how to critically appraise literature. This chapter aims to provide readers with an understanding of these topics and suggest where they may deepen their knowledge. It should also help them assess (grade) the strength of evidence to support the different aspects of their clinical practice.

2.2. What is evidence-based practice?

One of the best and earliest examples of evidence-based practice is Florence Nightingale's work during the Crimean War (1853–56). Having observed the unsanitary conditions and suffering of the casualties under her care, she undertook some simple research regarding her patients' basic hygiene, applied careful statistical analysis to the results, and improved her patients' outcomes.[1]

To communicate the high number of unnecessary deaths, she created, with the help of William Farr, her famous "rose diagram," which was instrumental in the passing of the strict 1875 Public Health Act.

From its humble beginnings, practice evolved from an evidence-based model where seniority, fashion, and personal opinion directed clinical practice.[2] True evidence-based medicine began in 1972 with Archie Cochrane's book, *Effectiveness and Efficiency: Random Reflections on Health Services.*[3]

By the mid-1990s, the use of clinical evidence received formal recognition when Sackett et al. (1996) defined it this way:

> Evidence-based medicine is the conscientious, explicit, and judicious use of current best evidence in making decisions about the care of individual patients. The practice of evidence-based medicine means integrating individual clinical expertise with the best available external clinical evidence from systematic research. The term individual clinical expertise can be defined as the proficiency and judgment that individual clinicians acquire through clinical experience and clinical practice. Increased expertise is reflected in many ways, especially in more effective and efficient diagnosis and in the more thoughtful identification and

4

compassionate use of individual patients' predicaments, rights, and preferences in making clinical decisions about their care. Best available external clinical evidence, is derived from clinically relevant research, often in the basic sciences of medicine, but especially from patient-centred clinical research into the accuracy and precision of diagnostic tests (including the clinical examination), the power of prognostic markers, and the efficacy and safety of therapeutic, rehabilitative, and preventive regimens. External clinical evidence invalidates previously accepted diagnostic tests and treatments and replaces them with new ones that are more powerful, more accurate, more efficacious, and safer.[4]

These principles were not meant to be exclusive to medicine. The use of the term evidence-based had by then already migrated into clinical practice and nursing and appeared in the *British Dental Journal* as an opinion paper as early as 1995.[5]

Since then, the principles of EPB have been accepted by many professions other than those involved in healthcare.

The basic principles and benefits of EBP are summarised in Table 1.

What is evidence-based practice?	Benefits of evidence-based practice
It is the use of current best evidence in making decisions about the care of individual patients. Practitioners closely consider what they are doing.	Patients are being offered the best treatment. Treatment decisions are easier to justify.

Table 1. Basic principles and benefits of evidence-based practice (EBP)

The approach to evidenced-based practice can be summarised in four stages:

1. The formulation of a precise, structured, clinical question about an aspect of patient management;
2. A literature search, and articles which may address or answer the question;
3. The subsequently appraised evidence; and
4. Monitoring changes and repeating the whole process. Audits and surveys may be used to corroborate the findings.

Stages 1,2 and 3 are addressed in chapter 3.

2.3. What is clinical expertise, and how does it fit into EBP?

Sackett et al. (1996) defined clinical expertise as "The proficiency and judgment that individual clinicians acquire through clinical experience and clinical practice."[4] The problem with this early definition is that it does not address the original reason evidence-based medicine was conceived in the first place—namely, to put knowledge in the place of unchallenged wisdom based on power in the form of seniority or eminence within an organisation.[6] Also, the quantity of experience a clinician possesses cannot be the only criterion that defines expertise but should also encompass the quality of the discipline being practised.

Expertise-based evidence presented in opinion papers, anecdotal reports, editorials, or case reports is placed at the bottom of the hierarchy of evidence pyramid as it is the most susceptible to bias (see Figure 2). The conventional model identifies clinical expertise as an internal component of the evidence-gathering process.

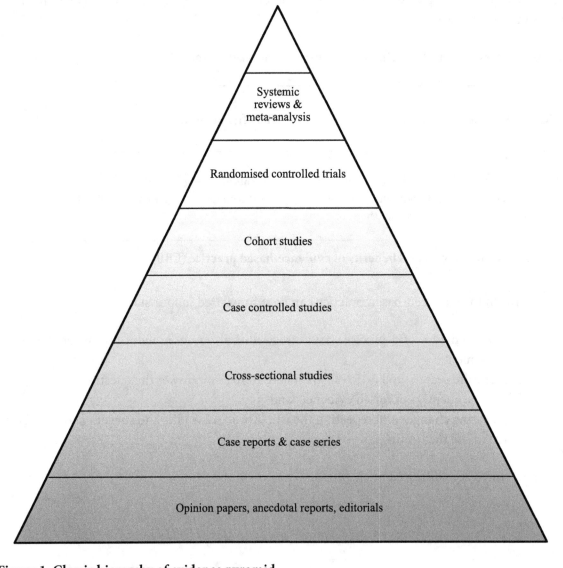

Figure 1. Classic hierarchy of evidence pyramid

The second definition of expertise was presented by Haynes (2002):

> Clinical expertise includes the general basic skills of clinical practice and the experience of the individual practitioner. In addition, clinical expertise must encompass and balance the patient's clinical state and circumstances, relevant research evidence, and the patient's preferences and actions if a successful and satisfying result is to occur.[6]

The basic skills and experience are obtained in practice. Helpful information can only be obtained in practice by the use of appropriate and robust clinical studies. These studies and their strengths and weaknesses are outlined in this chapter.

The best available research evidence comes from externally sourced, clinically relevant research from the basic sciences and patient-centred clinical research studies. This external clinical evidence appraises formerly accepted diagnostic tests and treatments and supersedes them with more powerful, accurate, successful, and safer modalities.

This concept is presented in Figure 2

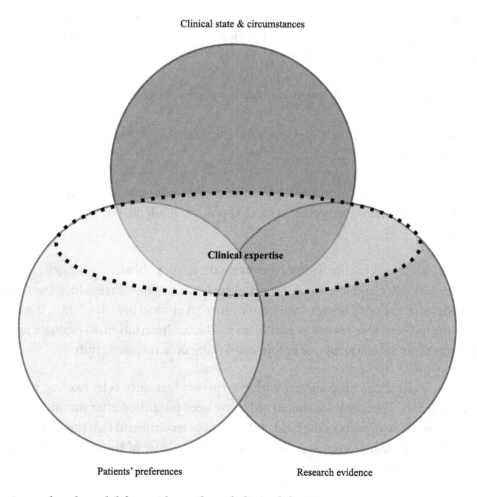

Figure 2. An updated model for evidence-based clinical decisions

The clinical state and circumstances *domain* refers to the clinical setting, facilities available to the patients and clinician, or the practicality of access to healthcare. Clinical expertise now sits outside the evidence process. It expands the role of clinical expertise to balance and integrate the three domains of clinical state, patient preferences, and research evidence.

One additional consideration regarding clinical expertise is that it can be divided into two groups, which separates clinicians wishing to undertake EBP from researchers:[7, 8]

Contributory expertise is held by those who know enough about the subject to make an original contribution to that domain.

Interactional expertise requires that a would-be expert discusses a particular domain's details so they are not conversationally separable from a contributory expert. However, they do not know enough to make an original contribution to the domain in question.

2.4. Critical appraisal

Once a research question has been developed, a search strategy created, and the literature search completed (see chapter 3), the clinician must critically appraise the results. Buccheri and Sharifi (2017) cited two definitions of critical appraisal:[9]

1. an objective, structured approach that results in a better understanding of a study's strengths and weaknesses;[10]
2. to identify evidence that comes from rigorous, reliable, unbiased, and methodologically appropriate research.[11]

Findings may be challenging to integrate into clinical practice as real-life practice seldom mirrors the ideal research situations. However, critical appraisal, if adequately undertaken, can detect flaws in studies.

Critical appraisal refers to the systematic evaluation of published research regarding its appropriateness, validity, and relevance. A critical evaluation of the current literature is necessary for a comprehensive understanding of the basis of current clinical practice. Thus, it is essential to undertake a formal literature review as part of an academic dissertation, to evaluate new or novel clinical innervations or treatments, or before embarking on a research study.

The primary way clinicians keep abreast with the current literature is by reading peer-reviewed professional journals. The literature should only have been published after submitted papers were refereed by two or more experts in the field. Referees may recommend that the paper be redrafted and resubmitted, rejected, or even accepted unchanged. Because of this process, the journal can maintain a reputation for publishing new, reliable, high-quality research.

However, the reader must never forget that evidence presented in published papers may not be robust despite peer review. Many will contain errors in methodology, statistical analyses, and their conclusions. Furthermore, because of the production time for books, audiotapes and videotapes, and CDs, these are less likely to have up-to-date information. They also may suffer from author bias.

No one study is likely to obtain results sufficient to merit a hypothesis or clinical technique's acceptance or rejection. Therefore, the relevant published papers on the topic need to be evaluated critically, and individual papers need to be appraised and weighed in the context of the overall knowledge pool. Critical analyses of all documents and other sources of information is essential.

The main issue is time, with thousands of health sciences-related studies being published every year. However, the online journals and resources listed at the end of this chapter, such as Evidence-Based Dentistry, The Centre for Evidence-Based Medicine and The Centre for Evidence-Based Dentistry, offer summaries of relevant, well-conducted research, as well as critical appraisal tools.

Another helpful resource is the blog 'The Dental Elf', which undertakes and publishes critical appraisals of current systematic dental reviews.

The critical-evaluation process aims to assess each study's relative merits as detailed in the published paper so that patients receive treatment based on the best available clinical evidence. Generally, only studies published in peer-reviewed journals should be considered when undertaking critical evaluation. However, where research is limited, it is acceptable to search the grey literature (such as conference abstracts, preprint archives, and opinion papers).

By utilising an appropriate critical appraisal tool, the clinician will be able to systematically

- Reduce the number of inappropriate studies requiring an appraisal;
- Focus on the most relevant papers;
- Distinguish between opinion and valid evidence;
- Assess the internal and external validity of the study; and
- Identify any bias present within the study.

There are four stages of critical appraisal:

1. Abstract and introduction;
2. Methodology;
3. Results;
4. Discussion and conclusion.

2.4.1. Abstract and introduction

It is essential to rapidly reduce the number of papers from the initial search by screening the introduction or abstract. If the paper does not fulfil all three of these points, reject it.

The key areas to look at:

- Does the paper's research question or hypothesis relate to your research question?
- Ideally, no paper should be older than ten years unless it is the only or a key reference paper.
- The paper should have been peer-reviewed.

2.4.2. Methodology

For those papers that fulfil the above criteria, it is time to access the full text and appraise the methods section. The first stage is to establish what kind of study design will be appraised. The primary study designs are

- A systematic review (SR);
- Diagnostic accuracy;
- Prognosis;
- Randomised controlled trials (RCTs);
- Observational qualitative study; and
- Individual patient data meta-analysis.

There are differences between the study methodologies that required changes to the appraisal methods employed. The Centre for Evidence-Based Medicine (CEBM) has critical appraisal worksheets available to download regarding these different study designs (https://www.cebm.ox.ac.uk/resources/ebm-tools/critical-appraisal-tools).

Areas to appraise within the methods section:

- Did the study have a registered protocol?[12] For a systematic review, the protocol should be registered on PROSPERO (https://www.crd.york.ac.uk/prospero/).
- Was a reporting guideline used to develop the study? If so, how well was it followed? Reporting guidelines can be found on the EQUATOR (Enhancing the Quality and Transparency of Health Research) network website (https://www.equator-network.org/).

They include

- o Randomised trials—Consolidated Standards of Reporting Trials (CONSORT)[13]
- o Observational studies—Strengthening the Reporting of Observational Studies in Epidemiology (STROBE)[14]

o Systematic reviews—Preferred Reporting Items for Systematic Reviews and Meta-Analyses (PRISMA)[15]

o Diagnostic/prognostic studies—Standards for Reporting Diagnostic Accuracy (STARD)[16]

o Clinical practice guidelines—Appraisal of Guidelines, Research and Evaluation (AGREE)[17]

Other considerations include

- The clarity of the exclusion/inclusion criteria for the study;
- How potential confounding variables and biases were managed;
- Whether the statistical methods were clearly described and appropriate to the research question (the blog Students 4 Best Evidence, run by the Cochrane Centre for Evidence-Based Medicine, has a comprehensive section on medical statistics. See https://s4be. cochrane.org/blog/topic/statistics/); and
- Whether the study has good internal/external validity. (Validity refers to how well the results of the study represent real-world outcomes. For example, was the study a simulation study using phantom head models rather than actual patients? Even though the study may be of high quality, it does represent a real patient.)[18]

2.4.3. Results

- Were the results presented in a way that would allow a reanalysis of the data? Reanalysing the primary data rather than just accepting the effect size can be useful, for example, if it has been presented as a relative value instead of an absolute value. A doubling of a tiny improvement in outcome could still be quite small.
- Were the charts clear and well presented?
- Were any of the results statistically significant, and if so, were they clinically significant? It is essential to determine how large the effect size was and if the study was adequately powered? Power refers to the probability that a statistical difference is a real difference. This is nicely summarised in the blog post No power, no evidence (see https://s4be. cochrane.org/blog/2014/01/21/no-power-no-evidence/).
- Be aware of surrogate and composite endpoints being substituted instead of direct endpoints. A surrogate outcome is a substitute endpoint (such as using a marker die to represent bacterial contamination); adding several endpoints together to create a new endpoint is called a composite endpoint.[19]

2.4.4. Discussion and conclusion (applicability)

- Were the authors able to answer their research question?
- Did the authors attempt to present weak results or nonsignificant results as evidence of a trend towards significance?

- Were any limitations in the study design discussed?
- Were there any conflicts of interest?

Critical appraisal means the researcher must go beyond just reading the abstract when reviewing the literature. An excellent way to proceed for anyone wishing to undertake further research is to take a little time to understand the various types of study designs in quantitative and qualitative research. It is also vital to gain a sound footing in basic medical statistics, as sometimes research papers have been known to "spin up" weak results until they reach statistical significance.[20]

On a final note, when starting a critical appraisal, use a high-quality checklist to standardise the appraisal process from the start.[21] A literature review may offer conflicting views on treatments and treatment modalities.

Critical appraisal

---

1. **The clinical question (abstract and introduction)**
   Has a clear question been formulated and stated?
   Question whether the studies are relevant to the study question.

2. **The methodology**
   Address, and if necessary, criticise the way statistics have been used.
   Assess the risk of bias due to the study design or how it was carried out.

3. **The results**
   Are the results clearly stated?
   Do they relate to the aims of the study?

4. **The applicability**
   How relevant are the results to everyday situations?

5. **Is the report clearly written?**

Table 2. The stages of critical review

2.5. The outcome of critical appraisal

Table 3 outlines the deficiencies that may be identified by critical appraisal.

Deficiencies identified by critical appraisal

Identified deficiency	Consequences
Poor literature review	Basis of study ill-founded
No stated aim or hypothesis	No direction to study
Wrong methodology	Conclusions not relevant to stated concepts
Poor sampling methods	Can lead to selection bias, and lack of internal and external validity
Small sample size	Bias; lack of statistical power

Poor selection of apparatus	Measurement errors can occur
Poor study design	Possible lack of internal validity
Poor controls	Possible lack of internal validity
Observer bias	Rosenthal effect i.e.high expectations lead to improved performance; lack of internal and external validity
Subject expectations	Hawthorne effect (modify an aspect of their behaviour in response to their awareness of being observed); lack of internal and external validity
Poor descriptive statistics	Difficulty in interpreting the empirical finding
Inappropriate statistics used	Conclusions not appropriate or relevant
Conflicts of Interest	This can lead to selection and reporting bias
Deviation from protocol	Lack of internal and external validity
Statistical versus clinical significance	Can result in ineffective and therefore harmful treatments; benefit unmeasurable in clinical practice

Table 3. Deficiencies which may be identified by critical appraisal

2.6. Validity and reliability

During a critical appraisal, validity and reliability should also be considered.

2.6.1. Validity is the extent to which the item within a study is being measured accurately and how closely it represents those items outside the study. Validity can be divided into two broad categories.

- **Internal validity** is defined as "the extent to which the observed results represent the truth in the population we are studying and, thus, are not due to methodological errors."[18] When appraising literature for internal validity, one needs to focus on errors in the methodology, such as participant selection, handling missing data, intention-to-treat, or the appropriateness of the statistical analysis. A recent paper on dental research waste (Pandis et al. 2020) identified significant deficiencies in internal validity in dental research.[22]

  These were concerning:

  o Sample size adequacy ranged from 7.3 to 35.6 per cent of papers;
  o Adequacy of randomisation (9 to 68 per cent);
  o Blinding (12 to 70 per cent);
  o Missing data (17 to 98 per cent); and
  o Reports of conflicts of interest (8 to 39 per cent) and funding (22.5 to 78 per cent).

- **External validity** refers to whether the study results can be applied to patients outside the study. For example, external validity would be considered poor if the study population were on average 20 years old and from a high socioeconomic bracket, and the population outside the study were older than 60 years and from a low socioeconomic bracket.

2.6.2. Reliability

Reliability refers to the consistency and reproducibility of measurement within a study; this can be divided into three components:[23]

- **Homogeneity** represents the reliability of the measurement between test subjects;
- **Stability** is the test-retest reliability is assessed when an instrument is given to the same participants more than once under similar circumstances.; and
- **Equivalence** is assessed through inter-rater reliability (or a kappa score), when a test is repeated utilising different observers.

2.7. Effectiveness and efficacy

Efficacy can be defined as the performance of an intervention under ideal and controlled circumstances, whereas effectiveness refers to its performance under 'real-world' conditions[24] The balance of efficacy and effectiveness within research papers can sometimes be hard to determine; however, the differences can be neatly summarised in Table 4 below by Singal et al(2015)[25]

	Efficacy study	**Effectiveness study**
Question	Does the intervention work under ideal circumstances?	Does the intervention work in the real world?
Setting	Resource intensive ideal setting.	Real-world, everyday setting
Study population	Highly selected, homogenous population Several exclusion criteria	Heterogenous population Few to no exclusion criteria
Providers	Highly experienced and trained	Representative usual providers
Intervention	Strictly enforced and standardised No concurrent interventions	Applied with flexibility Concurrent interventions and crossover permitted

Table 4. Differences between efficacy and effectiveness studies

2.8. Hierarchy of research methodologies

When undertaking a critical appraisal of research literature, it is essential to try and structure the search into a hierarchy of evidence. This can be visualised through the hierarchy of evidence pyramid (Figure 1), which ranks the study designs on their methodological strength and precision.

Systematic reviews (SRs) and meta-analyses are at the top of the pyramid. SRs search for, filter, and bring together multiple primary research studies, appraise their quality, and synthesise the data. The results can be presented either as a meta-analysis, a statistical tool that combines the results of multiple scientific studies or in a narrative form if the data cannot be combined. If the information is not available as a systematic review, the researcher typically moves down a level through randomised control trials and cohort studies. Finally, expert opinion, anecdotal reports, and editorials sit at the bottom of the pyramid.

Resources

Apart from the links incorporated in this chapter, several others with good online access can help the busy practitioner find reliable evidence on topics of interest and download training materials. While those cited are UK-based, they provide an excellent source of health-related information relevant to clinical researchers worldwide.

One of these is the Centre for Reviews and Dissemination (CDR), part of the National Institute for Health Research (NIHR) at The University of York, which provides research-based information on the effects of healthcare and social-care interventions. It also undertakes systematic reviews evaluating research evidence on health and public health questions. Its monthly EBP newsletter, Effectiveness Matters, summarises reliable research evidence about the effects of essential interventions for practitioners and decision makers in health services (visit www.york.ac.uk/inst/crd/effectiveness_matters.htm).

Others include

https://www.rcseng.ac.uk/library-and-publications/library/blog/dissecting-the-literature-the-importance-of-critical-appraisal/.

https://s4be.cochrane.org/blog/2016/09/06/critical-appraisal-checklist/.

The Centre for Evidence-Based Medicine: https://www.cebm.ox.ac.uk/resources/ebm-tools/critical-appraisal-tools.

The Centre for Evidence-Based Dentistry: www.dentistry.dundee.ac.uk/centre-evidence-based.

The Dental Elf: https://www.nationalelfservice.net/dentistry/.

References

1   Mackey A, Bassendowski S. The history of evidence-based practice in nursing education and practice. *Journal of Professional Nursing.* 2017;33(1):51-55.

2   Isaacs D, Fitzgerald D. Seven alternatives to evidence-based medicine. *British Medical Journal.* 1999;319(7225):1618-1618.

3   Cochrane. "Archie Cochrane in his own words: Selections arranged from his 1972 introduction to *Effectiveness and efficiency: Random reflections on the health services,*" *Controlled Clinical Trials.* 1989;10(4):428–33.

4   Sackett DL, Rosenberg WM, Gray JM, et al. Evidence-based medicine: What it is and what it is not. *British Medical Journal Publishing Group;* 1996.

5   Richards D, Lawrence A. Evidence-based dentistry. *British Dental Journal.* 1995;179(7):270-273.

6   Haynes RB. Clinical expertise in the era of evidence-based medicine and patient choice. *Evidence-Based Medicine.* 2002;7(2):36-38.

7   Collins, H and R Evans. *Rethinking Expertise,* Chicago, IL: University of Chicago Press, 2008.

8   Wieten S. Expertise in evidence-based medicine: A tale of three models. *Philosophy Ethics Humanities Medicine.* 2018;13(1):2.

9   Buccheri RK, Sharifi C. Critical appraisal tools and reporting guidelines for evidence-based practice. *Worldviews on Evidence-Based Nursing.* 2017;14(6):463-472.

10   Duffy JR. Critically appraising quantitative research. *Nursing and Health Sciences.* 2005;7(4):281-283.

11   Melnyk BM, Fineout-Overholt E. Evidence-*Based Practice* in *Nursing* & *Healthcare*: A *Guide* to *Best Practice*: Lippincott Williams & Wilkins; 2015.

12   Stewart L, Moher D, Shekelle P. Why prospective registration of systematic reviews makes sense. *Systematic Reviews.* 2012;1(1):7.

13   Schulz KF. Consort 2010 statement: Updated guidelines for reporting parallel group randomised trials. *Annals of Internal Medicine.* 2010;152(11):726.

14   Von Elm E, Altman DG, Egger M, et al. The strengthening the reporting of observational studies in epidemiology (STROBE) statement: Guidelines for reporting observational studies. *Annals of Internal Medicine.* 2007;147(8):573.

15   Moher D, Liberati A, Tetzlaff J, et al. Preferred reporting items for systematic reviews and meta-analyses: *The Prisma statement. PLoS Medicine.* 2009;6(7):e1000097.

16   Bossuyt PM, Reitsma JB, Bruns DE, et al. Stard 2015: An updated list of essential items for reporting diagnostic accuracy studies. *British Medical Journal.* 2015:h5527.

17   Brouwers MC, Kerkvliet K, Spithoff K. The agree reporting checklist: A tool to improve reporting of clinical practice guidelines. *British Medical Journal*. 2016:i1152.

18   Patino CM, Ferreira JC. Internal and external validity: Can you apply research study results to your patients? *Jornal Brasileiro de Pneumologia*. 2018;44(3):183-183.

19   Fleming TR, Powers JH. Biomarkers and surrogate endpoints in clinical trials. *Statistics in Medicine*. 2012;31(25):2973-2984.

20   Khan MS, Lateef N, Siddiqi TJ, et al. Level and prevalence of spin in published cardiovascular randomised clinical trial reports with statistically non-significant primary outcomes. *Journal of the American Medical Association* Network Open. 2019;2(5):e192622.

21   Centre for Evidence-Based Medicine: critical-appraisal tools 2021, https://www.cebm.ox.ac.uk/resources/ebm-tools/critical-appraisal-tools.

22   Pandis N, Fleming PS, Katsaros C, et al. Dental research waste in design, analysis, and reporting: A scoping review. *Journal of Dental Research*. 2021 Mar;100(3):245-252. doi: 10.1177/0022034520962751. Epub 2020 Oct 15.

23   Heale R, Twycross A. Validity and reliability in quantitative studies. *Evidence-Based Nursing*. 2015;18(3):66-67.

24   Revicki DA, Frank L. Pharmacoeconomic evaluation in the real world. *Pharmacoeconomics*. 1999;15(5):423-434.

25   Singal AG, Higgins PDR, Waljee AK. A primer on effectiveness and efficacy trials. Clinical Transl Gastroenterology. 2014;5(1):e45-e45.

Chapter 3. Asking a Research Question and Literature Searching

FARBEY R., EATON K.A., AND SANTINI A.

3.1. Overview

This chapter will address the first three stages of a research project, which are

1. The initial idea (asking a research question and identifying aims);
2. Searching the literature; and
3. Refining the question and aims in the light of the literature search.

3.2. The initial idea

3.2.1. Asking a research question and identifying the aims of the study

When deciding upon a topic, the key factors are that it is interesting and important to the individual or group concerned and that it is feasible to perform. This may be within a variety of settings, including a clinic, hospital, school, or university. Most research questions that are relevant to healthcare are likely to be clinical.

3.2.2. Asking the clinical question

Evidence-based practice requires that clinicians draw upon the best available research to facilitate their decision making. The first step is to source the research literature relevant to the question. There are two types of questions that can be asked, and the type helps determine which resources to access in order to answer the clinical question:

- Background questions ask for general knowledge about a condition or specific topic; and
- Foreground questions ask for specific knowledge to inform clinical decisions or actions.

3.2.4. Background questions

Background questions ask for general knowledge about a disease or disease process and have two essential components:

1. A question root (such as who, what, or when) with a verb; and
2. A disorder, test, treatment, or other aspects of healthcare.

Examples include what causes mouth ulcers? Or, do antibiotic or topical antiseptic prophylaxis reduce the risk of bisphosphonate-related osteonecrosis of the jaw?

3.2.5. Foreground questions

Foreground questions ask for specific knowledge about managing patients with a disease and have three or four essential components. Asking a good research question is not easy, and any clinical question must be answerable.[1, 2] Sackett et al. (1997)[1] suggested using PICO, a mnemonic used to describe the four elements of a valid clinical foreground question:

> **Patient:** Describe as accurately as possible the patient or group of patients of interest.

> **Intervention** (or cause, prognosis): What is the main intervention or therapy you wish to consider?

> **Comparison** (optional): Is there an alternative treatment to compare? Including no disease, a placebo, absence of risk factors, and so on.

> **Outcome:** What is the clinical outcome?

For example, when PICO is applied to the question "Are resin-based composites as effective as amalgam restorations in adults?"

> **P** = Patients requiring a posterior class III cavity restoration;

> **I** = Placement of a resin-based composite restoration;

> **C** = Placement of an amalgam restoration;

> **O** = What are the survival rates of these two types of restoration?

It indicates that the question is answerable and forms the basis for a possible clinical study.

A well-defined research question is essential in planning and designing a suitable and appropriate method for all types of research studies. It should indicate the kind of research and where it should be undertaken and specify the precise objectives of the research study. In addition, PICO helps researchers confirm the validity of the study they plan to undertake.

A good research question has five essential characteristics (Table 1):

F	Feasible
I	Interesting
N	Novel
E	Ethical
R	Relevant

Table 1. The five essential characteristics of a good research question.

The ideal sequence of events is to identify and justify a research question and then identify the research aims. When writing up a dissertation, thesis or manuscript for publication, it should be apparent that there is a commonality of wording between the aims and the hypothesis and, importantly, the title of the research project. However, it should be remembered that studies such as case reports or qualitative studies are not designed to test a hypothesis but to generate hypotheses for future studies.

3.2.6. Aims and objectives

Aims are what is hoped to achieve. They are statements of purpose and are written in general terms. They summarise expectations of what will be accomplished by the project.

Objectives are the action(s) taken in order to achieve the aim(s). They are detailed statements that define outcome measures and are essentially a list of phases to be carried out to accomplish these outcomes.

Time should be taken to detail and record the project's aims and objectives before commencing the study. This will help in maintaining a focus as the study is developed. It is also helpful to write objectives as a series of strong positive statements and refer to them as the study develops.

A research hypothesis is formulated based on the aims of the project. There are two variants, the null hypothesis and the alternative hypothesis. A null hypothesis states that a measured quantity under investigation is zero. An example of a null hypothesis could be resin-based composites are not as effective as amalgam restorations in adults.

The alternative hypothesis is different to the null hypothesis; it states that there is some relationship. The alternative hypothesis can be stated depending on the nature of the hypothesized relationship. In particular, it can be two-sided, i.e. there is some effect, in an as-yet-unknown direction, or one-sided, in which the direction of the hypothesized relationship, positive or negative, is fixed in advance. Hypotheses will be explained further in the chapter about analysing data.

The first stages of a study are summarised in Table 2.

1. Identify and justify a research question Requires: • Knowledge of the subject • A comprehensive critical review of the current literature
2. Identify the research aims State a [null] hypothesis in the case of a quantitative research project A hypothesis is a proposal about the relationship between groups that are to be tested

Table 2 The first stages of a study

3.3. Searching the literature

The next step is to perform a literature search to source previous studies on the topic, the methods used, the results obtained, and to assess the quality of these studies. This section of the paper helps not only those who wish to embark on a research project but anyone who wishes to access the scientific literature before carrying out a review or systematic search. Investigating the background literature to similar or related studies is essential for the success of a research project and is vital not only for planning a project but when writing the introduction and discussion sections of any paper.

Papers in journals are the premier source as they represent the most up-to-date knowledge available. Books, monographs, and other printed material such as statistical and government publications are important, but due to a time lag between writing and publication, they can be less current than journal papers.

3.3.1. Accessing literature

Several databases can be used to access literature. They include

- MEDLINE, for obtaining references (post-1950) to biomedical literature;
- The Index to Dental Literature (IDL), the hardcopy equivalent to MEDLINE for searching dental references before 1950. It is now no longer published.
- The Internet, which can be an essential research tool.

Healthcare and dental libraries and online sources are all useful. However, the most helpful resource is undoubtedly the MEDLINE database which, over the last twenty years, has become the most widely used resource for rapid literature reviews. See also sections 3.3.5. and 3.5. of this chapter.

3.3.2. Journals

Journals are vital for keeping up-to-date and disseminating research findings quickly and efficiently to the scientific community. They include

- General journals, such as *Primary Dental Journal*, the journal of the College of General Dentistry;
- Specialty journals, such as the *International Endodontic Journal* or the *Journal of Orthodontics*, cover clinical and research aspects of various healthcare and dental specialities;
- Journals of a non-specialist nature, such as the *Journal of Dentistry* or *Journal of Dental Research*, are vital;
- National dental journals, such as the *Journal of the American Medical Association* or the *British Dental Journal*, which include clinical research, case reports and news items;
- Most journals occasionally publish review articles, which are brief histories or condensed reviews of a particular subject. Typically, a long list of references relating to publications on the same topic or similar topics is found at the end of review articles. See some of the papers that have been published in Dental Update; for example, Santini (2010) is a well-received publication and included more than 160 references on a currently relevant topic;[3]

Such reference lists can save researchers time when searching for background literature on the topic of their project. Fairly recently, several peer-reviewed journals have started to publish papers online as soon as they have been accepted, before they appear in hard copy. In addition, some new journals publish solely online. Both types enable new knowledge to be disseminated more rapidly than traditional paper-only journals.

Traditionally, journals were funded by subscriptions from their readers or a parent organization or association, for example, the British Medical Association for the *British Medical Journal*. Readers who were not members of the organization/association still have to pay a fee to access such journals or individual papers. However, if readers are not members but are students of staff members of universities, they can usually have access to subscription journals free of charge via their university library. Similarly, NHS clinicians (salaried by or working under contract to the NHS) can access many journals free of charge via the library at their local NHS hospital's postgraduate centre.

In the last twenty years, there has been a move to open-access publishing. The authors or their employer pays for the publishing costs, and their papers can then be accessed from the journal's website free of charge by all-comers.

3.3.3. Books, monographs, and official and statistical publications

Because books and monographs have a longer lead-in time to publication than journals, they may not be as up to date, but they can provide an introduction, general overview, or historical perspective. In addition to textbooks on specific subjects, research methods, statistical techniques, and planning, there are reference texts, such as *Clinical Periodontology* and *Implant Dentistry.*[4]

Such reference texts review all the published papers within the subject. Three excellent books for novice researchers are *How to Read a Scientific Paper,*[5] which sets out the basics of evidence-based medicine and includes a very useful chapter on searching the literature. *Critical Thinking: Understanding and Evaluating Dental Research*[6] explains how to understand and evaluate dental research and has an excellent chapter on searching the dental literature. *Statistical and Methodological Aspects of Oral Health Research*[7] advises on research methodology and methods.

Theses and dissertations are either published just by a university, or, in some cases may be published in association with a journal—for example, prior to 2016, in Sweden in association with the *Swedish Dental Journal*. Swedish dental schools often publish important new findings and should not be overlooked. However, they may not be easy to find as they are not listed on MEDLINE and may only come to light as a reference in a published paper.

Official and statistical publications include annual reports and statistics issued by government agencies and statutory bodies such as the Office for National Statistics (formerly the Office of Population Censuses and Surveys), which periodically publishes the definitive dental health surveys for the United Kingdom.[8] An excellent example of an influential (USA) government agency report is the Health Effects of Ingested Fluoride, published by the National Academy Press.[9] Finally, British and European standards change occasionally, and there are many governmental reports relating to dental equipment.

3.3.4. Peer-reviewed and non-peer-reviewed literature

As previously described in chapter 2, peer-reviewed (or refereed) literature has been screened by individuals knowledgeable about the topic of the paper, book, or thesis concerned. The reviewers usually are authorities with a track record of papers published on the subject. They are independent of the authors on whose work they are reporting. Peer reviewers assess the whole paper and report comments and suggestions to the journal editor, including whether or not they consider the manuscript worthy of publication. The process does not guarantee that the results and conclusions in the published work are either true or correct. However, the process provides a check on the work's quality and should help ensure that poorly conducted research or badly written papers are not published.

The term *non-peer-reviewed literature* includes free dental and other journals and magazines, daily and weekly newspapers, and online material (such as Wikipedia). In general, they should not be quoted in a scientific paper as they are not peer-reviewed and may contain opinions that cannot be supported with objective scientific facts.

3.3.5. Indexes and abstracts

Indexes and abstracts enable healthcare practitioners and researchers to identify relevant journal articles from the plethora of published articles and are, therefore, almost as important as the journals themselves.

- The Index to Dental Literature (IDL), the main printed index for dentistry until the very end of the twentieth century, is no longer published. It was published quarterly and cumulated annually and also listed dissertations, theses, and new book titles (prior to 1950).
- Index Medicus was published monthly and cumulated annually by the National Library of Medicine in the United States from the late-nineteenth century. It formed the basis of the computerized index MEDLARS, which allowed interactive computerized (online) literature searching, thereby revolutionizing medical and dental research methods. These paper-based indexes are now used for historical research purposes only.

3.3.6. Online literature searching: keywords

All papers should contain keywords. They are usually found immediately following the paper's abstract and summarise the main areas covered by the paper (e.g. dental caries, epidemiology, 12-year-olds, United Kingdom). Abstracts are found at the beginning of a paper and may often be available via MEDLINE. They should be used to identify the original paper. The use of keywords during searching enables easy access to papers on the same or similar topics. However, the use of keywords is not without problems because key words can only search for the exact word or phrase selected. Thus, only papers that listed crown as a keyword would be retrieved if the keyword crown was employed. In other words, searching using keywords is very precise and does not necessarily consider broader concepts.

3.3.7. Medical Subject Headings (MeSH)

To overcome the potential problems when keywords are used in a search, classification systems that group keywords as concepts have been developed. Perhaps the most widely used in healthcare research is the Medical Subject Headings (MeSH)[10] system. This has been produced by the United States National Library of Medicine and is used for indexing journal articles in several databases, including MEDLINE. The indexers review all accepted papers for inclusion in MEDLINE and apply subject headings appropriate to their content. The drawback with this approach is that although the classification is more intuitive than keywords, it can be open to human error if the topic area is new to the indexer.

3.4. MEDLINE

MEDLINE is the online counterpart to MEDLARS (MEDical Literature Analysis and Retrieval System) that originated in 1964. It is the major international reference database for online biomedical literature searching. It indexes the contents of journals in medical, dental, nursing, biomedical and allied sciences. Online literature searching involves interrogating a dedicated web server that stores the data. This has several advantages. More than one concept (thesaurus terms, subheadings, free-text words or phrases) can be searched simultaneously to achieve precise results virtually instantaneously. The search often includes abstracts, which give more information than the title and thus helps to identify the most relevant or valuable articles. A retrospective search enables researchers to check whether the proposed research topic has been previously undertaken, avoiding reinventing the wheel. Some sections generate information on specific topics weekly or monthly, keeping researchers up-to-date with recently published literature. This is particularly useful as a mechanism for updating researchers during the lifetime of their project. The web-based versions of MEDLINE, all derived from the same source at the National Library of Medicine in the United States, are available with sophisticated user interfaces (such as Ovid or ProQuest Dialog) or less sophisticated interfaces (PubMed).

Ovid is a division of Wolters Kluwer, a publishing and information services company based in Philadelphia, Pennsylvania, with offices worldwide, is one major vendor of MEDLINE on the web. Some consider the Ovid version of MEDLINE to be superior to the PubMed version, which is available free of charge, because it offers more flexibility and more powerful search capabilities. For this reason, many dental/medical libraries subscribe to Ovid for access to MEDLINE, although some libraries prefer platforms such as EBSCO Information Services or ProQuest that offer more sophisticated versions of Medline' to that provided by PubMed.

3.5. Assessment of the quality of the literature

Following the acquisition of its previous owners, Thomson Reuters, in 2016, Clarivate[11] now hosts Web of Science, the leading global citation database. Previously part of Thomson Reuters' Institute for Scientific Information (ISI), it lists thousands of scientific journals, of which several leading dental and oral surgery titles are included. The company selects the journals it lists. Journals that are listed by Web of Science are given an impact factor, which is calculated based on the average number of papers published in the journal cited for up to two years after publication. However, the reliability of the impact factor has been questioned,[12] and because of their relatively small circulation, dental journals have relatively low impact factors compared to other areas of science. Nevertheless, many universities and government research funding agencies use the impact factor as a guide when awarding funds to university departments.

Web of Science also produces Current Contents Connect (which includes Current Contents Clinical Medicine); it is derived from more than ten thousand journals indexed and is updated weekly and lists tables of contents from current issues of leading scientific journals. It also publishes other leading indexes, such as Science Citation Index.

3.6. Predatory journals

Authors should avoid predatory journals. The website www.predatoryjournals.com[13] defines them as "Journals that publish work without proper peer review and which sometimes charge large fees for publication. These journals and publishers cheapen intellectual work by misleading scholars, preying particularly on early career researchers. The credibility of scholars duped into publishing in these journals can be seriously damaged by doing so."

The website lists ten unethical practices which predatory journals may be guilty of. They are

1. Charging exorbitant rates for publication of articles in conjunction with a lack of peer-review or editorial oversight;
2. Notifying authors of fees only after acceptance;
3. Targeting scholars through mass-email spamming in attempts to get them to publish or serve on editorial boards;
4. Quick acceptance of low-quality papers, including hoax papers;
5. Listing scholars as members of editorial boards without their permission or not allowing them to resign;
6. Listing fake scholars as members of editorial boards or authors;
7. Copying the visual design and language of the marketing materials and websites of legitimate, established journals;
8. Fraudulent or improper use of ISSNs;
9. Giving false information about the location of the publishing operation; and
10. Fake, non-existent, or misrepresented impact factors.

The Ottawa Hospital Research Institute has produced checklists to help in the detection of predatory journals.[14] More recently, further advice on this topic has appeared online.[15]

3.7. Other Internet resources

The Internet provides access to dental sites devoted to dental and related topics, which offer a vehicle for collaboration and practical (not financial) research assistance. The following are useful Internet resources/websites:

- https://www.priory.com/dent.htm: Dentistry Online. A refereed academic journal that contains full-text articles only available on the Internet.

- www.bmj.com: The *British Medical Journal* (BMJ) permits free online access to its non-current issues.
- https://bda.247lib.com/bdalib/: The British Dental Association Library's online catalogue. Most libraries have their catalogues available on the Internet.
- https://england.nhs.uk/primary-care/dentistry/dental-commissioning/: The NHS Dental commissioning and policy webpage links to various Department of Health dental policies and guidelines.
- https://www.nice.org.uk/guidance: The National Institute for Health and Clinical Excellence (NICE) offers current guidance to clinical issues, including ones affecting dentistry, such as antibiotic prophylaxis against infective endocarditis. Within its website is included NHS Evidence and the British National Formulary.
- https://pubmed.ncbi.nlm.nih.gov/: The National Library of Medicine's free MEDLINE service, PubMed. This publicly available Medline searching facility offers simple or more sophisticated advanced searching. It also offers users the ability to create automated alerts on search strategies.
- https://www.thecochranelibrary.com: The Cochrane Library is available free of charge to UK residents. There are research in progress and completed research projects on all known biomedical subjects within its various databases, including dentistry.
- https://www.nihr.ac.uk: The National Institute for Health Research (developed by the Department of Health) offers a useful link to biomedical research bodies in all spheres.
- www.evidence.nhs.uk: National Health Service (NHS) Evidence (formerly the National Library for Health).
- www.biomedcentral.com: BioMed Central (BMC) is a pioneer of open-access publishing. It contains an evolving portfolio of high-quality, peer-reviewed journals, including oral and dental research.
- www.scholar.google.com: Google Scholar links to several major authoritative sources yielding numerous literature references and is searchable using advanced search criteria such as exact phrase by author, publication and date.
- www.nature.com/bdj: The *British Dental Journal* (BDJ) and Evidence-Based Dentistry (EBJ) are both available to British Dental Association (BDA) members. Notably, apart from the current contents of these journals, there are also full-text backfiles spanning many years. In addition, several science papers per issue of the BDJ are only available via its website and are not published in the paper version.

https://www.ebscohost.com/nursing/products/cinahl-databases: CINAHL databases are the most widely-used research tools for nurses, students and allied health professionals. CINAHL is hosted by EBSCO Health and does include some dental and related literature.

- https://www.elsevier.com/en-gb/solutions/embase-biomedical-research: Embase covers the most important international biomedical literature, including dentistry, from 1947 to the present day, and all articles are indexed in depth.

- https://europepmc.org/: Europe PMC (Europe PubMed Central) is an open-access repository covering worldwide life-sciences literature with 37.6 million abstracts; 6.3 million full-text articles; 24,317 books and documents; and 187,161 preprints.
- BrowZine is an app for Android and Apple smartphones and devices. It is accessible through membership of many leading worldwide academic institutions. In addition, it offers users access to a panoply of full-text journals, including ones on dentistry and oral surgery.

3.7.1. Access points for sourcing dental literature

The BDA Library (64 Wimpole Street, London W1G 8YS. Tel: 020 7563 4545, e-mail: library@bda.org) offers its members the most comprehensive dental library in Europe. The BDA Library:

- Holds two hundred "live" journal titles, together with a large number of ceased publications;
- Has an impressive book stock;
- Loans books by post to members;
- Holds a variety of eBooks and e-Journals, accessible remotely to BDA members via the web;
- Has a range of DVDs on dental subjects;
- Offers a free MEDLINE searching service;
- Can provide photocopies of journal articles (subject to provisions of the Copyright Act 1988); and
- Has an online library catalogue (https://bda.247lib.com/bdalib/) that can pinpoint books, monographs, theses, or pamphlets on any subject.

Postgraduate medical centre libraries are extremely useful as centres for studying and researching. However, they are generally underrated and underused by general dental practitioners and dental care professionals. Most British universities with dental schools have excellent library facilities. In addition, anyone carrying out postgraduate research under the official auspices of a university has access to its library services.

The library of The Royal College of Surgeons of England

(35-43 Lincoln's Inn Fields, London WC2A 3PE. Tel: 020 7869 6556, email: library.athens@rcseng.ac.uk) has comprehensive dental collections, both historic and modern. subscribing members and fellows of the college, including diplomates of the faculty of dental surgery and faculty of general dental practice (UK), are eligible to join the library and then use its facilities, including extensive online resources. Opening hours are from 09:30-17:30, Monday to Friday. An online library that is available to Fellows and members of the college.

The library of the Royal College of Surgeons of Edinburgh Nicolson St, Edinburgh, EH8 9DW.

Tel: +44 (0)131 527 1632 Email: library@rcsed.ac.uk
Website: www.library.rcsed.ac.uk

Fellows, members and affiliates of the college have access to use the well-resourced medical and surgical library, with all the latest in texts, journals and electronic resources.

The library of the Royal College of Physicians and Surgeons of Glasgow, 232-242 St Vincent Street, Glasgow, G2 5RJ Telephone: +44 (0)141 221 6072 Email: library@rcpsg.ac.uk

The Royal Society of Medicine (1 Wimpole Street, London W1G 0AE. Tel: 020 7290 2940/2941 or email: library@rsm.ac.uk) holds the United Kingdom's most extensive medical library with some dental material. It offers its members excellent library facilities, including access to many biomedical databases, such as MEDLINE, Embase, DH-Data, Allied and Complementary Medicine (AMED) and the BrowZine full-text journal app. These can also be accessed remotely within the members-only section of the RSM website.

The British Library at St Pancras (96 Euston Road, London NW1 2DB. Tel: 01937 546546 or email: customer-services@bl.uk) offers a Science Reading Room that contains a wealth of information and resources to assist in research. In addition to its printed resources, it also offers readers access to online databases, electronic books, and journals. The Medicine and Life Sciences section is located on the second floor. To use the reading rooms, it is essential to obtain a reader pass, which is available to anyone conducting bona fide research. Any sizeable public library can often obtain virtually any literature for non-medical/dental subjects from the British Library as an interlibrary loan request.[16, 17]

The National Library of Scotland (George IV Bridge, Edinburgh, EH1 1EW Tel 0131 623 3700 website www.nls.uk email enquiries@natlibscot.uk It is necessary to obtain a reader ticket before using the actual site. Some resources are only accessible from a computer at the main site –others can be accessed remotely whose main residence address is in Scotland. Access by people residing out with Scotland might be possible upon application.

3.8. Refining the initial idea into a research question

Having performed a literature search, the researcher must consider whether the methodologies and results of previous studies on the same or related topics make it necessary to revise the initial idea (research question) and aims and objectives.

3.8.1. Involvement of other parties

Researchers must be aware of the need to consult with and involve other parties. Patient and public involvement (PPI) was mentioned in chapter 1. PPI may not be crucial for many MSc research projects which involve questionnaire surveys of dentists and other dental professionals. However, it is crucial for funded research as several funding bodies will not fund health services research (where practice-based research will sit) that has not evidenced PPI involvement in research design and informing the research question.

3.8.2. The James Lind alliance

The James Lind Alliance (JLA; jla.nihr.ac.uk) is a non-profit making initiative established in 2004. It brings patients, carers, and clinicians together in priority setting partnerships (PSPs) (jla.nihr.ac.uk/priority-setting-partnerships) to identify and prioritize the top ten unanswered questions or evidence uncertainties that they agree are the most important for a wide range of healthcare areas, including oral and dental health.[18] If researchers intend to seek external funding for their research, they should check to see if their research topic falls within the priority setting partnership's (PSP) top priorities for oral and dental health.

The JLA aims to make sure that health-research funders know the issues that matter most to the people who need to use the research in their everyday lives.

3.8.3. Priority-setting partnerships (PSPs)

The Oral and Dental Health PSP was established to find out the most important research questions about dental care and what keeps people's mouths, teeth, and gums healthy.

The PSP was instigated from observations that few large-scale clinical studies were being conducted in the United Kingdom (as evidenced by the size of the NIHR oral and dental portfolio), that much oral and dental research in this area was fragmented and could be more ambitious, collaborative, and multi-centred. There was also a perception that research funders did not prioritize oral and dental research and that funding calls could be better targeted to key areas.

The Oral and Dental Health PSP top ten was published in December 2018. It was as follows:

1. What is the best way to prevent tooth decay and reduce oral health inequalities at a community or population level?
2. How can access to dental services be improved for the general public?
3. What are the most effective ways of increasing early detection/diagnosis of oral cancer?
4. How can access to dental services be improved for people with additional needs?
5. How can dental health professionals work with other health professionals to help improve oral health?
6. How can basic oral hygiene be achieved for people with additional care needs?
7. How to improve communication between dental teams and patients/carers?
8. Is there a role for dental health professionals in treating oral health problems to improve general health?
9. What is the best way to prevent gum disease and reduce oral health inequalities at a community or population level?
10. What role do digital technologies play in the provision of dental care?

The following questions were also discussed and put in order of priority at the workshop:

11. What is the best way to treat dentally anxious patients?
12. What are the best ways of managing oral conditions associated with cancer treatment?
13. Do dental care professionals have a role in screening and treating general health problems?
14. What is the best way for dental teams to manage gum disease?
15. What are the barriers/enablers to maintaining a healthy mouth (across different populations and settings)?
16. How can people be encouraged to reduce sugar consumption for oral and general health?
17. What are the most effective ways of managing potentially malignant disorders (e.g. oral lichen planus)?
18. What is the best way to prevent gum disease in individuals?
19. What is the best way to manage teeth missing for any reason (e.g. tooth decay, trauma, developmental conditions) and at any age?
20. What is the best way to prevent tooth decay in individuals (of all ages)?
21. Is cleaning in between teeth needed for maintaining good oral health?
22. What interventions are best at managing tooth grinding/clenching?
23. Is the home use of a daily mouthwash helpful in maintaining good oral health?
24. What are the long-term health effects (including harms) of tooth whitening?
25. Should dental professionals recommend e-cigarettes?

Once this stage has been completed, the study can then be designed (planned), as will be described in detail in future chapters.

3.8. A Final Comment

It should be remembered that once accessed, literature needs to be critically appraised. Chapter 2 has dealt with this aspect. Chapter 2 has dealt with this aspect. In addition to the resources outlined in chapter 2, a paper comprehensively dealing with critical appraisal of the literature: "Dissecting the literature: the importance of critical appraisal" is available on the Royal College of Surgeons of England website [19]

References

1   Sackett DL, Richardson WS, Rosenberg W., Haynes RB. Evidence-based Medicine: How to Practice and Teach EBM. New York: Churchill Livingstone, 1997.

2   Straus SE, Glasziou P, Richardson WS, Haynes RB. Evidence-Based Medicine: How to Practice and Teach EBM. 5th ed. New York: Elsevier 2019.

3 Santini A. Current status of visible light activation units and the curing of light-activated resin-based composite materials. *Dental Update*. 2010;**37**: 214-216, 218-220,223-227.Lang NP, Lindhe J, eds. Clinical Periodontology and Implant Dentistry, 6ᵗʰ ed. Oxford, Wiley-Blackwell; 2015

4 Greenhalgh T. How to Read a Paper: The Basics of Evidence-Based Medicine and Healthcare. 6ᵗʰ ed. Oxford: Wiley-Blackwell; 2019.

5 Brunette DM, editor. Critical Thinking: Understanding and Evaluating Dental Research. 3ʳᵈ ed. Batavia, IL: Quintessence: 2020.

6 Lesaffre E, Feine J, Leroux B, Declerck D, editors. Statistical and Methodological Aspects of Oral Health Research. Oxford: John Wiley; 2009.

7 Kelly M, Steele J, Nuttall N, Bradnock G, Morris J, Nunn J, et al. Adult Dental Health Survey: Oral Health in the United Kingdom 1998. London: Stationery Office; 2000.

8 Subcommittee on Health Effects of Ingested Fluoride. Health Effects of Ingested Fluoride. Washington, DC: National Academy Press; 1993.

9 Medical Subject Headings (MeSH) Section. Home page online, accessed 6 July 2020), https://www.nlm.nih.gov/mesh/meshhome.hl.

10 Clarivate Web Of Science. Home page on the Internet. https://clarivate.com/webofsciencegroup (Accessed 1 October 2020).

11 European Association of Scientific Editors (EASE). Statement on inappropriate use of impact factors, accessed 1 October 2020, https://ease.org.uk/impact-factor-statement/.

12 Predatory Journals: definition and criteria to detect them, accessed 3 January 2021, www.predatoryjournals.com.

13 Ottawa Hospital Research Institute Centre for Journalology., www.ohri.ca>journaloology accessed 13 July 2021

14 How to detect a potential predatory deceptive journal, accessed 29 January 202.www.medrxiv.org/content/10.1101/19005728v1.full.pdf.

15 Stevens J. How to use libraries and modern information sources. *Dental Update*. 1990;**17**:250-253.

16 Marlborough HS. Using dental library services. *Dental Update*. 1996;**23**:20-24.

17 James Lind Alliance. What is it and its aims? www.jla.nihr.ac.uk accessed 13 July 2021.

18 Morrison K. Dissecting the literature: the importance of critical appraisal, 8 December 2017, Royal College of Surgeons of England, accessed 5 October 2021, https://bit.ly/3nikfsu.

Chapter 4. Designing Studies Part 1— Introduction and Quantitative Study Design

SANTINI A.

4.1. Overview

There are many types of study and aspects of their design. They are covered in multiple chapters and provide the fourth step in a research study. They are on the topics of

- Introduction and quantitative study design;
- Randomised controlled studies;
- Qualitative studies;
- Designing systematic reviews;
- Sampling ;
- Questionnaire design: and
- Screening and diagnostic testing.

When designing studies, the need for PPI, where relevant, must be considered, together with the principles of equality and inclusion. For example, when recruiting subjects for a study, there must be no discrimination of any sort, including gender, ethnicity, and language spoken, so that the research findings are generalisable and applicable to all.

After an introduction, this chapter describes the different types of quantitative study designs.

4.2. Introduction

The design of a clinical study is a complex matter. However, choosing an appropriate study design or methodology is crucial for success. It should refer back and apply to the stated aims and objectives.

It follows that the researcher should understand the strengths and weaknesses of different research designs. Consequently, clinical researchers must have in-depth knowledge of research designs and how to judge the quality of research through critical appraisal.[1]

There are several ways of classifying research studies that can be confusing to the early research worker. Broadly, they may be quantitative, qualitative, or mixed.

A **quantitative study** consists of a mathematical analysis of the research topic. The research outcomes will result from an assessment that measures variables numerically to produce data that can be analysed statistically.

A **qualitative study** seeks to answer questions, such as why or how. When designing a research question for a qualitative study, the researcher will need to ask a why or how question about that research topic. Qualitative research requirements typically include interviews with people to ask for their opinions and may involve the use of print, internet texts, and audio and visual media.

Mixed studies include both quantitative and qualitative aspects.[2]

4.2.2. Types of study

When the broad type of study and the specific aims and objectives have been identified, deliberation should be given to the "so what?" test. Essentially, this test emphasises why the research is expected to add new or useful knowledge. As previously described, the acronym FINER—feasible, interesting, novel, ethical, and relevant—reflects the five essential characteristics of a good research question and should be asked before designing a study.

The primary design methodologies are experimental, observational, prospective, retrospective, and cross-sectional studies. In addition, a clinical study can also be classified as a prognostic, survival, or diagnostic study.

Initially, the researcher should decide whether to take a passive and observational role or an active and interventional role, whereby an intervention to a controlled situation is applied and the effects measured. Research evidence's strength depends on how data were obtained, and an appropriate study plan is pivotal to obtaining robust evidence.

Good systematic reviews generate the highest level of evidence. However, systematic reviews and randomised controlled trials are not necessarily the best means of conducting clinical research as they were developed mainly to answer questions related to interventions or therapy.

Cohort studies or case-control studies are frequently more relevant studies to investigate disease, diagnosis, or prognosis. Individual case reports, case series, and expert opinion can also be considered, but they generate a lower level of evidence.

4.3. Basic research designs

Five types of basic research designs are described in Table1:

Experimental	Observational	Prospective studies	Retrospective studies	Cross-sectional studies
The researcher controls the intervention	Researcher observes patients	Longitudinal studies; gathering new data over time	Looking back and collating existing data	Observations at one point in time

Table 1. Basic Research Designs

Three types of studies are listed in Table 2:

Correlational studies	A correlational study is non-experimental, requiring the researcher to establish relationships without manipulating or randomly selecting the research subjects.	What is the relationship between gender and eating disorders?
Experimental studies	An experimental study requires the researcher to manipulate and randomly select the subjects of the research.	In vivo: Are eating disorders related to the consumption of fast food?
Mixed studies	A mixed study integrates qualitative and quantitative studies. The research determines the *why, how, what, where,* or *when* of the research topic.	What are the attitudes and feelings expressed by individuals who follow different diet patterns?

Table 2. Types of study

In **experimental studies**, the researcher manipulates and randomly selects the research subjects and compares any differences in the outcome measures between the experimental group and a control group where no intervention has been undertaken.

As shown in Table 3, experimental studies can be further divided into controlled or uncontrolled studies. However, uncontrolled studies provide weak evidence compared to controlled studies.

Experimental studies	
Controlled	**Uncontrolled**
A comparison group is used	No comparison group is used. • Limited use for formulating evidence-based practice • Useful as pilot studies • It can be used to investigate the safety of a new intervention and identify unanticipated effects. • Gather baseline data for the planning of more definitive trials

Table 3. Controlled and uncontrolled experimental studies

Observational studies can be subdivided into observational descriptive studies and observational analytical studies. In observational descriptive studies, the researcher observes one person or a group of people and then compiles a report.

In observational analytical studies, comparisons between the similarities and differences between two or more population groups are observed and reported.

In identifying an appropriate study design or methodology, the researcher should first consider the specified research question. Table 4 provides examples of research questions matched to study types.

"What might cause a disease or make individuals more likely to get it?" **Cohort study:** Subjects are chosen based on different exposure and followed to see if they get the disease.
"What is the extent and nature of a condition in the population?" **Cross-sectional study:** A randomly selected representative sample of people is surveyed to answer a question.
"Which medical intervention works best?" **Randomised controlled trial:** Participants are allocated by chance to different interventions then followed and outcomes assessed.
"What might have caused a disease or made individuals more likely to have got it?" **Case-control study:** People with an illness are matched to those without it and earlier exposure to different environmental factors compared.
"Is this a new condition or course of progression or recovery not recognised before?" **Case report/case series:** A description of the medical history of one or several patients.

Table 4. Research questions matched to study types

The research design will include listing the outcome measures obtained in the course of the study.

A dichotomous design will consider the absence or presence of disease; an interval design deals with counts of equal units (e.g. the number of days off sick or continuous design with units such as blood pressure, weight, height measurements).

The statistical tests employed in testing the study hypothesis will be predicated on the design. Therefore, it is essential to discuss and choose an appropriate design with a statistician before starting the study. Choosing the wrong design can lead to data being unusable for statistical purposes.

4.4. Preclinical research

Preclinical research takes place before clinical trials or testing in humans. Therefore, it should be completed before the main trial can begin. During preclinical research, feasibility and iterative testing are performed and scrutinised for their eventual suitability in the main trial. Preclinical research studies' main goals are to profile and determine whether a treatment, technique, method or product is ultimately safe for human use. The two types of preclinical research are in vitro and in vivo (Table 5).

In vitro	In vivo
In vitro research uses cells or biological molecules outside their normal biological context. • Traditionally: in solution or artificial culture medium, in test tubes and Petri dishes. • Modern techniques: a range of techniques used in molecular biology.	In vivo studies the effects of various biological entities on whole living organisms, usually plants, animals or humans, opposed to a partial or dead organism.

Table 5. Types of preclinical research

Preclinical studies test a drug, procedure, or medical treatment using laboratory models or animals. At present, for ethical reasons, animal studies are less frequently used.

Preclinical studies should occur before any testing is conducted in humans; they should establish a full clinical trial's potential value and viability. In addition, it is vital to ensure that human research subjects are protected from potential harm, as described in Chapter 12.

Usually, preclinical studies are not extensive. However, they should be designed to provide information on such aspects as dose and toxicity levels. After preclinical testing, researchers review their findings and decide whether the drug, treatment, or technique should be tested on people.

The differences between preclinical and clinical research are shown in Table 6

Preclinical research	Clinical research
Undertaken: Before clinical trials in humans.	Undertaken: As a comparison test of a product or treatment. The comparison can be made against • a placebo • previously accepted treatment modalities
Involving: • Iterative testing • Collection and analysis of data regarding drug safety	Involving: • Collection and analysis of data regarding drug safety • Measurement of outcomes concerning efficacy, dosage, effectiveness, compliance, and cost-effectiveness

In order to	In order to
• Profile and determine a product or treatment safety on humans.	• Establish the strength and nature of the effect of an intervention
	• Confirm a causal link between intervention and effect

Table 6 Fundamentals of preclinical and clinical research

4.5. Clinical research

Clinical research is used to determine the efficacy, effectiveness, and safety of medications, devices, diagnostic products, and treatment regimens intended for human use. Therefore, it should be differentiated from clinical practice. In clinical practice, recognised and well-established treatments are used, while in clinical research, the evidence is collected with the prospect of establishing a new treatment. Linking the two is the concept of evidence-based medicine, which can be defined as the well thought out and beneficial use of current best research evidence in patient care decisions.

Clinical trials consist of four phases:

1. Phase 0
2. Phase I
3. Phase II
4. Phase III
5. Phase IV

A clinical trial is only done when there is good reason to believe a new test or treatment may improve patient care. Following the successful outcome of a preclinical trial, a succession of clinical trials is undertaken to evaluate if tests or treatments are safe for and work in humans.

Phase 0

Phase 0 aims to understand how a drug is managed and affects the body. Only a minimal dose of a drug is administered to no more than ten to fifteen subjects.

Phase I

Phase I aims to find the best dose of a new drug with the most negligible side effects. Again, the drug is administered to no more than ten to fifteen subjects, starting with very low drug doses. Then, different cohorts of patients are progressively given higher drug doses until severe side effects halt the study or the preferred outcome is expressed. Only when a drug is deemed safe will it be progressed to be tested in phase II clinical trial.

Phase II

Phase II trials further assess the safety of the drug, in addition to observing if the drug works in practice. Phase II trials are done in sizable groups of patients. Combinations of drugs are often tested. At this point, a new drug is hardly ever compared to the current standard-of-care drug. If a drug is satisfactory and effective, testing proceeds to a phase III clinical trial.

Phase III

In phase III, the new drug is compared to the current accepted standard-of-care drug. More than one hundred patients are enrolled in this phase of the trials. An assessment is made of the side effects of each drug and which drug functions best. Phase III trials are often randomised; a control group gets the standard-of-care treatment, while the other groups get a new treatment. Randomisation is needed to make sure that the people in all trial arms are alike. A computer program is often used to assign people to the trial arms randomly (see chapter on qualitative studies).

Patients are not informed as to which group they are allocated. At this stage, a trial may be prematurely ended if the new drug's side effects are too severe or if one group has demonstrated much better results, even if these better results are obtained with the standard-of-care treatment. Federal Drug Agency (FDA) approval for using a new drug by the general public is customarily granted only after phase III clinical trials.

Phase IV

FDA approval of a new drug is not granted until testing is carried out on hundreds or thousands of patients. This is to facilitate a better understanding of the short-lived and long-lasting side effects and safety.

Evidence hierarchies categorise the importance and robustness of diverse types of biomedical research. There is no universally accepted hierarchy of evidence, though there is broad agreement on the relative strength of the principal types of research. For example, randomised controlled trials (RCTs) rank above observational studies, the critical justification being that RCTs come closest to identifying causality and eliminating bias.

4.6. Designing case reports and case series

The concepts of case reports and case series are not well defined, nor is there a clear distinction in the medical literature between these two subclasses. Both are types of observational studies. However, neither has a specific research design. This chapter defines a case report as the smallest publishable unit in the medical literature, while a case series aggregates several similar cases.

A case series is regarded as including more than four patients. Four patients or fewer should be reported individually as case reports. Also, case studies is considered a synonym for case reports, and clinical series is synonymous with case series (see Table 7).

Case reports (case studies)	Case series (clinical series)
Case reports are an invaluable first-hand source of evidence in medicine and a tool most often used in practice to exchange information and generate an expanded search for evidence.	A case series traces patients with a specific disease or similar prescribed treatment. Their medical records are then examined for exposure and outcome.
Four patients or fewer should be reported individually as case reports.	More than four patients are reported as case series.

Table 7. Case reports and case series

Case reports and case series have a high sensitivity for detecting novelty. As such, new diseases and unexpected effects, adverse or beneficial, are often detected for the first time. In this respect, they have a role to play in medical education. Good case reporting requires a sharp focus to illustrate why a specific observation is valuable in the setting of existing knowledge.

4.6.1. Case reports

In the medical sciences, case reports are studies that deal with the symptoms, signs, diagnosis, treatment, and follow-up of an individual patient. They usually describe an uncommon or unique occurrence. They may contain a literature review of other reported cases. However, these literature reviews are seldom extensive due to editorial requirements of short manuscript length in journals that accept case reports. Case reports are deemed anecdotal evidence. Due to their methodological limitations and lack of statistical sampling, they are placed at a low level in the evidence hierarchy, together with case series.

Limited though their conclusions may be, case reports may contribute significantly to the advancement of healthcare. Types of case reports are described in Table 8:

Those that show
- An unexpected association between disease and symptoms
- An unexpected event in the course of observing or treating a patient

Those that explain
- The possible pathology of a disease

Those that signal
- An adverse effect
- A unique or rare feature of a disease
- A unique therapeutic approach
- A positional or quantitative variation of the anatomical structures

Table 8. Types of case reports

Single or multiple cases are a valuable source for future research on diagnosis, treatment effectiveness, causes, and disease outcomes. They have a valid place in medical research and evidence-based medicine in that they facilitate the detection of new diseases and possible undesirable treatment effects. By providing a construct for case-based learning, they can play a part in medical education.

Advocates of case reports suggest a high sensitivity for detecting novel or unusual cases that may be submerged in the collective approach adopted in a cohort, survey or randomised controlled trial (RCT). An oft-stated attribute of the humble case report is that different aspects of the patient's medical situation (e.g. patient history, physical examination, diagnosis, psychosocial aspects, and follow-up) can be identified compared to RCTs. The latter, placed at the evidence hierarchy's pinnacle, usually assess a few variables and rarely reflect the complete picture of a complicated medical situation. Therefore, the case report remains one of the cornerstones of medical progress, providing many new ideas and avenues for future research in medicine, as shown in Table 9.

Case reports in medical research and evidence-based medicine

Can facilitate
- recognition of new diseases;
- adverse or unexpected effects of treatments; and
- unusual disease trajectories (such as rapid recovery, non-response to treatment).

Can help
- understand the clinical spectrum of rare diseases;
- understand unusual presentations of common diseases;
- generate study hypotheses, including plausible mechanisms of disease; and
- guide the personalisation of treatments in clinical practice.

Table 9. The beneficial roles of case reports in medical research and evidence-based medicine

Case reports offer the possibility of speedy publication. As a kind of rapid short communication, they are particularly attractive to early-career researchers or busy clinicians who may not have the time or resources to conduct large-scale research. Several journals specialise in publishing case reports.

The CARE (CAse REport) guidelines, including a reporting checklist, have been drawn up to aid in the robust reporting of case reports. See Appendix 1 for complete details.

In common with all manuscripts, publication in a case report of any personal information about an identifiable living patient requires the patient or guardian's explicit consent. Signed informed consent from patients, relatives, or guardians should accompany case report manuscripts. If the patient is dead, authors should seek permission from a relative, ideally the next of kin. When signed consent from a deceased patient, guardian, or family is not obtained, proof must be available to show that thorough attempts have been made to contact the family. The paper should also have been satisfactorily anonymised not to cause harm to the patient or the patient's family.

4.6.2. Designing case series

Case series progress from case reports. A clinical characteristic is identified in case reports, which presents a thought-provoking, infrequent, or educational set of conditions. Next, a case series traces patients with a similar identifiable disease or prescribed treatment. This group's medical records are then studied for exposure and outcome.

When selecting a theme for a case series, researchers use information-oriented sampling instead of random sampling. The resultant group of cases may then satisfy reasoned findings and explanations based on this knowledge of circumstances.

The relevance of case series research depends on the researcher's ability to convert the investigation from a descriptive account of what happened into a research communication of meaning, significance and value and consequently add to existing knowledge. They can be retrospective or prospective and usually involve fewer patients than more powerful case-control studies or RCTs.

The validity of a case series may be compromised by selection bias. Reports as to the causality of any observed correlations will have a selection bias in that they are likely to be based on patients from one location, such as a hospital or clinic. Due to the lack of a control group exposed to the same range of variables, the internal validity of a case series is usually low. In a case series report, the observed outcomes may be wholly or partly due to intervening causes. A placebo effect, Hawthorne effect, Rosenthal effect, time effects, and practice effects are only some of the intervening effects that can influence the internal validity of case series reports. Calculating the difference in effects between two treatment groups, which are assumed to be exposed to a very similar array of such intervening effects, allows the effects of these intervening variables to cancel out.

Case series and reports are in-depth studies of a situation rather than a comprehensive, statistically sound survey. They are helpful tools for refining a wide-ranging field of research into a defined researchable topic. A case series does not provide a comprehensive answer to a question. It is suggested that they are spinoffs, which can aid further development and hypothesis creation on a subject. Case series have also been used as a teaching method and in professional development.

A deliberate attempt is made to isolate one small study group or one particular population in a case study. Table 10 sets out an approach to designing a case series:

Choose the subject and relevance, **and then plan and design how to address the study by ensuring that**
- all collected data are relevant; and
- the study is focused and concise.

Moreover:
- There is no strict set of rules (unlike a scientific report);
- Draw up a shortlist of bullet points to be addressed during the study. Ensure that all research refers back to these;
- It is important to adopt a passive approach (questionnaire or survey); and
- Design the case report as an observer, not as an examiner.

Table 10. An approach to designing a case series

In general, a case series does not generate a great deal of new information. As a research method or strategy, case series have traditionally been viewed as lacking thoroughness, precision, and objectivity when compared with other research methods. Researchers should be cautious and precise in stating their research design and be highly conservative in presenting conclusions to avoid this criticism. The statistics employed in a case series report are descriptive and are complemented by graphical displays of disease indicators over time or compared with the norm. A topic will be selected for a case series if it is considered important concerning a general problem. Ideally, the following type of generalisation would be valid: "If it is valid for this series, it may be valid for all cases." Both case reports and case series help suggest possible answers to how and why questions, and in this role it can be used for exploratory or descriptive research.

The pros and cons of case series research are set out in Table 11:

Pros	Cons
• Researchers can focus on specific and interesting cases. • Try to test a theory with a typical case. • Examines a particular topic that is of interest • Facilitate recognition of new diseases and adverse effects of treatments • **Quick and cheap**	Methodologically limited (e.g. the lack of statistical sampling)
Facilitate an understanding of: • The clinical spectrum of rare diseases • Unusual presentations of common diseases • **Facilitate recognition of new diseases and adverse effects of treatments**	Restricted topic: Essential to realise that a case study cannot be generalised to fit a whole population or ecosystem.
• A useful tool whether testing scientific theories and models work in the real world • Help generate study hypotheses	
New and unexpected results may arise, leading to research taking new directions	
Offers more representative responses than a purely statistical survey	
Case studies can have a substantial effect: • Provide interesting themes than purely statistical surveys • The general public pays scant attention to pages of statistical calculations.	

Table 11. Pros and cons of case series research

4.7. Designing cross-sectional studies

Cross-sectional studies are observational studies that involve data collection from a population, or a representative subset, at one specific point in time, without follow-up. Cross-sectional studies are intended to provide data on a whole population under study, compared to case-control studies, which typically include solitary individuals with a specific characteristic. Occasionally, they can include a minority sample of the rest of the population.

Their suitability to demonstrate variables and patterns of distribution renders them helpful in evaluating the prevalence of acute or chronic conditions or to answer questions about the causes of disease or the results of an intervention.

Table 12 sets out the fundamentals of cross-sectional studies:

Variables measured at one point in time: • Normally no follow-up   • No distinction between predictors and outcomes
Provides descriptive information about the prevalence
Their use eliminates problems associated with   • Dropouts   • Time constraints   • Expense   as compared to follow-up studies.
Yield weak evidence for causality
Not best suited for studying uncommon diseases   Require large sample sizes (cf. case-control studies)

Table 12. Fundamentals of cross-sectional studies

In public health planning, they play a role in estimating the prevalence of an outcome or disease of interest for a given population.

By collecting data on individual characteristics, including exposure to risk factors, together with information on outcomes, cross-sectional studies make available a "snapshot" of the outcome and the characteristics at a precise point in time. A carefully designed cross-sectional study can provide an analytical approach that identifies or illuminates possible causal pathways, which can be further tested in RCTs.

They may also be described as censuses in that they are a significant source of information about the health of a population at the time they were conducted.

Cross-sectional studies may include the collection of specific data. Questions about past events or data initially collected for other purposes are frequently used. However, the difficulty some participants have in recalling past events may contribute to bias.

They are not the most suitable design for studying rare diseases, especially if this involves collecting data on a sample of individuals from the general population. However, a cross-sectional approach may be appropriate if the sample to be studied is drawn from the population of rare-diseased patients rather than the general population.

The use of routinely collected data allows extensive cross-sectional studies to be made at little or no expense. This is a significant advantage over other forms of epidemiological study. A natural progression follows from low-priced cross-sectional studies of routinely collected data that propose hypotheses to case-control studies, which then test these findings in detail, to cohort studies and RCTs. The latter is considerably more expensive and time-consuming but may give more robust evidence. In a cross-sectional survey, a specific group is investigated to see whether a specific activity is related to health, for example, the relationship of smoking to oral cancer.

A frequent problem in longitudinal studies and RCTs is due to "loss to follow-up," when subjects, for several reasons, fail to re-attend, thus minimising the amount of helpful information collected. However, this is not a problem in cross-sectional study design, as follow-up is not typically incorporated in the design.[5]

The advantages and disadvantages of cross-sectional studies are outlined in Table 13:

Advantages	Disadvantages
• Relatively inexpensive and take little time to conduct; • Can estimate the prevalence of the outcome of interest because the sample is usually taken from the whole population; • Many outcomes and risk factors can be assessed; • Useful for public health planning, understanding disease aetiology and the generation of hypotheses; • There is no loss to follow-up; • Use of routine data: large-scale, low-cost.	• Difficult to make causal inferences; • Only a snapshot: the situation may provide differing results if another timeframe had been chosen; • Prevalence-incidence bias (also called Neyman bias): especially in longer-lasting diseases, any risk factor that results in death will be under-represented among those with the disease.

Table 13. Advantages and disadvantages of cross-sectional studies

While cross-sectional studies allow the acquisition of wide-ranging knowledge about respondents, who may or may not possess or be affected by a particular disorder, they minimise the information on the outcome measures of interest on which the study is predicated. Therefore, it is always advisable before the study to consider what information might be relevant.

Associations between outcomes and long duration exposures are difficult to determine, let alone prove, using cross-sectional studies.[3]

4.8. Designing case-control studies

A case-control study analytically compares subjects with a specific disease, termed the "cases," with subjects without the disease termed "controls." The proportion of each group with a history of a particular exposure or characteristic of interest is then compared.

Case-control studies aim to decide on study controls that are typical of the population producing the cases. Controls provide an estimate of the exposure rate within the population.[4]

A case-control study makes comparisons between participants with a specific condition and those who do not have the specified condition. The researcher first identifies subjects who exhibit a particular health outcome, the second group without. The prevalence of each of the two groups to the exposure to a likely risk factor is then compared. A higher prevalence of exposure among cases with a health outcome than controls suggests a risk factor for the outcome under investigation. Ideally, controls should come from the same population from which the cases have originated. Whenever possible, controls should be matched for age, gender, and socioeconomic groupings.

The exposure status is established after a disease has been developed; it can result in recall bias when the two groups describe occurrences differently. Poor study design or poor or inadequate collection of exposure and outcome data are the leading causes of bias.

Because the disease and exposure have already occurred before the commencement of a case-control study, there may be a discrepancy in reporting exposure information between cases and controls based on their disease status. In addition, people who have a disease are more likely to remember past exposures differently.

Interviewer or observer bias occurs when the recording of exposure information differs due to the investigator's knowledge of an individual's disease status. Selection bias is an inherent problem in case-control studies and can give rise to non-comparability between cases and controls. Selection bias can also occur when participants are included or excluded from a study because of a presenting feature related to exposure to the risk factor under evaluation. An essential requirement is to select study controls that are representative of the target population. Selection bias may occur when patients selected as controls are unrepresentative of the target population.

A particular problem occurs when cases and controls are recruited solely from hospitals or clinics. Hospital patients are apt to have different characteristics from the population at large. If these characteristics are linked to the studied exposures, then the estimated exposure among controls may differ from the reference population. As a result, a biased estimate of the association between exposure and disease will take place. Selection bias may also be introduced in case-control studies when exposed cases are more likely to be selected than unexposed cases.[9]

Essential considerations when considering case-control studies are set out in Table 14:

Hypothesis
A clearly defined theory established at the outset of the study.
Case definition
The case definition is determined at the investigation's inception to ensure that all cases included in the study are based on the same diagnostic criteria.
Source of cases
The source needs to be clearly defined.
Measuring exposure status
In case-control studies, the extent of exposure is established after the development of the disease, and as a result, is predisposed to both recall and observer bias.

Table 14. Essential considerations when reviewing case-control studies

Nevertheless, case-control studies are regularly performed compared to other study designs; they are easier to perform.[4]

The stages in their design are set out in Table 15

Matters referring to case selection
Clear hypothesis
The beginning of a case-control study should begin with the formulation of a clearly defined hypothesis.
Case definition
Essential that the case definition is clearly formulated at the outset of the investigation. All cases included in the study should be based on the same diagnostic criteria.
Source of cases
The source of cases must be clearly defined. Cases may be drafted from various sources, such as hospitals, clinics, GP registers, or population-based.

Selection of cases

A fundamental problem in case-control studies is obtaining a comparable control group.

- Controls are used to estimate the prevalence of exposure in the population which gave rise to the cases.
- The ideal control group comprises a random sample from the general population that gave rise to the cases. However, unfortunately, this is not easy in practice.
- If there is no actual association between exposure and disease, the cases and controls should have the same exposure distribution.
- The source of controls is dependent on the source of cases.
- To reduce bias, controls should be selected to be a representative sample of the population that produced the cases, e.g. if cases are selected from a defined population such as a hospital register, controls should be obtained from the same hospital register.

Table 15. Stages in designing a case-controlled study

Case selection to ensure that the study population is representative, and to limit bias is essential. Table 16 lists methods to try to ensure this happens. Finally, table 17 presents key issues in case-control studies:

- Controls are obtained from the same population as the cases. Therefore, their selection should be separate from the exposures of interest.
- Ensure that controls do not include individuals with an outcome related to the exposure(s) being studied.
- Controls are not required to be in good health; inclusion of sick people is sometimes appropriate, as the control group should represent those at risk of becoming a case.
- Controls can have the same malady or syndrome as the experimental group but with a different rating or seriousness.
- Consequently, the power to detect an exposure effect is smaller because the difference between the cases and the controls is smaller.
- An increase in study numbers will increase the power of the study.
- The numbers of cases and controls do not have to be equal.
- Controls are often easier to find than actual cases.
- Increasing the number of controls above the number of cases, up to a ratio of about 4:1, is a cost-effective way to improve the study.

Table 16. Tips on case selection

- Data are collected retrospectively and may give rise to bias.
- The collection of retrospective data has the potential of introducing the possibility of recall bias.
- Recall bias is the tendency of subjects to report events differently between the two groups studied. For example, people who have a disease may be more likely to remember exposures more readily than those without the disease.

Table 17. Key issues in case-control studies

Case-control studies may use incident or prevalent cases (Table 18):

Incident cases	Prevalent cases
Cases recently diagnosed in a defined period.	Cases in which the outcome has been under investigation for some time.
Strength of incident cases:	**The weakness of prevalent cases:**
The recollection of past exposure(s) may be more precise among recently diagnosed cases.	The use of prevalent cases may give rise to recall bias as prevalent cases may be less likely to report past exposure(s) accurately.
The chronological of exposure and disease is easier to assess	Interpretation of results based on prevalent cases may prove more problematic.

Table 18. Incident and prevalent cases

The selection of controls in case-control studies is fundamental to the study concerned. Details of this process are set out in Table 19:

The aim is to select study controls representative of the population which produced the cases. The collection of exposure data should be the same for cases as for controls.
A problem is the selection of a comparable control group. • Controls estimate the prevalence of exposure in the population which gave rise to the cases. • Ideally, the control group is a random sample from the general population that gave rise to the cases. • To minimise bias, controls should be selected to represent the population that produced the cases. • The potential for selection bias is a particular problem when cases and controls are recruited exclusively from hospitals or clinics because they tend to have different characteristics than the general population. • The potential for selection bias may be minimised by opting for controls from more than one source, such as using both hospital and neighbourhood controls. • Selection bias can be introduced when exposed cases are more likely to be selected than unexposed cases.

Table 19. Selection of controls in case-control studies

Methods used to ascertain exposure status are set out in Table 20:

• Standardised questionnaires; • Biological samples; • Interviews with the subject; • Interviews with a spouse or other family members; • Medical records; • Pharmacy records; and • Employment records.

Table 20. Methods used to ascertain exposure status

In case-control studies, it is essential to avoid bias.[7] Common sources of bias in case-control studies are set out in Table 21:

Their retrospective nature renders case-control studies particularly susceptible to bias, which may be introduced due to poor study design or during the collection of data.
Recall bias
Cases and controls may have a different recollection of past exposures.
Interviewer/observer bias
The logging of exposure information is dependent on the investigator's knowledge of an individual's disease status.
Selection bias
Selection bias can occur • if control individuals are unrepresentative of the population that produced the cases; and • if cases or controls are included or excluded from a study because of some displayed characteristic related to exposure to the risk factor under evaluation.

Table 21. Common Causes of Bias in Case-Control Studies

The advantages and disadvantages of case-control studies are set out in Table 22:

Advantages	Disadvantages
• Cost-effective compared to other analytical studies, e.g. cohort studies; • Case-control studies are retrospective studies. Cases are identified at the commencement of the study. Therefore there is no long follow-up period or prolonged exposure to risk compared to cohort studies; • Valid for the studying of diseases with long latency periods; • Useful for the study of rare diseases.	• Markedly prone to bias, especially selection, recall and observer bias; • The selection of a comparable control group is problematic; • Case-control studies are limited to observing or assessing one outcome; • Unable to estimate incidence rates of disease (unless the study is population-based); • A wrong option for the study of rare exposures. • The temporal sequence between exposure and disease may be challenging to determine.

Table 22. The advantages and disadvantages of case-control studies

Table 23 sets out the strengths and weaknesses of case-control studies:

Strengths	Weaknesses
• Suitable for rare diseases. • It can be conducted in a short time. • Multiple exposures can be explored. • Inexpensive.	• Relies on recall and historical data on exposure. • Temporality and causality can be difficult to establish. • Allows cases and controls to be compared.

Table 23. Strengths and weaknesses of case-control studies

A final word about case-control studies: although they cannot prove causality, they may be able to demonstrate a statistical association that indicates a possible causal pathway.

4.9. Designing cohort studies

A cohort study is a longitudinal observational study. The investigated population consists of individuals who do not have a disease but are susceptible to acquiring a particular disease or health outcome. A cohort study design is suitable for assessing associations between multiple exposures and multiple outcomes. They are particularly suitable when studying rare exposures or exposures for which randomisation is not achievable for practical or ethical reasons. Features of cohort studies, types of cohort studies, and key characteristics of cohort studies and their strengths and weaknesses are described in Tables 24, 25, 26, and 27.

> - A group of patients or subjects with a common characteristic or experience within a defined period, e.g. born within the defined period, are subject to a medicine, vaccine, or pollutant, or to undergo a particular medical strategy.
> - The comparison group may be the general population from which the group is acquired. It also may be another similar group considered to have had little or no exposure.
> - Within a cohort, it is appropriate to compare subgroups with each other.
> - It analyses risk factors and uses correlations to determine the absolute risk of a subject contracting a disease or suffering an adverse outcome.
> - It can either be conducted prospectively or retrospectively from archived records and questionnaires.

Table 24. Features of cohort studies

Descriptive
Describes the occurrence of outcome over time
Analytical
Analyses the association between independent variables (risk factors) and dependent variables (outcomes)
Prospective
The researcher - Defines the sample - Measures characteristics that may predict subsequent outcomes - Follows the sample, measuring outcomes over time.
Retrospective
The researcher - Defines the sample (positive cases) - Identifies and records relevant risk factors (e.g. past behaviour, exposure to risks) - Establishes associations between outcome and risk factors.

Table 25. Types of cohort study

The Key characteristics of cohort studies are outlined in Table 26:

At the starting point of the study,
- Subjects are identified;
- An assessment is made of their exposure to a risk factor.

Over a defined timespan,

- The frequency of the outcome is measured and related to exposure status. This is frequently the incidence of disease or death. The effect of exposure on the outcome can be expressed as a relative risk.

Table 26. Key characteristics of cohort studies

Advantages	Disadvantages
• Possible to study multiple exposures and multiple outcomes in one cohort. • Rare exposures can be studied. • Demonstrates an appropriate temporal sequence between exposure and outcome. • Permits the direct calculation of incidence rates in both the exposed and unexposed groups. • Permits multiple outcomes to be assessed in the same study. • The combined effect of multiple exposures on disease risk can be determined. • As a cohort study usually has broader inclusion criteria and fewer exclusion criteria than an RCT, results may be more generalisable to clinical practice. • Provides an indication of the incubation or latency period for communicable or noncommunicable diseases, respectively. • Relatively uncommon exposures can be studied.	• Not possible to establish causal effects, as the exposure has not been allocated randomly; the possibility that association found may be due to other variables that differ between exposed and non-exposed subjects. (Confounders). • Potential large sample size requirements. • Long follow-up periods and the need to reassess exposure. • Potential losses to follow-up. • Possible outcome misclassification. • Potential exposure misclassification.

Table 27. Advantages and disadvantages of cohort studies

Randomised controlled trials (RCTs), although ranked higher in the hierarchy of clinical intervention studies than cohort studies, are frequently impossible to undertake for either practical or ethical reasons. Therefore, a cohort study often represents a suitable observational study design to answer various research questions in these situations.

4.9.1. Prospective versus retrospective cohort studies

In a prospective cohort study, the exposure is assessed at baseline, and the researcher follows the subjects over time to study the development of disease or mortality. Outcomes, such as developing a disease, are measured during the study period and compared to potential risk or protection factors. The number of observed outcomes should not be too small to be statistically insignificant or impossible to differentiate from those arising by chance. A good study design will reduce bias causes, such as the loss of individuals to follow up during the study. Prospective studies, in comparison to retrospective studies, by and large, have fewer potential sources of bias and confounding.[6]

The strengths and weaknesses of prospective cohort studies are set out in Table 28:

Strengths	Weaknesses
• A temporal relationship is established • Multiple outcomes can be studied • Suitable for rare exposure situations • A robust strategy for assessing incidence (the number of new cases in a specified time) • The researcher defines and applies the outcome criteria • Independent variables are measured before the dependent variables are collected and a time frame established • This reduces the chance of independent variables being influenced by knowledge of outcome variables	• Challenging to select and maintain a non-exposed group • Prone to "loss at follow-up" for long induction times • Changes can take place over time in both the exposure and outcome assessment • Expensive

Table 28. Strengths and weaknesses of prospective cohort studies

Selection bias can be introduced in a prospective cohort study by an inadequate response if non-response is selective (i.e. different in those with both exposure and an increased risk of developing the disease). In addition, the loss to follow-up can be a source of further bias. When selective loss to follow-up occurs, such attrition is never completely random.

In a retrospective cohort study, the researcher starts the study once the outcome has already been established. Then exposures to suspected risk or protection factors concerning this are measured. However, retrospective studies are criticised as sources of error because confounding and bias are more common than in prospective studies.

In both types of cohort studies, even when confounding and bias should be reduced as much as possible, unknown effects in unknown directions can arise. Nevertheless, cohort studies remain an effective study type yielding highly generalisable results if this fact is borne in mind in the designing process.

The strengths and weaknesses of retrospective cohort studies are set out in Table 29:

Strengths	Weaknesses
• Time-efficient and elegant, as questions are answered using existing data • Useful in studying rare conditions and those with low incidence, even in the presence of risk factors	• Uses past data often collected for other purposes, not specifically for the question under current investigation • Patients who have died or recovered may not be included in the cohort, thereby introducing selection bias

Table 29. Strengths and weaknesses of retrospective cohort studies

The differences between cohort studies and case-control studies are set out in Table 30. Identification of cases and controls in case-control studies are listed in Table 31. Finally, the methods used to measure exposure status are listed in Table 32.

Cohort studies	Case-control studies
Cohort studies are generally but not exclusively perspective; the opposite is true for case-control studies. • the outcome is measured after exposure • Are a source of accurate incidence rates and relative risks • may expose unsuspected associations with outcome • best for common outcomes • expensive • should involve large participant numbers • it takes a long time to complete • prone to attrition bias • prone to the bias of change in methods over time.	Case-control studies are usually but not exclusively retrospective; the opposite is true for cohort studies. • the outcome is measured before exposure • controls are selected based on not having the outcome • good for rare outcomes • relatively inexpensive • smaller numbers required • quicker to complete • prone to selection bias • predisposed to recall or retrospective bias.

Table 30. Cohort Studies Versus Case-control Studies

In Table 31, we see methods used to measure exposure status:

• Biological samples; • Interviews with the subject; • Interviews with a spouse or other family members; • Medical records; • Employment records; and • Pharmacy records.

Table 31. Methods used to measure exposure status

References

1   Koretz RL. Considerations of study design. *Nutrition in Clinical Practice* 2007, 22(6):593-598.

2   Creswell J. Research design; qualitative and quantitative and mixed methods approaches. London: Sage; 2009.

3   Mann CJ. Observational research methods. Research design II: cohort, cross-sectional, and case-control studies. *Emergency Medicine Journal* 2003;20:54-60.

4   van Stralen KJ, Dekker FW, Zoccali C, Jager KJ.Case-control studies--an efficient observational study design. *Nephron Clinical Practice*. 2010;114(1): 1-4.

5   Sedgwick P. Cross-sectional studies: advantages and disadvantages. *British Medical Journal* 2014;348 f7707 ng JW, Chung KC. Observational studies: cohort and case-control studies. *Plastic Reconstruction Surgery* 2010;126(6):2234–2242.

6   Geneletti S, Best N, Toledano MB, Elliott P, Richardson S. Uncovering selection bias in case-control studies using Bayesian post-stratification. *Statistics in Medicine* 2013;32(15):2555-2570.

Chapter 5. Designing Studies Part 2— Randomised Controlled Trials

SANTINI A.

5.1. Overview

After a brief introduction, this chapter will cover the following aspects of randomised controlled trials (RCTs):

- Design features;
- Selection of patients;
- Clinical trials;
- Sampling methods;
- Randomisation;
- Blinding; and
- Reporting the results of RCTs.

5.2. Introduction

A randomised controlled trial (RCT) is a clinical study in which the people being studied are randomly assigned to different treatments. RCTs are generally considered to be the gold standard for a clinical trial. They are often used to test the usefulness, success or efficacy of various medical therapies or procedures. Before any intervention, after they have been recruited and assessed for suitability, patients are randomly assigned into groups. One of which will be a control group. After a defined follow-up period, data are collected and analysed.

5.3. Design features of a randomised controlled trial (RCT)

The key features of the design of an RCT will now be discussed, highlighting the importance of the validity of findings and emphasising the errors related to bias, confounding, and chance.[1]

In an RCT, subjects are randomly assigned to one of two groups: one, the experimental group, receiving the intervention that is being tested, and the other, the comparison or control group, receiving an alternative current conventional treatment. The two groups are then followed up to see if there are differences in their treatment outcomes. In some RCTs, three groups (two tests and one control) may be recruited. The trial results and subsequent analysis are used to assess the effectiveness of the intervention, which is the extent to which treatment, procedure, or service does patients more good than harm. RCTs are the most stringent way of determining whether a cause-effect relation exists between the intervention and the outcome.[1]

This chapter discusses various key features of RCT design, with particular emphasis on the validity of findings. Of course, there are many potential errors associated with health research. However, the main ones to be considered are bias, confounding, and chance.

Bias is defined as a departure of outcomes from the truth. For example, an error in study design will result in bias. There are several types of bias. Selection bias occurs when the studied groups differ systematically in one or more respects. Observer or information bias occurs when there are differences in the way evidence is collected.

A confounding variable is an unquantified third variable that affects the assumed cause and the assumed effect. A good example relates to the hospitalisation of older patients. Generally speaking, older patients are likely to be hospitalised because of their age. However, suppose a new drug is being investigated but is less likely to be prescribed to older patients, and the study's outcome of interest is access to a hospital. In that case, older patients for unrelated reasons may experience the outcome of interest, such as access to a hospital, where the perceived association between the drug and the likelihood of being admitted to a hospital would be confounded by age.

Chance is a random error that advances the notion that there is an association between an intervention and an outcome. Random error is reduced using large sample sizes. The results of any research project are affected by these types of error, resulting in the inaccuracy of the study's interpretation, conclusions, and generalisability. A well-designed RCT will minimise if not eradicate any adverse impact resulting from these errors.

Design strategies

A well-designed study allows researchers to show how manipulating one set of variables, the independent variables, produces changes in the second set of variables, the outcome or dependent variables. Studies should be designed to ensure that all variables other than the independent variables are controlled. The outcome variables are due to variations in the independent variables and no other factors. This is not easily achieved outside a laboratory setting. Clinical studies, of which RCTs are one type, nearly always take place in clinics and hospitals, and researchers should design studies that control extraneous variables in these environments. Between-group designs always include groups that receive a defined intervention, a test group, and another that receives either no active treatment (placebo) or a comparison treatment (usually the standard treatment for that condition, known as treatment as usual, or TAU). This is the control group.

Many study designs, including non-randomised controlled trials, can detect associations between an intervention and an outcome. However, they cannot rule out the possibility that the outcome measure was affected by a third factor. In experimental clinical studies, the researcher actively changes independent variables and monitors the outcome by measuring the outcome or dependent variables. RCTs are designed primarily to assess clinical interventions in clinical locations and to minimise third-factor effect or bias. They are the most demanding way to determine a cause-effect relation between treatment and outcome, often used to test the efficacy or effectiveness of various medical intervention types, frequently medications, within a patient population.

RCTs are increasingly used in other public services, such as educational research and criminology, within an increasing recognition of the value of the evidence-based policy.[2,3]

The features of a well-designed RCT are set out in Table 1. The general requirements for RCTs are set out in Table 2.

1. To ensure the generalisability of results, the sample population should approximate the tested hypothesis. In addition, sufficient patients must be recruited to result in a high probability of detecting a clinically significant difference between treatments if a difference truly exists.
2. There should be effective subject-randomisation for both the intervention and control groups to eliminate selection bias and minimise confounding variables.
3. Both groups should receive identical treatments undertaken in all particulars except for the tested intervention. To achieve this, subjects should be blinded to which group they are being assigned.
4. Investigators measuring outcome measures should be blinded to treatment allocation.
5. The intention to treat analysis policy should be followed where patients are analysed within their group, regardless of whether they underwent the intended intervention or not.
6. Analysis should centre on testing the a priori hypothesis rather than "trawling" to find a significant difference.

Table 1. Features of a well-designed RCT

Population	The researcher defines the population he or she wishes to study.	These steps are common in all clinical trials.
Sample	A sample population is selected using an appropriate sampling method.	
Assignment	The sample population is assigned to different intervention groups. However, all subgroups must be mainly the same. Differences would make it difficult to attribute the cause to outcome measurements.	In RCTs, one or more groups receive an active intervention. One group gets a control intervention missing the active factor. This preferably is a placebo or no-treatment group.
Intervention treatment	To ensure blinding, the researcher administers the treatment/s (independent variable) to the various groups, including any placebo.	The treatment/s must be administered in an unbiased manner.
Outcome measurement	The study is assessed by analysis of the outcome measures (dependent variables).	Dependent variables can be measured: • Before and after the intervention period (pre/post-testing). • Only after the intervention period (post-testing). • On multiple occasions.

Table 2. General requirements for RCTs

The first step in the initial design stage of an RCT is the assessment of subjects for eligibility. This is realised by stating and employing a set of *a priori* inclusion and exclusion criteria. For example, all outpatient clinic attendees may be one inclusion criterion, adjusted by excluding the non-recruitment of children or pregnant women. These eligibility criteria are preferably applied before the study population's random sampling to achieve the required study numbers. The second and third steps involve randomising the participants before the study begins and allocated to alternative treatments or interventions under study. The two or more groups are followed in precisely the same way; data are collected and finally analysed.

Randomised controlled trials may be classified by

- Study design (Table 3)
- The outcome of interest (Table 4)
- Hypothesis (Table 5)

Parallel group	Each participant is randomised into a group. All participants in any one group receive or do not receive a specific treatment.
Crossover	Over time, each participant receives or does not receive specific treatment in random order.
Cluster	Pre-existing groups (such as towns, areas, and schools) are randomly selected to receive or not to receive a specific treatment.
Factorial	Each participant is randomised to a group that receives or does not receive specific permutations of treatment.

Table 3. Randomised controlled trials by study design

Classification of randomised controlled trials by outcome of interest	
Explanatory	Explanatory RCTs test efficacy with highly selected participants and highly controlled conditions.
Pragmatic	Pragmatic RCTs test effectiveness in everyday practice. Participants are not highly selected, and conditions are accommodating.

Table 4. Randomised controlled trials by outcome of interest

Superiority trials	Most RCTs are superiority trials, in which one intervention is hypothesised to be statistically significantly superior to another.
Non-inferiority trials	This type of RCT is established whether a new treatment is worse than a reference treatment.
Equivalence trials	In this type of RCT, the hypothesis is that there is no statistical difference between two different treatment modalities.

Table 5. Randomised controlled trials by hypothesis

The remainder of this chapter will focus on the elements of the traditional randomised controlled trial: the selection of participants, approaches to randomisation, blinding, measuring baseline variables, intervention, and control.

Though generally considered the gold standard for a clinical trial, RCTs are not without disadvantages (Table 6):

Advantages
Considered the most reliable scientific evidence because their design reduces causality and bias.
It may be combined in systematic reviews, which are increasingly used as a basis for evidence-based practice.
Return on investments may be high and offset initial high costs.
Disadvantages
Limitations of external validity: • Location (what works in one locality/country may not be relevant in another). • Patients' characteristics (inclusion/exclusion of patients with better-than-average prognoses or based on sex, age, and other criteria). • Study procedures may be unrealistic and difficult to achieve in the real world. • May use composite outcome measures not standard in clinical practice.
It can be costly. Time required: • Trials may take several years to complete. • Data not made available for extended periods. • Maybe less relevant at the time of publication.
Difficulty in studying rare events. RCTs with a considerable sample size would need to compensate for: • Infrequently occurring events (e.g. sudden infant death syndrome) • Uncommon adverse outcomes (e.g. rare drug side effects)
Erroneous belief in a therapeutic effect • Misunderstanding by participants of the difference between research and treatment. • Evidence suggests that many participants believe they will always receive the best treatment (despite informed consent).
Limited variables • Usually study a limited number of variables and often only one. • Rarely reflects the entire nature of a complicated medical scenario.
Statistical errors • RCTs are subject to both type I and II errors. • Sample size of many "negative" RCTs may be too small to arrive at negativity conclusions.

Table 6. Advantages and disadvantages of randomised controlled trials

5.4. Selection of patients

A target population, appropriate and accessible to the study, is selected after exclusion and inclusion criteria have been defined as in any clinical trial.

Inclusion criteria are a list of conditions that a person must have in order to be incorporated in a sample population.

Exclusion criteria are a list of criteria that, if met by a subject, lead to that subject not being allowed into the sample population, even if he or she meets the inclusion criteria.

Exclusion criteria fall into three main categories:

1. A participant is too unwell to participate in the study. An ethical concern is that a participant with a comorbid illness may not receive beneficial treatment and opportunities if included in a study and may put patients at risk. Subjects who are too unwell are therefore often excluded from sample populations.
2. A participant may become unwell during the study. For ethical reasons, exclusion criteria may exclude patients who are well but may become ill in the study, should they take part. For example, patients with allergies or intolerances to the medicines prescribed in the study or taking medication that may interact with the study medicines fall into this category.
3. A participant has a confounding factor. Study conclusions can arrive at the wrong decisions when confounding factors are present. To avoid this, subjects with confounding factors are excluded from the sample population. As a result, confounding due to these factors will no longer be a problem.

In many clinical studies, outcome rates are often much lower than predictable at the beginning of the trial. Therefore, studies should be planned so that the prerequisite sample size can be recruited from a large, easily reached population. The time factor and available funding are the two most common constraints in achieving an appropriate sample size.

It is usually not practicable to include every person in a target population in a study. As an alternative, a sample population is recruited, representative of the target population.

Table 7 describes the effects of inclusion and exclusion criteria if they are inappropriate:

Inclusion criteria	Exclusion criteria
• Power of the study: defined inclusion criteria should allow sufficient numbers of participants to be enrolled such that the study has adequate power to identify an effect on the outcome; • High-risk patients: inclusion of this type of patient may reduce the numbers required; • The most significant benefit: the inclusion of patients who are likely to benefit most from treatment can result in smaller and shorter studies.	Unnecessary exclusion criteria may • Make sufficient recruitment numbers difficult; • Increase the cost of recruitment; • Increase the complexity of the study; • Reduce the generalisability of results.

Table 7. Effects of inclusion and exclusion criteria

5.5. Clinical trials

Confusion can occur between the terms "randomised controlled trial" and "randomised clinical trial." The differences are summarised in Table 8:

Randomised controlled trial	Randomised clinical trial
Reserved for studies that have a control group: • Placebo-controlled (no treatment) • Positive-controlled (previously tested treatment)	No mention of a control group. Can refer to comparisons of multiple treatment groups without controls. Not all randomised clinical trials are randomised controlled trials.

Table 8. Differences between randomised controlled trials and randomised clinical trials

There are several legitimate reasons why patients should be excluded from a clinical trial, and some are listed in Table 9:

1. Treatment could potentially be harmful:
  • Risk of adverse reactions;
  • Risk of allocation to no-treatment (placebo) group.
2. Treatment is likely to be ineffective because the patient has
  • A low risk for the outcome;
  • A disease that is not likely to respond to the study treatment;
  • Current treatment is likely to interfere with study treatment outcomes.
3. The patient is likely to be uncooperative or adhere to treatment plans.
4. The patient is unlikely to complete the study and attend follow-up.
5. Other practical reasons:
  • Language barriers
  • Cognitive reasons
  • No telephone number.

Table 9. Reasons patients should be excluded from a clinical trial

The researcher must record sufficient information about the participants:

- To demonstrate that the randomisation process has worked and a balance between the control and intervention groups.
- To be able to contact patients and so reduce loss to follow-up.
- To allow judgment by others as to the generalisability of the outcome measures.
- To identify major clinical characteristics and prognostic factors to enable predetermined subgroup analysis.

5.6. Sampling methods

When recruiting a sample for a study, the principles of equality and inclusion must be followed.

Five standard techniques are used to obtain a sample from a population. They are as follows:

1. Simple random sampling: Every person in the target population has an equal chance of being selected. Researchers usually have to access a database holding details of the target population. Random sampling is also known as representative sampling or proportionate sampling because all groups should be proportionately represented.
2. Systematic sampling: Every nth member of the target population is selected once the first person has been chosen randomly. This is known as quasi-random sampling. It usually obtains a representative sample of the population.
3. Stratified sampling: Subjects in the target population are put into subgroups depending on one or more characteristics, such as age, social class, or ethnicity. A sample is drawn from each of the subgroups, usually at random. This guarantees that people with specific characteristics are represented in the sample population.
4. Cluster sampling: The target population is divided into similar and representative clusters. Some of these clusters are exhaustively sampled; other clusters are not used.
5. Convenience sampling: Sampling is undertaken by selecting people as they appear and often choosing whether to be included in the sample. It is the easiest and potentially most dangerous. Good results can be obtained, but the data can be seriously biased.

The researcher must record sufficient information about the participants

- To demonstrate that the randomisation process has worked and a balance between the control and intervention groups;
- To be able to contact patients and reduce loss to follow-up;
- To allow judgment by others as to the generalisability of the outcome measures.[4]

5.7. Randomisation

Randomisation is a central feature of RCT design. At its simplest, it refers to allocating study subjects by chance to be included in either an intervention group or a control or comparison group. As randomisation is pivotal to a clinical trial, every effort must be made to undertake it correctly and with care. It is also crucial that the researcher(s) cannot influence the allocation of participants. In RCTs, it should occur before the study commences.

It is undertaken to eliminate, so far as possible, factors that could affect outcomes other than the intervention factor. Performed correctly as a method of experimental control, it safeguards against both selection bias and accidental bias. In addition, it should produce comparable groups by eliminating bias in treatment assignments, such as subject or researcher preference. Finally, it permits probability theory to express the likelihood of chance as a source for differences in outcome measures between groups.

The benefits of randomisation may be summarised as eliminating selection bias, balancing the groups concerning many known and unknown confounding or prognostic variables, and permitting statistical tests based on an assumption of the equality of treatments. In general, a randomised experiment is an essential tool for testing the efficacy of a treatment.

The advantages of randomisation are set out in Table 10:

Maximises statistical power
Equal numbers in groups tend to increase statistical power, though this is not always true (Dunnett's procedure)
Permits using probability theory to express the likelihood that differences in outcome measures between treatments arose by chance alone.
Expedites blinding of the identity of treatments from participants, researchers and analysts.
Minimises selection bias
Selection bias may occur if researchers can enrol participants preferentially between treatment groups (consciously or otherwise).
Selection bias is highest if previous treatment assignments are known (unblinded studies) or can be guessed.
Adequate randomisation reduces these risks.
Minimise allocation bias and confounding
Can occur if covariates that affect outcome measures are not equally distributed between groups.

Table 10. The advantages of randomisation

There are two processes involved in randomising patients to different interventions. The first is to choose a randomisation procedure to generate an unpredictable sequence of allocations. This may be a simple random assignment of patients to any group at equal probabilities; it may be "restricted" or "adaptive."

A second and more practical issue is allocation concealment. This refers to the rigorous safeguards taken to ensure that patients' group assignments are not revealed before their definitive allocation to respective groups. Non-random, systematic group assignment methods, such as alternating subjects between one group and the other, can cause contamination and a contravention of allocation concealment. As a result, randomisation goals are seldom fully met, and no one randomisation method fully addresses the problems associated with randomisation. Therefore, researchers must be diligent and select the most appropriate procedure for each study, with full consideration given to its advantages and disadvantages.

No single randomisation technique is ideal in all circumstances. Researchers should select one with due attention to the study design in question.

The preferred approach is simple randomisation of participants in equal ratios to the different groups. Simple randomisation works well for large clinical trials with participant numbers above one hundred. It is imperative to select a method that will produce interpretable and valid results (Table 10). Online software is available to generate randomisation codes using block randomisation procedures.

For small-to-moderate clinical trials with participant numbers below one hundred and without covariates, block randomisation helps achieve balance. For example, the randomisation method is preset to ensure that of the first n cases, exactly half are assigned to the intervention group and half to the control group. On the other hand, for small-to-moderate clinical trials with several prognostic factors or covariates, the adaptive randomisation method could help provide a means to achieve treatment balance.

Table 11 sets out the advantages and disadvantages of simple randomisation:

Advantages	Disadvantages
• The most common and basic method of simple randomisation is a coin, based on a single sequence of random assignments. • A random number table found in a statistics book, or computer-generated random numbers, can also be used. • Maintains complete randomness of the assignment of a subject to a particular group. • The approach is simple and easy to implement in clinical research. • In large-scale clinical research, simple randomisation can be reliable in generating similar numbers of subjects among groups.	• Randomisation results could be problematic in clinical research with small sample sizes, resulting in an unequal number of participants among groups.

Table 11. Advantages and disadvantages of simple randomisation

The advantages and disadvantages of block randomisations and covariate adaptive randomisations are set out in Tables 12 and 13.

Advantages	Disadvantages
• They are designed to randomise subjects into groups that result in equal sample sizes. • It is used to ensure a balance in sample size across groups over time. • Blocks are small and balanced with predetermined group assignments, which keeps the numbers of subjects in each group similar at all times.	• Groups may be generated that are rarely comparable in terms of specific covariates that could confound the data and may negatively influence the clinical trial results. • Any such imbalance could introduce bias in the statistical analysis and reduce the power of the study. • To avoid this, sample size and covariates must be balanced in clinical research.

Table 12. Advantages and disadvantages of block randomisation

Advantages	Disadvantages
• Covariate adaptive randomisation produces fewer imbalances than other conventional randomisation methods and can successfully balance significant covariates among control and treatment groups. • It is recommended as a valid alternative randomisation method for clinical research. • A new participant is sequentially assigned to a particular treatment group in covariate adaptive randomisation by considering the specific covariates and previous participants' assignments. • Covariate adaptive randomisation uses the method of minimisation by assessing the imbalance of sample size among several covariates.	• Covariate adaptive randomisation methods may lead to treatment assignments, sometimes becoming highly predictable. • This predictability stems from the ongoing assignment of participants to groups wherein participants' current allocation may suggest future participant group assignment. • The complicated computation process of covariate adaptive randomisation increases the administrative burden, limiting its use in practice.

Table 13. Advantages and disadvantages of covariate adaptive randomisation

Stratified randomisation controls for the possible influence of covariates that would jeopardise the conclusions of the clinical research. The simplest example is when males and females are known to react differently to an intervention. They are therefore randomised separately to ensure an equal gender balance in both groups. Using stratified randomisation, the researcher must identify specific covariates who understand each covariate's potential influence on the dependent variable. Stratified randomisation is achieved by generating a separate block for each combination of covariates, and subjects are assigned to the appropriate block of covariates. After all, subjects have been identified and assigned into blocks; simple randomisation is performed within each block to assign subjects to one of the groups.

The advantages and disadvantages of stratified randomisation are set out in Table 14:

Advantages	Disadvantages
• A relatively simple and helpful technique, especially for smaller clinical trials. • Addresses the need to control and balance the influence of covariates. • It can be used to balance groups in terms of subjects' baseline characteristics (covariates).	• Tends to be complicated if many covariates must be controlled. • This works only when all subjects have been identified before group assignment; this is rarely applicable as clinical subjects are usually enrolled one at a time continuously. • When baseline characteristics of all subjects are not available before the assignment, using stratified randomisation is difficult.

Table 14. Advantages and disadvantages of stratified randomisation

One potential problem with small to moderate-size clinical research projects is that simple randomisation (with or without taking stratification of prognostic variables into account) may cause an imbalance of important covariates among treatment groups. The imbalance of covariates is important because of its potential to influence the interpretation of research results.[5]

5.8. Blinding

The term blinding or masking refers to withholding information about the assigned interventions from people involved in the trial whom this knowledge may influence. Blinding is an essential safeguard against bias, particularly when assessing subjective outcomes. For example, researchers can look more closely at outcome measures in the untreated group or make a diagnosis more frequently in unblinded studies.

Double blinding is where both study subject and researcher remain unaware of which group any particular subject has been randomly assigned to. It is undertaken to eliminate, as much as possible, any preconceived ideas (on the part of both researchers and participants) which could influence outcome measures. Often it requires the administration of placebos to control subjects that look and taste the same as the intervention medication but are identifiable through labelling of the batches from which they are sourced. Key features of double-blinding are set out in Table 15.

Single blinding occurs when it is impossible to blind either the researcher or the subject for practical or ethical reasons, for example, when a new surgical procedure is radically different from the standard method. In some circumstances, blinding is not possible. The reasons for this should be clearly stated in the study protocol and any study reports on completion.

In double blinding, neither the researcher nor the patient knows whether the patient is in the experimental or control group throughout the study.	
Most useful • When the control group is receiving an identical placebo drug or "pretend" intervention	Ethical problems • Surgical trials: few participants would agree to "pretend" surgical interventions. • Is it ethical to deny one group potentially life-saving drugs?

Table 15. Key features of double blinding

In some studies, for technical or ethical reasons, intervention blinding may be impossible. In such circumstances, the study should be designed to limit and standardise other potential co-interventions as much as possible and blinding personnel responsible for collecting and deciding outcome measures.

5.9. Reporting results of RCTs: the CONSORT 2010 statement

The flow diagram from the CONSORT 2010 statement is at Table 16. Inadequate reporting of trials is common and impedes the use of trial results in healthcare research and practice. Complete and transparent reporting of results of clinical trials is essential for assessing the quality of healthcare.

CONSORT 2010 Flow Diagram

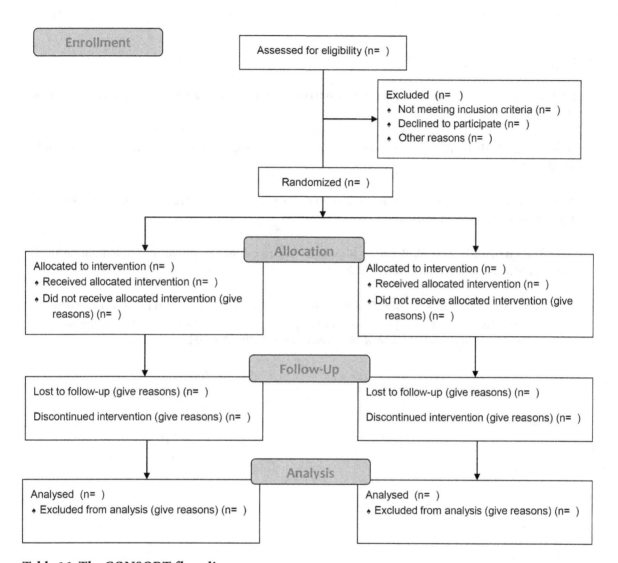

Table 16. The CONSORT flow diagram

A series of reporting guidelines have been developed. The pioneering first framework was the CONSORT (consolidated standards of reporting trials) statement in 1996, which provided recommendations for publishing randomised controlled clinical trials, the gold standard to assess healthcare interventions. However, it should be noted that although the statement has been received positively overall, concerns have been raised that such publication guidelines may be too prescriptive and may impede the creativity of research.

The CONSORT 2010 statement is an evidence-based set of recommendations for reporting RCTs. The checklist contains twenty-five items focusing on "individually randomised, two-group, parallel trials," the most common RCT type. It is recommended that the statement be read in conjunction with the CONSORT 2010 explanation and elaboration for essential clarifications on all the items. See Appendix 1 for the CONSORT checklist.

References

1   Sibbald B, Roland M. Understanding controlled trials: Why are randomised controlled trials important? *British Medical Journal*, 998;316:201.

2   Brocklehurst P, Hoare Z. "How to design a randomised controlled trial," *British Dental Journal*. 2017; 12;222:721-726.

3   Bhide A, Shah PS, Acharya G. A simplified guide to randomised controlled trials. *Acta Obstetrica Gynecologica Scandinavia*. 2018;97:380-387.

4   Lake S, Kammann E, Klar N, Betensky R. Sample size re-estimation in cluster randomisation trials. *Statistics in Medicine*. 2002. 30;21:1337-1350.

5   Penić A, Begić D, Balajić K, Kowalski M, Marušić A, Livia Puljak L. Definitions of blinding in randomised controlled trials of interventions published in high-impact anaesthesiology journals: a methodological study and survey of authors. *British Medical Journal Open*. 2020; 10: e035168.

Chapter 6. Designing Studies Part 3—Qualitative Study Design

REED D., SANTINI A.

6.1. Overview

This chapter addresses the following aspects of qualitative research:

- Introduction to qualitative research;
- Qualitative philosophical approaches;
- Qualitative methodologic approaches;
- Data collecting methods in qualitative research;
- Analysing qualitative data; and
- Addressing criticism of qualitative research

This chapter is intended to introduce qualitative research and, as such, provides signposts to essential further research and reading.

6.2. Introduction to qualitative research[1, 2]

Qualitative research is the study of "things," often but not always in their natural settings, attempting to make sense of, or to interpret, phenomena in terms of the meanings people bring to them. Qualitative research is intended to penetrate the more profound significance that the research subject ascribes to the topic being researched. It involves constructivist or interpretive, naturalistic approaches to a subject matter and prioritises the data contributing to important research questions or existing information. The purpose of interpretivist enquiry is to understand and interpret behaviour rather than to predict causes and effects from which to generalise. For an interpretivist researcher, the priority is to understand reasons, meanings, drivers and other subjective experiences located in a specific context.

The features that constitute sound qualitative research are different to those that constitute sound quantitative research, and therefore qualitative research requires adopting a particular mind set. Moreover, this different mind-set requires a different set of credibility indictors and techniques when constructing a qualitative research proposal; Table 1 provides a helpful comparative table.

Credibility Indicators	Quantitative	Qualitative
1. **Have subjectivities been acknowledged and managed?**	**Objectivity**—conclusions based on observable phenomena; not influenced by emotions, personal prejudices, or subjectivities	**Neutrality**—subjectivities recognised and negotiated in a manner that attempts to avoid biasing results/conclusions. **Subjectivities** declared and transparent—acceptance and disclosure of researchers subjective positioning and how it might affect the research process, including conclusions drawn
2. **Has the true essence been captured?**	**Validity**—concerned with truth value, i.e. whether conclusions are correct, in addition to whether methods, approaches, and techniques related to what is being explored.	**Authenticity**—concerned with truth and value while recognising that multiple truths may exist. Also concerned with describing the deep structure of experience/phenomenon in a manner that is "true" to the experience.
3. **Are the methods approached with consistency?**	**Reliability**—concerned with internal consistency, i.e. whether data/results collected, measured, or generated are the same under repeated trials.	**Dependability**—accepts that reliability in social studies may not be possible, but attests that methods are systematic, well documented, and designed to account for research subjectivities.
4. **Are arguments relevant and appropriate?**	**Generalisability**—whether findings and conclusions from a sample, setting, or group are directly applicable to a larger population, a different setting, or another group.	**Transferability**—whether finding and conclusions from a selection (rather than a numerically calculated sample), setting, or group that lead to lessons learned that might be germane to a larger population, a different setting, or another group.
5. **Can the research be verified?**	**Reproducibility**—concerned with whether results/conclusions would be supported if the same methodology was used in a different study with an identical/similar context.	**Auditability**—accepts the import of the research context and therefore seeks full explication of methods to allow others to see how and why the researcher arrived at their conclusions.

Table 1. Credibility indicators for judging quantitative & qualitative research[3]

Qualitative research is used to understand people's underlying reasons, opinions, and motivations by collecting and analysing non-numerical data to appreciate ideas, notions, perceptions, opinions, or experiences. It is a means of highlighting trends in thought and opinions and investigating a problem in greater depth. Some typical methods include interviews, focus groups, participation observations, and a review of pre-existing material. The sample or selection of data sources is typically small and thus not intended to be analysed for statistical significance or produce generalizable conclusions.

A qualitative study, like a quantitative study, must have a detailed protocol prepared before the study. A question that specifically addresses a problem should be included in the protocol. This question details the study's aim at the onset of the study and should be well-matched for use with qualitative methods.[4, 5]

6.3. Qualitative philosophical approaches[4, 5]

A qualitative approach is a wide-ranging philosophy of how to conduct a particular style of research. Qualitative researchers do not usually start with the objective of testing a previously formulated theory. Alternatively, conceptual understanding is built up from the ongoing collected data. In qualitative studies, conceptual understanding is inductively derived from the data, and understanding is built and updated as new data are collected and compared with existing data. The consequence is understanding that elucidates the investigated phenomenon.

As new observations lead to new associations, revisions can be made to the core concept and more data collected. At the culmination of the study, there should be a comprehensive, if not an exhaustive, explanation for the phenomenon in question.

Undertaking qualitative research requires the investigator to adopt a relativist philosophical stance, that is, an acceptance that human action is rooted in subjective meaning systems, which emerge from society rather than the laws of nature. The investigator seeks to create understanding through one of two main inter-related stances. In real-world research, final understanding is usually created through adopting either an interpretistic stance, when the final outcomes largely focus on the researcher(s) views (this is termed an *etic* approach when the investigator emphasises what they consider important). Alternatively, by adopting a constructivist stance, where final outcomes are derived between the investigator(s) and interaction, corroboration and confirmation from the research participants or data source (this is also referred to as an *emic* approach— investigating how local [to the subject being studied] people think).

Conclusions are derived through inductive reasoning. Inductive is a term used to describe something that leads to something else. When applied to reasoning, information is collected, and conclusions are drawn from what is observed.

Inductive reasoning works by moving from specific observations to broader generalities and theories. Inductive reasoning begins with specific observations from which patterns and regularities are detected and formulated into tentative explanations, conclusions or possible theories. Inductive reasoning, by its very nature, is more open-ended and exploratory, especially at the beginning.

Robust qualitative research relies on a coherent link between the philosophical underpinning, the type of reasoning, and the methodological framework. This is depicted in Figure 1:

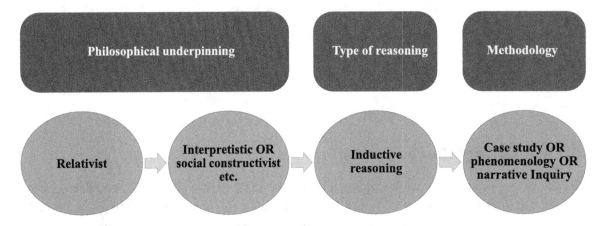

Figure 1: The characteristics of the qualitative philosophy and methodology[6]

6.4. Qualitative methodologic approaches

The methodological framework provides the structure of the study. Embedded in the methodology is the acceptance that data collection and analysis

- are iterative and evolving;
- require researchers to use their skills to question, listen, and look for clues and evidence, and then weigh the evidence to make judgements;
- are considered intuitive and common sense in nature; and
- are context dependant.

All of these points need to be considered and embedded within the research proposal. Therefore, it is no surprise that there are various methodological frameworks, each containing subtle but significant differences, each intended to facilitate a specific purpose. A selection of the common qualitative methodological approaches that might be particularly useful in practitioner research is outlined below.

6.4.1. Case study

In practitioner research, case study methodology is frequently used. It is important to note that case study, in the context of research methodology, is a term used to refer to a close-up, in-depth look at a particular group within a particular bounded area or context. Occasionally the terms case reports or case series might be used. Using case study in a methodological sense requires an in-depth and detailed account, which commences with a clear statement that defines what constitutes "the case" under investigation.

A case study is beneficial for underexplored areas; the methodology offers a straightforward structure that can be applied to a particular area or group. Case studies have a high sensitivity for detecting novelty, they permit the discovery of new diseases and unexpected effects, adverse or beneficial, and the study of mechanisms and thus play an essential role in dental education. Theorists credited with guiding what constitutes a sound case study framework are Yin,[7] Thomas,[8] and Starman.[9]

6.4.2. Grounded theory

Grounded theory aims to discover or construct theory from data systematically obtained and analysed using comparative analysis. Grounded theory involves the collection and analysis of data. The theory is "grounded" in actual data, which means the analysis and development of theories happen after collecting data. It was introduced to legitimise qualitative research. Grounded theory is a structured yet flexible methodology. This methodology is appropriate when little is known about a phenomenon. The aim is to produce or construct an explanatory theory that uncovers a process inherent to the inquiry's substantive area. A significant characteristic of grounded theory is that its goal is to produce a theory that is grounded in the data. Contemporary theorists credited with guiding what constitutes a sound grounded theory study framework are Glaser and Strauss[10] and Charmaz.[11]

6.4.3. Phenomenology

The phenomenological philosophical movement originated in the twentieth century; its main objective is to investigate and describe phenomena as consciously experienced by the participants. The general purpose of a phenomenological study is to understand and describe a specific phenomenon that answers the question, "What is the 'meaning' of one's lived experience?" The researcher seeks subjects willing to describe their thoughts, feelings, and interpretations that combine to provide the "meaning" that the participant gives in terms of his or her experience of a particular phenomenon under investigation. Contemporary theorists credited with guiding what constitutes a sound phenomenological study framework are Moustakas,[12] Smith, Flowers, and Larkin,[13] and Paley.[14]

6.4.4. Ethnography

Ethnography is a research approach in which people are observed in their cultural setting. The goal is to produce a narrative account of that specific culture, ethos or background. It investigates how people interact with one another and with their social and cultural environment. The aim is to learn from, rather than study, community members, to describe and interpret a cultural or social group or system. A variation of this is autoethnography, the study of one's own culture. Contemporary theorists credited with guiding what constitutes a sound ethnographic study framework are Hammersley,[15] Fetterman,[16] and Gobo.[17]

6.4.5. Ethnomethodology

This is a qualitative research methodology which gathers observations of everyday interactions. These observations can also include interviews and documentary data to produce detailed and comprehensive accounts of different social phenomena. It ignores the what and concentrates on the how, the implicit rule that people understand and generates order. Contemporary theorists credited with guiding what constitutes a sound ethnomethodology study framework are Have[18] and Liberman.[19]

6.5. Narrative research

Narrative research is a term that covers a range of similar but subtlety different range of methodologies that have a common aim of capturing the accounts of participants, either the written or spoken words or visual representation of individuals, characteristically focusing on the lives of individuals as told through their own stories. Contemporary theorists credited with guiding what constitutes a sound ethnographic study framework are Riessman,[20, 21] Squire et al.,[22] and Goodson et al.[23]

A summary of typical practice-based approaches to qualitative research is given in Table 2:

Type of Approach	Methodology
Case Study	A clearly defined particular bounded area to understand that bounded area, including how participants understand and comprehend their experiences related to that area.
Grounded theory	Data are collected on a topic of interest and theories created inductively
Phenomenology	A phenomenon or event is explored by describing and interpreting participants' meaning of a particular lived experience.
Ethnography	Researchers aim to learn from rather than study groups or organisations to describe, interpret, and understand their cultures, philosophies, and values.
Ethnomethodology	Investigators understand from observations of everyday interactions and produce detailed and comprehensive accounts of how the implicit rule that people understand generates order.
Narrative research	Participants' accounts are studied to understand their recall of perceptions of their life experiences.

Table 2. Summary of methodological approaches to qualitative research

6.6. Other things to consider as part of the qualitative methodological framework[24, 25]

6.6.1. Reflexivity

Reflexivity is important in qualitative research because the researcher can introduce bias in various ways that can modify a study, including the choice of data gathering methods, data collection and analyses, and the reporting of the outcome measures. Reflexivity is the process in which the researcher reflects on how to provide more effective and impartial analysis. It involves examining and consciously acknowledging the researcher's assumptions and preconceptions which may therefore shape the outcome. All qualitative research is contextual, between two or more people within a detailed time and place. The integrity of the findings increases when researchers define the circumstantial associations between themselves and the participants (reflexivity) and their relationship, insider/outsider positionality, and status. The researcher is responsible for concisely and unambiguously attending to these issues so that the reader can evaluate the research.

6.6.2. Bracketing

Bracketing is a qualitative research method to reduce a researcher's preconceptions' potential adverse effects. It involves the identification and temporary setting aside of the researcher's assumptions.

6.6.3. Relatability rather than generalisation, transferability, or applicability

Generalisability refers to the extent to which the findings from a sample can be generalised to an entire population (provided that the sample is representative for the population) regardless of context. This is often at variance with the intended purpose of qualitative research. The terms "transferability," "relatability," or "applicability" are often used. Transferability refers to the extent to which the findings found in a specific context can be transferred to another, very similar context. The concept of relatability or applicability refers to the degree of relatedness on whether knowledge gained from one context is relevant to, applicable to other contexts, or the same context in another time frame. It assumes a role similar to transferability. The act of relatability, making the relationship link, is the reader's responsibility who seeks to apply theory elsewhere and the original researcher. Although the researcher might make suggestions to whom the research might be of interest or relevance.

6.6.4. Congruence

To demonstrate the proper application of research methodology, it is expected that there is congruence between the research question, aim, the philosophical stance and principles, the methodological framework, the methods of data collection, and the analytic process. Therefore, the researcher must detail the rationale and justification for every decision and every step taken concerning how the research is conducted.

6.7. Data collecting methods in qualitative research[4, 5, 6, 24]

There are various data collection methods in qualitative research. The method of data collection selected for a particular study should be cognisant of the methodology. The most common qualitative data collection methods include recording what has been seen, heard, or come across using comprehensive field notes, one-to-one talks between the researcher and the participant in which the researcher asks the participant questions, questioning and encouraging discussion among a group of participants, distributing questionnaires among participants, accumulating previously recorded data in the form of texts, images, audio or video recordings, not necessarily made by the current researcher.

These are summarised in Table 3:

In-depth interviews (audio-recorded and transcribed) • **Structured interviews** aim to focus on specific areas in order to find answers to predetermined questions. However, the interviewer is in control, so this technique is less naturalistic. • **Semi-structured interviews** follow a topic guide but allow for open-ended answers and follow-up of points raised. • **Unstructured interviews** aim to discuss a limited number of topics in great depth, with no structure or preconceived plan. The interviewee is in control.
Focus groups • The researcher interviews groups of people with something in common. The people are free to talk to each other in the group. The data arises from the interaction between group members rather than between the researcher and the group. Focus groups can provide data on the group's cultural norms and help exploratory research into issues of concern to the group. However, focus groups are not naturalistic, some participants can dominate the discussions, and there are issues around confidentiality. Delphi committees are a type of focus group.
Participant observation • The researcher not only observes a group but adopts a role within the group from which to participate in some manner, usually over an extended period. This method allows for data to be collected on naturally occurring behaviours in their usual contexts. However, there can be a conflict between a researcher's dual role as a researcher and a participant. An added danger is that the researcher might end up over-identifying with the group, impairing analytical objectivity.
Review of pre-existing data • Pre-existing data can be documents, recordings (video or audio), image depictions (photographs, paintings, cartoons or other images), objects of art, or data from previous research available for further analysis.

Review of artefacts

- Cultural artefacts offer an insight into: technological processes, economic development and social structure, among other attributes.
- Social artefacts do not have a physical form, neither do social artefacts need to be of historical value (i.e. items created a moment ago can be classified as social artefacts).
- Artefacts can be referred to under three main groupings:
  - Primary artefacts: Used in production, e.g. electric toothbrushes
  - Secondary artefacts: Related to the primary artefact, e.g. User's manual
  - Tertiary artefacts: Representation of secondary artefact, e.g. a photograph of the user's manual.

Table 3. Common sources of qualitative data

6.8. Sampling or selecting[6]

It is common for the term sample to be used in qualitative research when technically the data gathered are not a sample but a selection. In quantitative research, the sample is a term that indicates a percentage of a larger population and aims to represent that population, and this usually involves a power calculation (see chapter 8). However, in qualitative research, it is usual and acceptable to select particular data sources. Selection is the deliberate or purposeful choice of a specific group. Not intended to be representative of a wider population. Purposeful sampling or selection is commonly used in qualitative research to identify and select information-rich cases related to the phenomenon of interest. The researcher consciously selects subjects who have knowledge or experience of the area being investigated.

Purposive selection may not represent a larger population; however, this does not mean that subjects are drawn arbitrarily or without any specific purpose in mind. Purposive selection/sampling is used in qualitative studies where the researcher's objective is in-depth, idiographic understanding rather than more general understanding.

Types of purposive selection/ sampling are described in Table 4:

Sample/Selection type	Description
Maximal variation selection/sampling	Those seeking to understand how a phenomenon is seen and understood among different people, in different settings and at different times. The researcher selects a small number of units or cases that maximise the diversity relevant to the research question. Links to heterogeneous selection/sampling.
Extreme (or deviant) case selection/sampling	The selection of unusual cases of the phenomenon of interest or cases that are considered outliers, exceptions to the rule emerging from the analysis.
Typical selection/sampling	Selecting cases that are not in any way atypical, extreme, deviant, or unusual

Theory or concept selection/sampling	The process selects occurrences, events, periods, or people based on their positionality, relationship, or exemplification of theoretical constructs. Thus, theoretical selection/sampling is a linked component in grounded theories.
Homogeneous selection/sampling	One particular subgroup—similar characteristics to allow a deeper exploration.
Critical selection/sampling	Selecting a small number of important cases is likely to provide the maximum information and have the maximum effect on the development of knowledge.
Opportunistic selection/sampling	Opportunistic or emergent selection/sampling occurs when the researcher makes selection/sampling decisions during data collection. This commonly occurs in field research. The observer gains more knowledge of a setting and makes decisions that take advantage of events as these occur.
Snowball selection/sampling	Data are collected from a member(s) of the target population, who then provides information to enable the location or contact other members of that population they know.
Confirming or disconfirming selection/sampling	Selection of confirming and disconfirming cases, usually when part of the data collection and analysis has been completed. Serve to provide further depth to patterns emerging from data analysis or disconfirm (with the selection of disconfirming cases). In addition, it can aid in establishing limitations of research findings.

Table 4. Types of commonly used types of purposive selection /sampling in qualitative studies

Other ethical considerations related to qualitative research are covered in the chapter on ethics.

6.9. Analysing qualitative data[26, 27, 28, 29]

Qualitative data analysis is employed at the end of the data collection phase. It entails looking for similarities or differences and then identifying patterns, commonly referred to as themes.

6.9.1. Common types of qualitative data analysis

To demonstrate the proper application of data analysis, it is necessary to select a type of data analysis that congruent (align) the research question and the purpose or aim of the research project.

6.9.2. Thematic analysis (TA)

Thematic analysis is one of the most common analytic techniques. Building on the definition of theme provided earlier, thematic analysis requires the investigator to look for the relationships between the different themes in order to gain a deeper understanding with regards to the relevance the data have to the research question being asked. A thematic analysis follows the basic principles of coding data and then, depending on the model of TA being followed, grouping data into categories and then into themes. Collected data are abstracted and compared to all the other collected data to compose a provisional understanding. Initial ideas and concepts are tested, and new data sources are found. The outcomes of the process are indicative of trends the investor(s) identify within the data. The investigator(s) are expected to substantiate a particular theme by using extracted quotes from the transcribed contributions that participants have made.

However, it is incumbent on the qualitative researcher to select the analytic process most consistent with the research question and aim. The focus of the study will determine the selection of the appropriate process. Examples of the various types of qualitative analysis are listed but not explained in detail in Table 5. It is beyond the scope of this manual to describe the types of qualitative analysis, other than thematic analysis, but merely to draw readers' attention to their existence. For details of all types of qualitative analysis, readers are referred to *The SAGE Handbook of Qualitative Analysis.*[2]

Types of Analytic Processes	Purpose
Thematic analysis	Coding and categorising to indicate trends
Narrative analysis	Iterative and related to story building
Content analysis	Linguistic (words or text) quantification
Discourse analysis	Explores language—how the language used portrays social or historical contexts
Conversational analysis	Explores the structures of speech
Semiotics	Interpretation of signs and symbols
Hermeneutics	Interpretation of text and literature looking at alternative viewpoints. In some professional fields the term has been expanded to mean interpretation in general, rather than related to documents … hermeneutics spiral/circle … double hermeneutics.
Grounded theory	Inductive—generates theory from data

Table 5. Examples of various types of qualitative analysis

Having selected the type of data analysis to be conducted, it is necessary to follow a model to process the data.

6.9.3. Model of Data Analysis[24, 26, 27, 28, 29]

To demonstrate sound data analysis, the researcher must identify a model, i.e. a set of stages congruent with the methodology and methods underpinning the project and then demonstrate fidelity to that model. Typically, models for data analysis of qualitative research include the following stages:

1. Immersion: Data must first be prepared and organised, which involves transcribing interviews or compiling field notes. The data should then be studied, reviewed, and examined for patterns or repeated ideas.

2. Coding: Coding is an iterative process that requires a constant comparison and re-examination of the transcripts. The codes are regularly occurring strands detectable within the transcriptions or data sources. Data sources are usually coded line by line. As a new code became apparent, the previous coded data sources are re-examined to check for and then absorb a new code that might have been newly noticed. The codes are numerically listed, given titles, and short definitions to clarify what would be considered under each code and what would be more appropriately allocated an alternative code. The codes (strands) identify the relationship involved in the elite knowledge acquisition process, from initial primary socialisation to secondary, tertiary, and then professional socialisation. Once established, the codes are then grouped into categories.

3. Categories: The next stage in the analytical process is grouping the codes into categories. Categories are codes that have a shared relationship. Categories are formed by examining the codes and identifying how the codes could be most appropriately grouped. Not all codes are mutually exclusive, and on occasion, codes cross the boundaries of more than one category. As with the coding stage, the categories are given label definitions. In some models of qualitative data analysis, the categories stage is omitted, and coding links directly to themes.

4. Themes: Data are then brought together into unified, integrated and all-encompassing themes. Themes move beyond categories and descriptions into explanation and interpretation of data related to the investigated issues. Usually, themes are configurations of commonly occurring patterns across the data. A theme would be presented as a title, with a definition (what the theme is or is not) and then an explanation of the data which support the assertion that it is possible to identify the theme. It may be possible to detect how themes interact or relate. Simply listing key points from individual participants could not be defined as a theme—because the list is not commonly occurring across several participants.

6.9.4. Computer use in qualitative data analysis

Qualitative research studies produce large amounts of data that need to be proficiently managed. Computer packages, such as NVivo, offer data management efficiency and provide a mechanism for storing and retrieving material. Locating cases, statements, phrases, or even words is facilitated, replacing labour-intensive methods. However, certain disadvantages have been highlighted in using a computer programme, including quantifying qualitative data: analysis instead of a qualitative review, e.g. counting occurrences, giving more weight to more frequent events, and ignoring isolated incidences. It is necessary to weigh up the benefits and suitability of using electronic analytic tools, as there is a risk of reducing qualitative research methodology's acknowledged strength and the degree of insight and experience it deploys to develop new understandings of the world. Computer packages require the researcher to learn the programme, and despite some helpful YouTube tutorials, this can take time. It is up to the investigator to determine if this might be an investment worth making.

6.10. Addressing criticisms of qualitative research[3, 4, 5, 6]

In terms of rigour, several criticisms of qualitative research need to be mitigated through a robust research design and standards for qualitative research.

Subjectivity: Qualitative research cannot be replicated mainly due to the researcher's key role in analysing and interpreting data. Interpretations of the same data can vary due to the researcher's decisions regarding what is important and what is irrelevant.
Unreliability: Qualitative research is prone to be unreliable because of uncontrolled factors that affect the data in a real-world setting.
Limited generalisability: It is difficult to draw generalisable conclusions due to data bias and unrepresentativeness to the broader population. Small samples are frequently used to gather detailed data about specific contexts and can contribute to limited generalisability.
Labour-intensive: Data analysis is often checked or performed manually; increasingly sophisticated software is used to manage and record large amounts of text, reducing labour insensitivity.

Table 6. Summary of criticisms of qualitative research qualitative research

6.11. Verifying outcomes[3, 26]

Given the criticisms frequently levelled at qualitative research, it is necessary to establish credibility in qualitative research through clear and well-defined verification techniques. This can be achieved through a process of triangulation, which refers to using multiple sources in qualitative research to develop or verify a comprehensive understanding of phenomena through amalgamating information from different sources.

To accomplish this, the research is undertaken from multiple perspectives; this could take the form of using several facilitators, different locations, or multiple individuals analysing the same data. Related to improving understanding more than additional verification, these can be data-led or investigator-led.

Typical examples of verification techniques are detailed in Table 7:

Technique	Explanation
Inter-rater reliability	This is using co-researchers (or supervisors for MSc students) to corroborate (usually but not always) independently the analysis and subsequent findings.

Peer Review	An external person conducts checks the research process, critically reviewing all aspects of the methodology.
Member or participant checking	Two ways: Firstly, permitting participants to confirm that transcripts are an accurate basis on which analysis can commence. Secondly, and arguably the most important, permitting participants to comment on the analysis and to confirm they have not been misinterpreted or their contribution misrepresented.
Prolonged engagement:	Emersion within a context sufficient to understand the culture, the context, and to build trust and rapport.
Persistent observation:	Evidence of engaging with the situation beyond a preliminary, superficial level
A full explication of methods	A complete rationale and a detailed, precise explanation of what was done in terms of data collection and why…
Fully auditable	Permitting an independent "other" to review the process and provide documentation of that process.
Saturation	Keep data collecting until no new information emerges. To end data collection when satisfied additional data no longer adds richness to understanding or aids in building theories. This can be difficult to prove.

Table 7. Examples of verification techniques

6.12. Conclusions

Qualitative research is intended to contribute to understanding rather than predict causes and effects from which to generalise. Consequently, the features that constitute robust qualitative research are different to those that constitute thorough quantitative research. Therefore, to conduct sound qualitative research, the investigator(s) must adopt a specific mindset and adopt a particular set of techniques and credibility indicators when constructing and conducting the study.

References

1   Lincoln, Y. and Guba, E. (1985) Naturalistic Inquiry. CA: Sage.

2   Denzin, N. And Lincoln, Y. (eds.) (2018) The Sage handbook of qualitative research, 5th edn. Los Angeles: Sage Publications, 2017.

3   O'Leary, Z. (2021) The essential guide to doing your research project. 4th edn. London: Sage.

4   Pope, C. and May, N. (2020) Qualitative Research in Healthcare. Oxford: Wiley Black and Son Ltd.

5   Robson, C. and McCartan, K. (2016) Real World Research. 4th edn. Chichester: John Wiley and Son Ltd.

6   Reed. D. (2021) 'The principles of qualitative research' (PowerPoint Presentation). WKBL8820—Research Skills. The University of Kent. January 2021.

7   Yin, R. (2018) Case Study Research and Applications: Design and Methods. 6ᵗʰ edn. London: Sage.

8   Starman, A. (2013) The case study as a type of qualitative research. *Journal of Contemporary Educational Studies.* 1: 2013. pp. 28-43.

9   Thomas, G. (2015) How To Do Your Case Study. 2ⁿᵈ edn. London. Sage

10   Glaser, B. and Strauss, A. (2000) Discovery of grounded theory: strategies for qualitative research. Oxford: Routledge.

11   Charmaz, K. (2014) Constructing grounded theory approaches. 2ⁿᵈ edn. London. Sage

12   Moustakas, C. (1994) Phenomenological Research Methods. London: Sage.

13   Smith, J., Flowers P. and Larkin, M. (2009) Interpretative Phenomenological Analysis (IPA): theory, methods and research. Oxford. Sage

14   Paley, J. (2017) Phenomenology as qualitative research: a critical analysis of meaning attribution. Oxford: Routledge.

15   Hammersley, M. and Atkinson. P. (2019) Ethnography: Principles in Practice. 4ᵗʰ Edition. Oxford: Routledge.

16   Fetterman, D. (2019) Ethnography: Step-by-step(Applied Social Research Methods).4ᵗʰ Edition. USA: Sage.

17   Gobo, G. (2008) Doing Ethnography. London: Sage.

18   Have, PT. (2004) Understanding Qualitative Research and Ethnomethodology. London: Sage.

19   Liberman, K. (2014) More Studies in Ethnomethodology. USA: State University of New York Press.

20   Riessman, C. (2008) Narrative methods for the human sciences. Thousand Oaks, USA: Sage.

21   Riessman, C. (2012) 'Analysis of personal narratives', in Gubrium, J., Holstein, J., Marvasti, A. and McKinney, K. (ed.) The Sage handbook of interview research: the complexity of the craft. USA: Sage, pp. 367-380.

22   Squire, C., Davis, M., Esin, G., Andrews, M., Harrision, B., Hyden, L. and Hyden, M. (2015) What Is Narrative Research? London: Bloomsbury.

23   Goodson, I., Antikainen, A., Sikes, P. and Andrews, M. (2017) The Routledge International Handbook on Narrative and Life History. London: Routledge.

24   King, N., Horrocks, C. and Brooks, J. (2019) Interviews in Qualitative Research. 2ⁿᵈ edn. London: Sage.

25   Dwyer, C. S. and Buckle, J. (2009) 'The space between: on being an insider-outsider in qualitative research', *International Journal of Qualitative Methods,* 8(1), pp. 54-63.

26   Reed. D. (2020) 'The principles of qualitative data analysis' (PowerPoint Presentation). WKBL8160 –Dissertation. The University of Kent. December 2020.

27   Saldana, J. (2021) The Coding Manual for Qualitative Researchers. 4th edn. London: Sage.

28   Green, J., Willis, K., Hughes, E., Small, R., Welch, N., Gibbs, L. and Daly, J. (2007) Generating best evidence from qualitative research: the role of data analysis. *Australian and New Zealand Journal of Public Health.* 31(6), 545-550.

29   Braun, V. and Clarke, V. (2013) Successful Qualitative Research, A Practical Guide For Beginners. London: Sage.

Chapter 7. Designing Studies Part 4—Systematic Reviews

SANTINI A.

7.1. Overview

After the introduction, this chapter considers the following aspects of systematic reviews:

- Strengths and weaknesses;
- Data sources for a systematic review; and
- Meta-analysis.

7.2. Introduction

Systematic reviews attempt to identify, appraise, and synthesise all the empirical evidence that meets specified eligibility criteria to answer a given research question. Systematic reviews use explicit methods to minimise bias to produce reliable findings that can be used to inform decision-making. They have been defined as reviews "of a clearly formulated question that uses systematic and explicit methods to identify, select, and critically appraise relevant research and to collect and analyse data from studies that are included in the review" (Section 1.2, *Cochrane Handbook for Systematic Reviews of Interventions*).

They are particularly valuable when the results of randomised controlled trials, conducted over several years on an important clinical question, remain inconclusive or contradictory. By providing a summary overview of the findings of several individual trials, a systematic review may come to reliable conclusions and highlight any gaps in the research evidence. Furthermore, when a systematic review does obtain previously unclear results, it may remove the requirement for further research, saving resources and, potentially, lives.

An excellent systematic review employs and reports a comprehensive search of all potentially relevant articles, published or unpublished. The search should use explicit, reproducible selection criteria to minimise bias in the selected body of evidence.[1]

The five steps to take when conducting systematic reviews are set out in Table 1:

- Definition of the research question;
- Literature search;
- Assessment of identified studies for eligibility, quality and findings;
- If possible, pooling of results; and
- Reporting results, including gaps and weaknesses and their implications, for practice.

Table 1. Five steps to follow when conducting a systematic review

A summary of the strengths and weaknesses of systematic reviews is set out in Table 2:

Strengths
• Summarises multiple studies to provide clinicians, healthcare providers and policymakers with a quick and reliable method of keeping up to date with quality research, thus aiding clinical and policy decision-making; • May remove or reduce the requirement for further primary research before a recommendation to change clinical practice; • Critically examining primary studies can improve understanding of inconsistencies and gaps in the research literature, suggesting new avenues of enquiry; • Application of specific and transparent selection criteria limits bias in identifying and rejecting studies; • Provides a more precise estimate of effect because of the methods used and numbers of participants involved; • By comparing results from different studies, generalisability, and consistency (i.e. low heterogeneity can be investigated); • Reasons for any heterogeneity can be identified, aiding in new hypotheses about specific subgroups of patients or treatment regimes.
Weaknesses
• Not a guarantee of quality: may be conducted poorly or be based on weak or few primary studies; • Maybe over-prescriptive in inclusion/exclusion criteria, resulting in a small study pool for analysis and the exclusion of potentially relevant studies; • It can be outdated due to the time and cost of conducting a comprehensive systematic review; • If studies using different interventions or patient groups are aggregated, important effects may be masked; • The findings of systematic reviews may conflict with those from large-scale clinical trials, possibly due to the inclusion in the systematic review of smaller, less reliable studies; • It may be affected by publication bias, including the under-utilisation of non-English language and unpublished research; • Likely to include studies published over several years or even decades and across different countries and health systems, potentially involving a range of undeclared differences in practice or culture.

Table 2. Strengths and weaknesses of systematic reviews

7.3. Data sources for a systematic review

A systematic review that relies on one literature database is open to the criticism that potentially relevant material may have been missed. Missing important material would increase the risk of bias and risk of unreliable conclusions. Therefore, the reported systematic review should clearly state the sources and follow-up policy employed in the search, which should include the following:

- Library databases (such as PubMed, PsycINFO, Embase, CINAHL, ERIC) selected for relevance to the research question;
- Hand searches of paper journals relevant to the subject, especially if more than twenty years old;
- Cochrane clinical trials register;

- Foreign-language literature;
- "Grey literature" (academic theses, internal reports, non-peer-reviewed journals, commercial files), often not available from electronic databases;
- References (and references of references) listed in primary sources but not found in the initial search (possibly because of their age);
- Other unpublished sources suggested by experts in the field, contacted personally; and
- Raw data or statistical summaries from published trials if required to pool results (e.g. standard deviations or confidence intervals), obtained by personal communication with authors.

7.4. Meta-analysis

A meta-analysis is an amplification of systematic reviews. In a meta-analysis, the results of several independent studies identified in a systematic review that have commonality—in other words, homogeneity in structure, including interventions and outcomes, are statistically combined and analysed. Thus, meta-analysis is based on a comprehensive, detailed, and systematic review of previous research that addresses the potential problems of homogeneity and the appropriateness of combining studies.

The essential questions relevant to the principles of a meta-analysis are set out in Table 3, and the features of a well and poorly designed meta-analysis are in Table 4:

- Was it appropriate to have combined the individual trials that comprise the meta-analysis?
- How robust is the result to changes in assumptions?
- Does the reached conclusion make clinical sense?
- Has the analysis contributed to rational decision-making and patient management?

Table 3. Essential questions relevant to the principles of meta-analysis

Well-designed meta-analysis	Poorly designed meta-analysis
Should objectively appraise the evidence. Should provide - A precise estimate of a treatment effect; - An explanation of heterogeneity between the results of individual studies.	May be biased, owing to - Exclusion of relevant studies; - Inclusion of inadequate studies; - The inappropriate combining of studies using different interventions or regimes (e.g. dosage, follow-up period, concomitant therapy).

Table 4. Features of well and poorly designed meta-analysis

If the steps in Table 5 are followed, misleading analyses can generally be avoided. These steps are identical to previously outlined steps for undertaking other types of research. Therefore, they are repeated here for emphasis.[3]

1. Review the literature relating to the study ↓ Formulate the problem.
2. Prepare a detailed research protocol to include • Objectives; • Hypotheses to be tested.
3. Detail methods and criteria for identifying and selecting relevant studies. Eligibility criteria for the data to be included must be defined at the outset. Define criteria relating to • Quality of studies; • Combinability of treatments; • Patients, outcomes, and lengths of follow-up.
4. Detail methods for collecting and analysing information.
5. Report the study.

Table 5. Steps to avoid misleading analysis

The issues to be considered when designing a meta-analysis are set out in Table 6:

1. Define essential inclusion criteria.
2. Include only controlled trials with proper randomisation of patients.
3. Include only studies that report on all initially included patients according to the "intention to treat" principle.
4. Include only studies with an objective, preferably blinded, outcome assessment.
5. Define a strategy for the identification of relevant studies.
   • Published results may suffer from publication bias.
   • Unpublished studies may differ from published results.

Table 6. Steps to be considered when designing a meta-analysis

7.5. Sources of data for systematic reviews

The data sources, data collection, standardisation of data, and the statistics for calculating overall effect are detailed below in Tables 7, 8, 9, and 10.

Electronic databases	Cochrane Collaboration	Citation indices
The exclusive use of electronic databases may miss some relevant studies.	• An extensive manual search of medical journals published in English and other languages. • Regarded as the best electronic source of studies.	Also, consider using • Citation indices • Bibliographies of review articles • Monographs.

Table 7. Sources of data

A standardised record form is needed for data collection. Use two independent observers to extract the data (reduces errors).

Use specially designed scales to rate the quality of the studies. Prepare materials in which observers are "blinded" to

- the names and institutions of the authors;
- the names of the journals; and
- sources of funding.

Table 8. Data collection

Standardisation of data		
For inter-study comparison: • Individual results must be expressed in a standardised format.	When the endpoint is continuous: • Use the mean difference between the treatment and control groups. • The underlying population value will influence the size of a difference. • Differences are often presented in units of standard deviation.	When the endpoint is binary: • The odds ratio allows for ease in combining data. • Testing the overall effect for significance.

Table 9. Standardisation of data

The simple arithmetic mean of the results from all studies: • May lead to misleading results; • Results from small studies are more likely to occur by chance but are given the same weight as more extensive studies; • Give small studies less weight.	• The weighted average of the results is used, in which the more extensive trials have more influence than the smaller ones; • The "fixed effects" approach considers that this variability between results is exclusively due to random variation; • The "random effects" approach assumes a different underlying effect for each study; • The "random effects" approach gives wider confidence intervals than the "fixed effects" approach; • Neither of these approaches is "correct"; • A substantial difference in the combined effect calculated by the "fixed" and "random effects" approaches occurs when markedly heterogeneous studies.

Table 10. Statistics for calculating the overall effect

Finally, a checklist for meta-analysis studies, including heterogeneity and sensitivity analysis, is summarised in Tables 11, 12, and 13.

- Carefully plan in advance, as for any other study;
- A written protocol;
- A comprehensive search for relevant studies;
- A precise definition of eligibility criteria for studies;
- Present results to allow a visual estimation of the degree of heterogeneity between studies;
- Agree on statistical methods for combining the data (there is no single "correct" method);
- Undertake a sensitivity analysis to assess the robustness of combined estimates to different assumptions and inclusion criteria.

Table 11. Checklist for a meta-analysis study

- It is not applicable to combine the results when studies differ significantly (for example, high heterogeneity);
- It is not easy to test heterogeneity across studies;
- When statistical testing indicates good homogeneity, the differences between studies are assumed to result from sampling variation. Therefore, a fixed-effects model is appropriate;
- When statistical testing shows that significant heterogeneity exists between study results, then a random-effects model is advised;
- Note: statistical tests lack power—can fail to reject the null hypothesis of homogeneity of results when, in fact, significant differences exist between studies;
- When a statistical test indicates heterogeneity, an attempt to investigate and explain this should be attempted.

Table 12. Checklist for heterogeneity

Sensitivity analysis can be performed

- To indicate whether the results from the meta-analysis are robust;
- To indicate whether the choice of statistical method is appropriate;
- To exclude poor-quality trials;
- To avoid publication bias likely to distort conclusions.

Table 13. Checklist for sensitivity analysis

References

1   Cumpston M, Li T, Page MJ, Chandler J, Welch VA, Higgins JP, Thomas J. Updated guidance for trusted systematic reviews: Cochrane Database of Systematic Reviews. 2019;3:10:ED000142.

2   Hasidic AB. Meta-analysis in medical research. *Hippokratia*. 2010;14:29–37.

3   Zeng X, Zhang Y, Kwong JS, Zhang C, Li S, Sun F, Niu Y, Du L. The methodological quality assessment tools for preclinical and clinical studies, systematic review and meta-analysis, and clinical practice guidelines are systematic reviews. *Journal of Evidence Based Medicine*. 2015;8:2–10.

Chapter 8. Designing Studies Part 5—Sampling

Santini A.

8.1. Overview

After an introduction, this chapter considers the following aspects of sampling:

- Types of random sampling;
- External and internal validity and generalisability;
- Sample size calculation;
- Bias; and
- Concealed allocation and blinding.

8.2. Introduction

In research, it is usually too costly, too inconvenient and often practically impossible to study the whole targeted population; a sample is therefore taken.

The sample size is the number of subjects selected from the general population, and it should be representative of the total population. The size and the method of sampling must be such that the researcher can make valid inferences about the target population from the sample. Basic sampling methods include incidental or convenience sampling (non-random), quota sampling and random sampling, each with advantages and disadvantages.

Random sampling is the preferred method as it tends to satisfy the aim of representativeness. Stratified and cluster, or area and systematic are also common types of random sampling methods. Features of representative and poorly representative samples are set out in Table 1 and basic sampling methods and random sampling in Table 2:

Representative samples	Poorly representative samples
• The researcher can generalise from the sample to the whole population. • Removes inconvenience and expense of studying the whole population.	• Any bias in selection methods leads to less validity in generalisation. • Results from a study cannot necessarily be transferred to the whole population.

Table 1. Features of Representative and Unrepresentative Sample

Basic sampling methods		
Incidental or convenience sampling (non-random)	**Quota sampling**	**Random sampling**
• Most commonly used; • Cheapest; • Easiest; • Participants may offer to take part (self-select); • Unlikely to be representative; • Bias is introduced when not representative.	• A quota of subjects of a specified type is recruited; • Ensures that relevant characteristics are reflected in the sample (e.g. gender, disease severity, treatment type); • Not random, so open to bias.	• All have the same chance of random selection • More expensive; • More likely to be representative of the whole population; • More difficult to achieve a reasonable response rate.

Random sampling	
Advantages	**Disadvantages**
• The size of sampling error (how representative the sample is) can be calculated because both population and sample size are known. • The required sample size is usually smaller because of the increased representation.	• To obtain an accurate random sample, the researcher must first obtain an all-inclusive list of the whole population. Unfortunately, this is often impossible as either no such list exists or it is continuously changing. • Cost due to planning and expenses, which increase with the size of the target population.

Table 2. Features of basic sampling methods and random sampling

8.3. Types of random sampling

Three types of random sampling—stratified, cluster or area, and systematic—are detailed in Table 3:

1. **Stratified**
Subgroups stratified, e. g. males and females in the target population.   **Advantages**   Set quotas for each subgroup (same approach as quota sampling).   • Proportional representation for all subgroups;   • Statistically robust as the exact representation of samples is known.   **Disadvantages**   • A complete list with all characteristics and proportions of subgroups is required;   • Gain in sample accuracy compared to simple random sampling is small;   • Cost.

2. Cluster or area

Subgroups of the population are used as sampling units rather than individuals. The subgroups, or clusters, are randomly sampled, and all members of the selected cluster are then included in the study. Clustering must be taken into account in the analysis, as the principle of all individuals having an equal chance of being selected is violated.

Advantages
- Effective
- Cost-effective;
- Complete list of individuals not required.

3. Systematic

Choosing from a list: for example, every fifth, tenth, and so on are selected for inclusion.

Advantages
- Usually produces a representative sample;
- Easy and convenient if a list of cases is available.

Disadvantages
- Not a proper random sampling method;
- It assumes that cases themselves are included and ordered in the list in a random fashion.

Table 3. Three types of random sampling

When a genuinely representative sample is obtained, the researcher can legitimately generalise from the sample to the population as a whole without the expense and inconvenience of studying the whole target population. Therefore, a sample is a subset of the target population, and "sampling" involves selecting this subset.

In any report of a research study, participants and how they are recruited must be clearly detailed. Exclusion and inclusion criteria should also be clearly defined. For ethical reasons, participant anonymity must be maintained with no means of identification given in the study protocol or report. Photographs of participants can only be published if they have given written consent.

8.4. External and internal validity and generalisability

The external validity of a study is the degree to which the experimental results of a research study can be applied to different groups of people, situations, and measures, i.e. the extent to which the results can be generalised to other settings. External validity is a function of the researcher and the study design, whereas generalisability is a function of the researcher and the user.

A study's validity is predicated by the experimental design and is one of the key factors when assessing the legitimacy of the results. Though unrelated to the project's basis, many factors can influence and invalidate the research findings.

Internal validity and external validity

Internal validity is affected by errors in the study design, such as not controlling all significant variables or data collection problems relating to research instruments (see Chapter 16).

Factors that affect internal validity, amongst others, are subject variability, population size, the time allotted for data collection or experimental treatment, and instrument sensitivity.

External validity is the degree to which the study findings apply to a larger population or other settings. Conversely, a lack of external validity means that the findings cannot be applied to a situation other than the one in which the research study was conducted.

Factors affecting external validity include population characteristics, the interaction of subject selection and the research study, clarity of the stated independent variables, the effect of the study environment, effects related to the researcher, data collection methods, and the effect of time. Controlling all possible factors that threaten the research's validity is a primary responsibility of every good researcher.

8.5. Sample size calculation

When a study produces inconclusive results, it may be due to insufficient numbers, i.e. small sample size, to achieve statistical significance of clinically relevant differences between groups. A flawed study design may result in a sample size that is too small. If efforts have not been taken to calculate a sample size before data collection, there is no going back; the researcher has wasted his time. Pertinent advice is to consult a statistician on the methodology and required sample size before starting any data collection.

It is often mistakenly assumed that increasing a sample size achieves more accurate results. This is because increasing the sample size reduces the chance of sampling error. However, as the sampling error is inversely proportional to the sample size's square root, doubling the sample size will only reduce the sampling error by a factor of $\sqrt{2}$ (i.e. 1.414).

Before calculating sample size, estimates of the target population's features and the likely pattern of the outcome measure in that population must be made. These include the population size, the prevalence of the condition (outcome measure) to be studied in the population, confidence intervals (margin of error), confidence level, and standard deviation (see chapter on data collection for further explanation). Additionally, researchers must determine the size of the difference between the study's intervention and control groups in the outcome measure, which will be considered clinically significant, and what power level is to be chosen. This is expressed as the alpha level.

The requirements when calculating sample size are set out in Table 4:

Population size	• How many are needed for the target group? • Populations are generally approximated.
Margin of error	• No sample is perfect. How much error will you accept? • Determined by confidence intervals. How much higher or lower than the population mean are you prepared to let your sample group fall?
Confidence levels	How confidently do you want the true mean to fall within the selected confidence interval? (Usually set at 90, 95, or 99 per cent.)
Standard deviation	How much variance is expected in the results? (Use of 0.5 usually leads to an appropriate sample size.)

Table 4. Requirements when calculating sample size

Several sample size calculators are available online such as that of the Australian Bureau of Statistics.[1] The total population and the required confidence level and confidence interval must be entered in the calculation template. For studies involving human subjects, the confidence level is usually set at 95% and the confidence interval at 0.05. Using these settings, for a population of 40,000 the required sample size would be 381.

A shortlist of statistical terms used in sample size calculations, and common descriptors is set out in Table 5. Also, see chapter on data collection for further details of statistical terms and tests.

Power	• The chance of finding a statistically significant difference if one exists; • A study with a power of 80 per cent has a 20 per cent chance of a type II error.
Probability	• The level at which differences between groups are significantly significant.
Type I error	• Frequently occurs in small groups; • Often no clinical significance despite statistically significant difference; • Can occur when the sample size is overpowered; • The null hypothesis was rejected in error.
Type II error	• Often a clinically meaningful difference does *not* produce a statistically significant difference; • Can occur when the sample size is underpowered; • The null hypothesis was accepted in error.
Common descriptors	
• Gender • Years of residence • Self-assigned ethnicity • Religion • Country of birth • Ethnic group • Parents' country of birth. Use the same descriptors as in the national census when possible.	

Table 5. Statistical terms used in sample size calculations

8.6. Bias

Researchers can unintentionally fail to document measurements accurately, and participants may display selective memory when reporting previous events. Both result in bias which skews the results and may happen at any stage of a research project. Therefore, it is vital to bear this in mind and think about how this might occur when the study is being planned.[2]

Experimental bias generates results that are not representative of what is intended to be measured and prevents generalisation beyond the study concerned. Consequently, the value of such results is diminished or wiped out.

Researcher bias occurs when a researcher unintentionally influences results, data, or a participant due to a subjective effect. For example, bias can be due to errors in the research method or the interpretation of data related to the researcher's behaviour, preconceived beliefs, expectancies, or aspirations concerning the expected results.

For example, a researcher may inadvertently prompt participants to act or answer in a particular way.

It is crucial to consider researcher bias as a possible issue in any research project.

8.6.1. Types of bias

When a sample population is obtained that is unrepresentative of the target population, it may bias results such that any results and conclusions drawn from the sample population cannot be generalised to the population as a whole.

Types of bias include

Selection bias

Selection bias occurs when the researcher enrols a sample population that is unrepresentative of the target population.[3]

Sampling bias

When some target population members are more likely to be selected for inclusion in a sample, sampling bias occurs. This can occur in several ways, and these should be considered when designing a study.

Berkson (admission rate) bias

When the sample population is taken from a hospital setting, hospital cases often do not reflect the rate or severity of the condition in the community population, as the association between exposure and disease is unrepresentative of the actual situation.

Diagnostic purity bias

When comorbidity is excluded in the sample population, the sample population may not reflect the real complexity of cases in the population.

Neyman bias c.f. (incidence-prevalence bias, survival bias)

Neyman bias occurs when the prevalence of a condition does not reflect its incidence. This bias occurs mainly in studies on rapidly progressive conditions when patients are included in a sample population but die before their data are collected. The overall result is that interventions are recorded on patients with milder forms of illness, but the study data are generalised to the whole target population.

Membership bias

When a group's membership is used to recruit subjects, the group might not represent the population. Group members may be more motivated to look after their health than the typical person in the target population. However, group members tend to follow trial protocols well, compared to "real-life people" who are less inclined to maintain their health and healthy lifestyle.

Historical control bias

When subjects and controls are chosen across time, temporal changes in definitions, exposures, diseases, and treatments can occur. The result is that such subjects and controls cannot be compared with one another.

Response bias

Response bias occurs when individuals volunteer for studies, but they differ in some way from the population. Volunteers are more motivated to improve their health, participate more readily, and adhere to trial conditions better. When designing a study selecting by advertising for volunteers in newspapers or social media might lead to a response bias.

8.6.2. Allocation and selection bias

Once a population sample has been recruited, the researcher should also be aware that the study design minimises allocation and selection bias. This can happen when subjects are allocated to different arms of a study. The group of subjects in each arm should be representative of the target population. Selection bias occurs during the allocation process when each arm's subjects are not representative of the target population. When researchers or participants decide which subjects go to specific groups, selection bias is unavoidable.

Information bias

Also termed measurement bias or misclassification bias, information bias is a subtype of bias due to a non-random error when measuring variables. The most common reason for it is insufficient clarity in the definition of the outcome of exposure.

Unfortunately, sampling errors can occur even if steps are taken to reduce the risk of selection bias. Large sample sizes and probability sampling help to minimise sampling error.

8.6.3. Confounding

Confounding implies a "mixing of effects." Clinical questions mainly address the relationship which exists between an exposure and an outcome. When a relationship between an exposure and an outcome is proven, there may be other reasons why they exist that affect this relationship. For example, a third factor, a confounder and its unrelated influence can influence the outcome of an experimental design. Essentially, it does not have a direct relationship between the exposure and the outcome, though its presence makes it look like a direct relationship between the two.

A positive confounder results in an association between two variables that do not exist. A negative confounder masks an association that is present. Researchers should accept that confounding may be an issue and design a study that will eliminate or minimise the possibility of their effect.

Confounding variables can wreck a study and produce worthless data. When designing a study, these considerations must be addressed before the formulation of a protocol.

8.7. Concealed allocation and blinding

Concealed allocation and blinding are related to keeping interventions secret. Concealed allocation is an element of the randomisation and allocation processes, which work towards the exclusion selection bias. Blinding, on the other hand, takes place after randomisation and aims to reduce observation bias.

Researchers should not know which group a subject will be allocated to. This strategy will help to eliminate selection bias. When the subjects in each sample population group are not representative of the target population, a selection bias results.

Concealed allocation means that the researchers cannot predict which group the next subject will be allocated to with any accuracy. Concealed allocation is a function of a randomisation strategy. A good study design will outline the concealment strategy. Conversely, if this is not listed in the methods and materials section, it must be assumed that randomisation may be deficient.

In a well-designed study, the people recruiting subjects should be different from those involved in and randomisation.

In research, blinding refers to a procedure where study participants are barred from knowing information that may influence them and is used to remove such bias.

References

1   The Australian Bureau of Statistics offers an online sample size calculator, which can be accessed on 31 March 2021 at www.abs.gov.au/.../home/Sample+Size/Calculator.

2   Dohoo IR. Prev Bias—is it a problem, and what should we do? *Veterinary Medicine*. 2014 ;113(3):331-337.

3   Tripepi G, Jager KJ, Dekker FW, Zoccali. Selection bias and information bias in clinical research. *Nephron Clinical Practice*. 2010;115:c94-99.

Chapter 9. Designing Studies Part 6—Questionnaires

Santini A.

9.1. Overview

This chapter deals with the various aspects of questionnaire design. They are

- The initial steps before developing and designing a questionnaire;
- Structuring a good questionnaire;
- Essential features of questionnaire design;
- Wording the questions;
- Piloting (pre-testing) questionnaires;
- Characteristics of reliability and validity of questionnaires; and
- Obtaining a reasonable response rate.

9.2. Introduction

More research, with increasing use of questionnaires, is being undertaken in healthcare to achieve research objectives. A questionnaire consists of a sequence of questions intended to acquire data from respondents. This usually involves the respondents being asked direct, specific questions by self-completing a survey form or interview.

Because questionnaires are comparatively low-cost and quick to acquire data from a large sample population, they are appealing. However, they are not without drawbacks.

A well-designed questionnaire is needed to achieve results. Since there is no ideal model on which questionnaires can be based, what constitutes good design differs enormously. A good questionnaire design requires realising the research objectives and delivering accurate information that can be evaluated, interpreted, and then generalised and applied to clinical situations.

Both researchers and respondents should find a questionnaire user friendly.[1]

9.3. The initial steps before developing and designing a questionnaire

It is essential to clarify the research question and the best way to collect data to answer this question in any study. An appropriate study design or methodology should refer back and apply to the stated aims and objectives. This is crucial for any study's success, not least one involving a questionnaire.

Before structuring a questionnaire, the researcher should decide what information is required, define the target respondents and choose the recipient's method for answering. Only when these three elements have been agreed on should the researcher progress to construct a questionnaire.

A preliminary decision to be made is whether the researcher wishes to gather qualitative or quantitative data. When the researcher wishes to analyse the gathered data statistically, a formal, standardised questionnaire is required. Qualitative data, also known as exploratory data, seek to understand a subject better or establish hypotheses.

When data are not statistically analysed, and the information is primarily qualitative, there is no need to use formal questions. Such a formal format may restrict dialogue and put off the respondents' from expanding on their views. So instead, there is often an introductory brief or remit in this type of questionnaire, followed by a short list of open-ended questions. Prompts may accompany these open-ended questions to encourage appropriate and helpful answers.

9.4. Structuring a good questionnaire

Questions should be formulated to measure the targeted population's opinions, experiences, and activities. The effort to obtain accurate random sampling and a high response rate will be worthless if the questionnaire is predicated on unclear or biased questions.[2]

Questionnaires can be classified, according to the nature of the questions, as quantitative or qualitative. For example, questionnaire answers acquired through closed-ended questions with multiple choice options are analysed by quantitative methods. Conversely, qualitative methods are used to analyse answers obtained by open-ended questions. This can involve discussions and critical analyses without using numbers or computations.

9.4.1. Closed-ended questions

Closed-ended questions enable researchers to generate data quickly. The researchers set the range of possible answers, not the respondents, and the depth and strength of potential responses are lower. Closed-ended items often frustrate respondents because researchers have not taken into account all potential responses. This potential problem can be overcome by answering "other," followed by "please specify."

9.4.2. Open-ended questions

When using open-ended questions or when the respondent is asked for personal comments, planning how the resulting data will be analysed is essential. The study design must give adequate time, skills, and resources for analysis, without which both the participants' and researchers' time will be wasted. If time or skill to analyse free-text responses is unavailable, do not include such questions in the survey design.

When questionnaires are administered by interviewing respondents, Each respondent should be given the same stimuli using the exact wording when asking the questions and asking them in the same order. Different interviewers must carry out and ask questions and consistently answer respondents' enquiries. To enable respondents to receive clarification on any issue, a set of proscribed questions and answers should be prepared for the interviewer.

Table 1 outlines the steps that should be taken in developing a questionnaire:

- Identify the required information;
- Identify the target respondents;
- Select the method for reaching the target respondents;
- Select the questions' subject matter;
- Develop the wording of the questions;
- Arrange the questions in a meaningful order and format;
- Trial the length of the questionnaire;
- Pre-test the questionnaire on a small sample population; and
- Work up and hone the final version.

Table 1. Steps to be taken when developing a questionnaire

Do not start designing a questionnaire by writing questions. Step one is to create a clear idea of the research aims and what the respondent will provide to meet these aims.

Questions should develop logically from the study's previously defined research question.

A summary of the rules of questionnaire design is outlined in Table 2:

- Begin with a clear idea of the research questions;
- Identify the key areas of interest relating to the study;
- Is a survey the best way to collect the data that will address the question?
- Design questions based on principles of survey design;
- Keep in mind how the responses to specific questions will be used in the analysis of the survey.

In writing each question, consider
- How will the answer be coded?
- How will it be analysed?
- How does it relate to the other questions under consideration?

Table 2. Rules of questionnaire design

9.5. Essential features of questionnaire design

Designing a questionnaire is complex, as questions can be formulated at different levels of detail and in different ways. Questions placed at or near the beginning of a questionnaire may influence responses to later questions. Pretesting or piloting is an essential step in the questionnaire design process. It gives the researcher an insight and better understanding of the recipients' response attitudes to the questionnaire in general and specific questions.

Before constructing a questionnaire, decide what information is required, define the target recipients, and choose the recipients' method. The population from which the researcher proposes to generalise the collected sample data must be well-defined. In addition, demographics of the target respondents, such as age, education need to be considered.

The stages in designing a questionnaire are listed in Table 3:

1. Decide on question content;
2. Develop the wording of the questions;
3. Organise questions in a meaningful way;
4. Read through and assess the length of the questionnaire;
5. Check that the layout is user-friendly;
6. Pilot the questionnaire.
7. Reassess the questionnaire; and
8. Agree on the final survey form.

Table 3. Stages in designing a questionnaire

When making decisions on which questions to include in a survey, critically evaluate their features. Do not be tempted to include questions that do not contribute to the previously established research design.

A well-designed and well-laid out questionnaire is crucial, and a range of people should easily understand it. However, above all, it must be user-friendly. Failure to achieve these criteria will unquestionably lead to low returns.

When designing a questionnaire, points to remember are set out in Table 4 and ideas for layout in Table 5.

1. Questions should have a conversational quality. They should be arranged to proceed from <ul><li>The broad to detailed;</li><li>The impersonal to personal;</li><li>The simple to complex.</li></ul>
2. The respondents' recollection and interest should be sustained by appropriate wording.

3. Avoid questions that
- are leading
- are challenging to answer
- are time-consuming
- are disconcerting
- are intimidating
- combine two questions (e.g. "How often do you smoke cigarettes or cigars?")
- contain a double negative.

Table 4. Points to remember when designing a questionnaire

- It should be easy to use, code, and maintain.
- Leave space between items.
- Use A4 size paper.
- Number the pages consecutively.
- Do not split questions into two pages.
- Use colour.
- Ensure that instructions are distinct from questions (e.g. by using italics, capitals, or colour).
- Maintain interest by the use of arrows and boxes.
- Consider precoding questions.
- Consider using a format that allows the form to be scanned by machine-readers.

Table 5. Ideas for a questionnaire layout

9.6. Types of questionnaires

Questionnaires can be

- Postal;
- Email;
- Internet;
- Face-to-face interview;
- Computerised self-administered;
- Telephone and video-linked; and
- In-house questionnaires.

9.6.1. Postal questionnaires

Respondents receive the questionnaire usually with a pre-paid envelope. The advantage of postal questionnaires is that respondents have and can take time to consider their answers.

The disadvantages are that they are expensive and time-consuming as the researcher has to wait until questionnaires are returned. In addition, a significant drawback is that the recipient may immediately discard the questionnaire without considering the subject matter due to the increasing use of research questionnaires.

An inadequate response to a postal questionnaire will reduce the study's statistical power and may introduce bias. To avoid a poor response rate, many disciplines have researched the various issues that can influence a portal return, including the questionnaire length, the colour of the envelope ink, including a stamped addressed envelope in which to return the questionnaire and financial incentives.[3, 4]

9.6.2. Email and internet questionnaires

Internet surveys use a web-based system to distribute questionnaires. This has the advantages of cost savings and easy distribution. A complete list of email addresses available for the target sample, such as membership lists of a professional body or university students, facilitates such a survey. However, it may limit the distribution to an unrepresentative sample.[5, 6] In addition, since the advent of the General Data Protection Regulations (GDPR), many organisations have refused to make lists of their members' email addresses available to researchers.

Nevertheless, such surveys are increasingly popular, and one commercial package in everyday use is SurveyMonkey.[7]

The advantages and disadvantages of postal and internet surveys are set out in Table 6:

Postal	
Advantages	Disadvantages
• They are frequently used for research • Lower costs than personal interviews • Eliminates potential interviewer bias • The envelope can be badged with a hospital or university logo.	• May result in a biased sample • The response rate may be low. • Delay of weeks for return of all responses • Higher costs than web surveys due to printing and postage costs.
Internet	
Advantages	Disadvantages
• They are frequently used for research • Low-cost (no postage, printing) • Fast • Can use filters/hidden sections • The initial approach is badged with a hospital or university logo • Anonymity: more honest responses? • Typed responses: increased legibility • Survey software simplifies coding and analysis.	• May result in a biased sample • Older/non-web users not reached • The response rate may be low. • The initial approach may have to be indirect due to GDPR. • Delay of weeks for return of all responses • Anonymity: non-responders unidentifiable? • Random respondents may reply if a survey is an open webpage.

Table 6. Advantages and disadvantages of postal and internet surveys

9.6.3. Face-to-face surveys

A face-to-face survey may be preferred when a specific target population is involved. More in-depth information can be sought by probing and observation of the respondent's behaviour. Respondents in a face-to-face interview may be more likely to answer sensitive questions or tolerate a longer questionnaire. Problems of a possible lack of literacy are reduced. However, the costs of face-to-face surveys are high, and training and calibration of interviewers are essential to reduce the possibility of introducing bias by leading the respondent towards specific responses. Because of these disadvantages, the early-career researcher may not be in a position to set up a study based on face-to-face interviews unless the study is small or a pilot. Telephone and video-link interviews remove the disadvantage of cost. However, they may also lose some of the benefits of face-to-face contact between the interviewer and the respondent. Therefore, training interviewers before telephone and video-link interviews is essential.[8]

Computerised self-administered questionnaires use computer technology to design the questionnaire and allow respondents to complete the survey with little assistance.

9.6.4. Telephone surveys

These occur when the researcher calls potential respondents by phone. The advantage of a telephone questionnaire is that the survey can be accomplished in a short time. The disadvantage is that it takes the researcher's time and is therefore expensive. In addition, people may not feel comfortable answering questions over the phone. Obtaining a good sample group to answer a questionnaire over the phone is a significant problem.

9.6.5. In-house surveys

The researcher visits respondents in their homes or workplaces. The advantage is that the researcher can focus the respondent's attention on the questions. The disadvantages include that they are time-consuming, expensive, and respondents may show a reluctance to the researcher being in their homes or workplaces.

9.7. Wording the questions

Survey questions can be classified as closed, open-ended and open response-option questions.

9.7.1. Closed questions

Closed questioning has significant advantages. The respondent is provided with an easy way of answering without thinking about how to express their answer. As a result, the respondent relies less on memory when answering a question. Answers are straightforwardly categorised, and analysis is facilitated. However, unless there is the possibility of adding additional information by adding the option "other, please specify" to a list of possible answers, they have the disadvantage of not letting the respondent give a different answer to the one suggested. They also regularly propose answers that respondents previously have not taken into account.

9.7.2. Open-ended questions

With open-ended questions, no answers are put forward, and the respondent is requested to answer the question in their own words. Open questions may produce unexpected results and generate original and valuable data. However, the data analysis is challenging when obtained through questionnaires with open questions.

The advantage inherent in an open question survey is that any options proposed by the researcher do not sway the respondent. Thus the issues which are significant to the respondent are frequently given. Data, thoughts and concepts not initially foreseen by the researcher may therefore be initiated. The respondent can modify their answers and can express the strength of their attitudes and views. However, the disadvantages are apparent, and their use should be carefully considered. Respondents may find it difficult to 'put their answers into words; therefore, their response may not fully describe their feelings or mindsets. They may not give a full answer simply because they may forget to mention salient points.

A significant disadvantage is a requirement for data, collected as verbatim remarks and observation, to be categorised and be codified. This presents chances for recording and interpreting errors in the answers given on the part of interviewers. It is also labour intensive and time-consuming. An example is when a question, such as "When were you last on holiday?" is put to a respondent, the answers can vary from "last week," "A year ago," "Just returned from holiday," and "I cannot remember the last time."

9.7.3. Multiple-choice questions

Respondents choose from a set of answers. The disadvantage is that the questionnaire may become unclear, puzzling, and tedious if there are too many answers to choose from, discouraging the respondent from completing the questionnaire.

9.7.4. Dichotomous questions

The respondents are given two options to choose from, yes or no. In many ways, it is the most straightforward form of a questionnaire from the respondent's perspective. However, often answers are not clear cut, and the answers yes or no may mask the absolute truth.

9.7.5. Scaling questions or ranking questions

The respondent is given the option to rank the available answers to the questions on a scale of a range of values (e.g. from 1 to 10).

It is beyond this chapter's scope to describe more than a few topics central to the wording of questions. However, sources for further consultation are given at the end of the chapter.

Some of the key issues to be considered when wording questionnaires are set out in Table 7:

Ask clear and specific questions the respondent will be able to answer.
Closed-ended questions should include all reasonable responses, and the response categories should be mutually exclusive.
Do not use "double-barrelled" questions. Instead, ask only one question at a time. Respondents find it difficult to answer questions that include more than one notion, leading to responses that are difficult to interpret.

Table 7. Key issues when wording questionnaires

A standard survey question has the "agree-disagree" structure. This has the disadvantage, as research shows that less informed respondents tend to agree with such statements. This is sometimes called an "acquiescence bias" since some respondents are more likely to acquiesce to the statement. Offering respondents a choice between alternative statements is a better format.

There is a natural tendency to want to be accepted and liked. This leads some respondents to give inaccurate answers to sensitive topics such as understating alcohol and drug use, tax evasion and racial bias while overstating charitable contributions, attending church and whether they intend to vote in an election. This tendency can lead to social desirability bias.

9.8. Arranging the questions in a meaningful order

The order in which questions are placed in the questionnaire is important. The placement of a question may affect the result more than the selection of words used in the question.

9.8.1. Opening questions

Questions occurring early in a questionnaire should not unintentionally influence how respondents answer succeeding questions. Opening questions should be easy to answer and of a non-threatening kind. The first question sets the survey's tone. The respondent's first experience of the survey should not be complicated or off-putting. A first question, challenging to understand, embarrassing, or beyond the respondent's comprehension or knowledge can result in the respondent taking little or no further interest in the survey. Engage the respondent with a comfortable and friendly first question.

9.8.2. The order of questions

Order questions so that one leads easily and naturally to the next. Set questions by topic or theme as respondents can feel confused or perplexed by questions fluctuating from one theme to another.

9.8.3. Variety of questions

Reduce the possibility of respondents becoming bored by varying the type of question. An occasional open-ended question distributed throughout the questionnaire may provide respite from many questions that have limited respondents' answers to pre-coded categories. Such open-ended questions will not be subject to analysis and are purely there to relieve tedium and monotony.

Whenever possible, the exact wording of commonly asked questions from standard surveys should be used rather than self-penned questions. Previously used questionnaires for similar topics are very helpful. They can often be used directly, and their reliability and validity have usually been established. Besides, such questions are valuable in comparing the study results with those from similar previous studies.

9.8.4. Closing questions

Many respondents become increasingly uninterested towards the end of a questionnaire and frequently give thoughtless or rash answers. Therefore, do not place questions of particular significance at the end of the survey; instead, place them near the start. However, possibly sensitive questions should be kept to the end to avoid respondents being antagonised and failing to complete the survey before necessary data are obtained.

Ample writing space should allow recording open-ended answers and cater to differences in handwriting between interviewers and respondents.

The aim of the questions generally determines the type of response format used. The characteristics of open and closed questions and their advantages and disadvantages are set out in Tables 8, 9, and 10.

- **There are** no answer choices to select from;
- The respondent must do more work in giving answers.

Examples
- How do you feel about your GP?
- What are the barriers to better health for yourself?

Advantages	Disadvantages
• Stimulates free thought • Not limited to the researcher's expected answers • Useful in both exploratory and qualitative studies.	• Demanding for the respondent • Answers may be incomplete, irrelevant, unclear. • It may be challenging to analyse using quantitative techniques. • Require content analysis, classification of answers.

Table 8. Characteristics, advantages, and disadvantages of open-ended question

Closed-ended questions with ordered choices
- answers provided
- may have gradations of a dimension of thought or behaviour
- The need to find an answer that most closely matches their beliefs.

Example
How often have you seen your GP this year?
- Never
- Once
- Twice
- 3–4 times

Advantages	Disadvantages
• Readily analysable • Helpful in assessing gradations of frequency or intensity (feelings, pain).	• May limit the range of answers to a single dimension • Forces answers in a specific way • Valid responses are easily overlooked, e.g. "never," "cannot remember," "I do not have a GP," or "I always go straight to A&E."

Visual analogue scales

A visual analogue scale may be appropriate if you believe that the character or attitude you wish to measure ranges across a continuum of values, e.g. pain, happiness or satisfaction. Instead of selecting a written response category or entering an open-ended response, the respondent indicates their answer with a mark on a line.

Mark the horizontal line to indicate how much pain you felt during the procedure.

Worst pain possible   No pain at all

|————————————————————————|

Advantages	Disadvantages
• It is easily transformed into an arithmetic value. • Useful to measure change within individuals • Easy to complete.	• May hide qualifications, e.g. "pain came and went" • Subjective, e.g. some respondents may be more likely to avoid extremes due to their personality rather than their experience • May distort ordinal responses to appear as an interval scale.

Table 9. Characteristics, advantages, and disadvantages of closed-ended questions with ordered choices

Closed-ended questions with unordered choices	
Example	
Which of the following has occupied most of your time in the past week?	

Digging in the garden
    Watching TV
    Working in the house
    Walking outside the house	

Advantages	**Disadvantages**
• Not limited to choosing among gradations of a single dimension • Helpful in selecting priorities (policy or decision-making).	• More difficult than ordered choices • Respondent forced to select an answer when more than one may be appropriate.
Partially closed questions	
Example	
Which of the following areas of expenditure do you want to have the highest priority in Anyburgh Hospital?	

Emergency department
    X-Ray department
    Laboratories
    Other (please specify)	

Advantages	**Disadvantages**
• Provides an "out" if certain responses are overlooked • "Other" responses will require classifying and coding a range of differing replies (including "do not know").	• Bias towards answering with one of the given options • "Other" may not add much. If "other" is used frequently, it may signal a faulty question (or responses)!

Table 10. Characteristics, advantages, and disadvantages of closed-ended questions with unordered choices

9.9. Piloting (pretesting) questionnaires

It is essential to pilot a questionnaire using a sample of people from the survey population to assess its response. Whether or not the survey will effectively achieve the desired results will only be ascertained after being used in conjunction with actual respondents. Therefore, it is expedient to pilot or pre-test the questionnaire before using it in a full-scale survey. In addition, piloting will aid the identification of any errors or slip-ups that need modifying or revising. A significant, though a small number of people should be included in a pilot to study potential variations within and across the population. The respondents chosen for the pilot survey should generally be characteristic of the type of respondent invited to participate in the main survey.

Piloting allows the identification of issues regarding readability and understanding in phrasing and overall arrangement. Pilot respondents should be monitored and interviewed closely. It is crucial to identify and subsequently avoid any inappropriate or problematic questions. A seldom undertaken but recommended task is to statistically evaluate pilot data to confirm that the analytic techniques can be used in the final data analysis.

The purpose of pre-testing or piloting a questionnaire is to establish whether

- the questions' wording will accomplish the desired results;
- the questions have been placed in the most appropriate and most effective sequence;
- the questions are appreciated and understood by all classes of respondent;
- additional or special questions are needed;
- some questions should be eliminated; and
- the instructions to interviewers are adequate.

After the questionnaire has been piloted and considered satisfactory, it remains for the layout-out of the questionnaire to be finalised. Questions should be suitably assembled and ordered and allocated numbers. If interviewers are to be involved, clear instructions for the interviewer on how to conduct the survey should also be included.

In addition to assessing the questions' clarity, piloting should test the procedures used in the questionnaire, such as the contact letter, second invitations, and any incentives. It is best to conduct pilot tests well before the survey to allow time for substantial changes to the questionnaire or procedures.

The questions which should be answered during a pilot are set out in Table 11:

- Are all the questions valid?
- Is the wording clear?
- Do different people have similar interpretations of questions?
- Do closed-ended questions have appropriate possible answers?
- Does the questionnaire give a positive impression?
- Is there any bias in the questions?

Table 11. Questions to be asked when piloting a questionnaire

A pre-pilot stage is advantageous. The pre-pilot may be relatively informal and based on convenience. For example, a draft questionnaire could be given to colleagues, friends or family members, asking them for comments on its ease of use, relevance, comprehensibility, repetitiveness, and missing issues. A more formal pilot study can then be performed with a cross-section of potential respondents, if possible, with differing ages, reading levels and socioeconomic groups. Based on the pre-pilot and pilot studies, the questionnaire may require redesigning, including shortening, to ensure user-friendliness and validity.

9.10. Characteristics of reliability and validity of questionnaires

Reliability and validity are terms that describe two completely different concepts, although they are often closely interrelated.

A valid questionnaire measures what it claims to measure. Frequently many are unsuccessful in achieving this. For example, a self-completion questionnaire that aims to quantity people's exercising habits may be invalid because the respondents' acquired data (answers) may differ from that undertaken. In addition, a survey developed and successfully used at a different time, country, or cultural context may not be a valid measurement of the studied group.

Table 12 sets out the characteristics of reliability and validity of questionnaires:

Various estimates of validity	Various estimates of reliability
• Face validity: Do the questions make sense? • Content validity: Do the questions express the underlying concept they were designed to reflect? • Criterion validity: Do responses to the questions agree with an objective criterion or gold standard for the underlying concept? • Construct validity: are the hypotheses concerning the relationships between the underlying concepts borne out by the responses?	• Test-retest: Does the same question have the same response over time? • Inter-rater: Do two interviewers with the same questionnaire get the same response? • Internal consistency: Do questions designed to evaluate the same concept obtain equivalent responses?

Table 12. Characteristics of the questionnaire: reliability versus validity

Reliability is an essential constituent of validity. However, on its own, it is not an adequate measure of validity. A test can be reliable but not valid, whereas a test cannot be valid yet unreliable. Reliability describes the repeatability and constancy of a test. Validity defines the final results' strength and whether the results accurately represent the real world. It relates to the questions' ability to encapsulate the fundamental notions being appraised. "Does the test measure what it is intended to measure?" and "What can be concluded about the person who gave a specific response?" are question types that relate to validity.

9.11. Obtaining a good response rate

The response rate is the percentage of respondents who completed and returned a survey questionnaire. A response rate of 60 per cent or more is usually deemed necessary for a study's results to be valid. To achieve this level of response, careful planning and survey design are required. For example, the questionnaire's brevity or offering incentives may increase response rates but do not guarantee an acceptable response rate.

Approaches that may improve response rates are set out in Table 13:

- University and charity sponsorship
- Pre-notification of respondents
- Sample size calculation
- Subject salient to the respondent
- Individualised approach
- Confidentiality assured
- Importance stressed
- Brevity
- Ease of completion
- Reminder(s), including a second copy of the questionnaire
- Upfront incentives provided
- Telephone follow-up
- A thank you letter/postcard to all, acting as a final reminder to non-respondents.

Table 13. Approaches that may increase response rates

9.12. Covering Letters

A covering (cover) letter should accompany all questionnaires and surveys. It is usually the first thing the respondent reads; it must be well written and formatted in an attention-grabbing manner. It may be included in the same envelope as the questionnaire. However, it has been shown that improved response rates are obtained if the cover letter precedes the arrival of the questionnaire.

Table 14 describes the content and format of a covering letter:

The content of the letter should:
- introduce and explain the survey
- introduce the lead researcher, their position and institution
- be simple, with no long sentences, jargon or abbreviations
- be no longer than **one** side of an A4 page
- be in a 12-point font size
- anticipate respondents' questions.

Format
- Use headed paper from your institution (with consent).
- **1st paragraph**: state the purpose and importance of the study and why you and your institution should be trusted.
- **2nd paragraph**: explain that confidentiality will be maintained and that participation is voluntary. Refer to the ethics committee and other approvals.
- **3rd paragraph**: re-emphasise study reason/justification and how the results will be used (e.g. possible benefit to patients, NHS.)
- **4th paragraph**: explain whether and how results will be made available.
- **Thank the participant for reading the letter and for completing the questionnaire.**
- Remind them to use the enclosed stamped or Freepost envelope, and refer to a deadline if there is one.
- Give contact details in case they would like further information.
- Sign off the letter personally, if possible, jointly with your supervisor or head of the department.

Table 14. Content and format of a covering letter

Returned questionnaires must be checked for completeness. A frequent error is the omission of some answers to questions. The researcher should return the incomplete questionnaire to the respondent noting that the omissions may have been made in error. The research's success depends on getting a complete set of results. However, answers to sensitive or difficult questions may have been intentionally omitted by the respondent. In this event, the respondent's views should be appreciated. However, despite researchers' best efforts, there are frequently different response rates for some questions. Therefore, when writing up the results of a questionnaire-based survey, the authors should give the number of responses to each question.

References

1   Rattray J, Jones M.C.J Essential elements of questionnaire design and development. *Clinical Nursing.* 2007; 16:234–243.

2   Greenhaugh T, Selecting, designing, and developing your questionnaire. Selecting, designing, and developing your questionnaire. *British Medical Journal* 2004 29; 328: 1312–1315.

3   Duncan A, Ruth Floate R, Clarkson J, Ramsay C. Three behaviour change theory-informed randomised studies within a trial to improve response rates to trial postal questionnaires. *Journal of Clinical Epidemiology.* 2020, 122:35–41.

4   Edwards P.J., Roberts I., Clarke M.J., Diguiseppi C., Wentz R., Kwan I., Coper R., Felix L.M., Pratap S. Methods to increase response to postal and electronic questionnaires. *Cochrane Database of Systematic Reviews* 8 July 2009 (3) MR000008

5   Rosenbaum J, Lidz CW. Maximising the results of internet surveys. University of Massachusetts Medical School Centre for Mental Health Services Research. Issue Brief 2007;4:1.

6   Dillman DA. Mail and internet surveys: the tailored design method. 3rd ed. Hoboken, NJ: John Wiley & Sons; 2007.

7   Surveymonkey is online commercial software. There are no fees for small and straightforward surveys. Surveys can be sent out via mobile, web, or social media. www.surveymonkey.com.

8   Dialling I. Face-to-face interviewing. In: Lavrakas P. Encyclopedia of survey research methods. SAGE Publications website. http://srmo.sagepub.com/view/encyclopedia-of-survey-research-methods/n174.xml

Chapter 10. Designing Studies Part 7—Screening and Diagnostic Testing

SANTINI A.

10.1. Overview and introduction

This chapter explains the features of screening and testing and how research studies into screening and testing are designed. It aims to help the reader

- Differentiate between screening and diagnostic testing;
- Calculate and interpret test characteristics;
- Understand what is meant by test accuracy;
- Understand the basic study design for evaluating test accuracy;
- Understand the meaning of sensitivity, specificity, positive predictive value, and negative predictive value, and evaluate them numerically.

10.2. The differences between screening tests and diagnostic tests

Screening tests are not diagnostic tests, and the difference between screening tests and diagnostic tests is often misunderstood. Screening trials evaluate new tests for detecting health conditions in people and the efficiency of new drugs or medical techniques. Screening tests are undertaken to assess if they can improve on currently used methodologies and at what cost. Thus, they differ from clinical trials, which are research studies that test how well new medical techniques work in patients.

Diagnostic tests establish the presence or absence of disease in order to make treatment decisions. A diagnostic test is carried out on symptomatic individuals or after a screen-positive confirmatory test has been obtained.[1]

Key differences between screening tests and diagnostic tests are set out in Table 1:

	Screening test	Diagnostic test
Objective	To detect a potential disease	To establish the presence or absence of disease

Population targeted	A target population of asymptomatic members of a population who are potentially at risk of disease is recruited. Usually, large numbers are screened.	Individuals who have symptoms of a disease are recruited to establish a diagnosis. Also, asymptomatic individuals who have had a positive screening test.
Test procedure	The test should be simple to administer and be acceptable to patients and administrating personnel.	The test may be invasive. However, this can be defended as it is crucial in confirming a diagnosis.
The threshold of a positive result	To not miss individuals with the disease, the threshold selected is towards the high sensitivity level.	Selected towards high specificity levels to reflect true negatives.
Significance of a positive result.	The suggestion of the presence of the disease This indicates that confirmation by further tests may be necessary.	The result specifies a definite diagnosis.
Price	The tests should be inexpensive as large numbers will need to be screened to detect a relatively small number of potential cases.	Higher costs for a diagnostic test may be warranted to establish a diagnosis.

Table 1. The differences between screening and diagnostic tests

A new medical test must first undergo a series of assessments before being introduced into general clinical use. The following questions should be asked: Is it effective? Does the test work in the laboratory? Is it clinically efficient? Does the test work in the patient population of interest? Will the test bring about health outcomes benefits?[2]

The word screening refers to testing for the early signs of disease in asymptomatic patients. The object is to detect patients who have a disease or condition so that the disease or condition can be treated before it progresses to an advanced stage.

10.3. Types of screening tests

A spectrum of screening tests exists and may be used on individuals or in population-wide mass screening. They include

Individual screening: In the United Kingdom, a spectrum of tests are available on the NHS, including blood pressure screening, breast cancer screening, cervical cancer screening, cholesterol screening, colorectal cancer screening, and dental check-ups, as well as routine blood tests to evaluate organ function, such as that of the kidneys, liver, thyroid, and heart.

Population-wide screening includes population-wide mass screening for tuberculosis to reduce mycobacterium tuberculosis transmission in the community. Population-wide screening for coronavirus (COVID-19) was introduced in many countries after the SARS-CoV-2 pandemic outbreak in 2020.

Both individual screening and population-wide screening generally target symptomless individuals. In contrast, diagnostic testing is performed on asymptomatic patients to establish if they have a specific disease or condition.

10.4. Diagnostic Accuracy Studies

A new test's diagnostic accuracy is evaluated to assess how well it discriminates between patients with or without a specific disease. The accuracy of an index test cannot be evaluated without a reference standard. At the commencement of a study, there should be a consensus that the reference standard to be used is more accurate than the index test. More than one acceptable reference standard would be appropriate for use in a test accuracy study.

The test accuracy is defined as a comparison between the disease conditions (target condition) estimated by a test of interest (index test) and the best estimate of the actual disease state (reference standard). It is an unequivocal acknowledgement that most tests make errors even if correctly performed.

A degree of pragmatism may be required when choosing an acceptable reference standard. The most accurate reference standard may not be feasible or ethical. Less accurate methods may have to be used. The reference standard may not always be a gold standard (vide infra); the use of a non-gold or imperfect standard may occur when there is no generally accepted reference standard for the target condition. However, using an imperfect reference standard produces a reference standard bias.[3]

Figure 1 describes a method for evaluating the diagnostic accuracy of a medical test with binary test results and dichotomised disease status:

All patients included in the study sample

Index test (new test)

Reference test (gold standard)

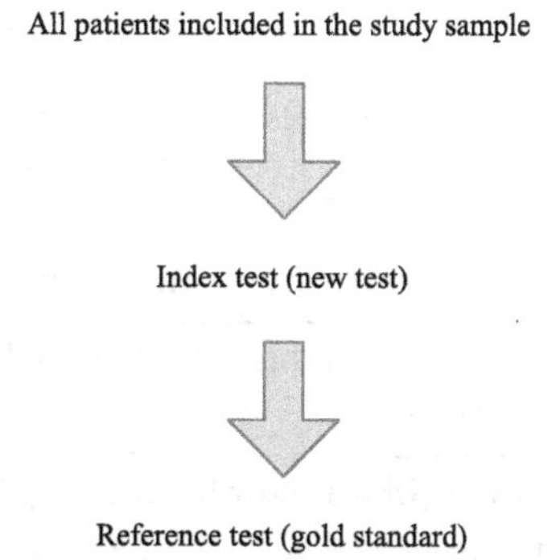

Index test	Reference test (gold standard)	
	Positive	Negative
Positive	True - positive	False - positive
Negative	False - negative	True - negative

All patients take the Index test (new test) and the Reference test (gold standard) simultaneously or within a short interval to avoid changes in the disease's status.

Figure 1. A method of evaluating the diagnostic accuracy of a medical test with binary test results and dichotomised disease status.

Depending on the test's resultant characteristics, including sensitivity and specificity standards, the new test's role when seeking a diagnosis can be determined. For example, it may be deemed better than any existing test, a possible replacement test or used as a triage test.

The primary measures of the diagnostic accuracy of a test are sensitivity and specificity. Other measures are predictive values, likelihood values, overall accuracy, receiver operating characteristic (ROC) curve, area under the ROC curve (AUROC) ROC surface, and volume under the ROC surface (VUS).

Definitions of the words and phrases used to describe diagnostic test characteristics are given in Table 2:

Sensitivity (true-positive rate)

The proportion of subjects who have the disorder (by the gold standard) has a positive result by the new test.

Specificity (true-negative rate)
is the proportion of subjects who do not have the disorder and give a negative test.
The positive predictive value (PPV)
is the proportion of subjects who give a positive test result and have the disease.
The negative predictive value (NPV)
is the proportion of subjects who give a negative test result and do not have the disease.
The likelihood ratio for a positive test result (LR+) is how much more likely a positive result is found in a person with, as opposed to without, the disease?
The likelihood ratio for a negative test result (LR-) is how likely a negative result is to be found in a person with the disease than not having the disease.
Accuracy of a test
This is the proportion of subjects who give the correct result.
A false positive is an error resulting from the incorrect indication of a disease's presence, i.e. the result is positive when, in reality, the patient is disease-free.
A false negative is an error resulting from the incorrect indication that the patient does not have the disease, i.e. the result is negative when, in reality, the patient has the disease.

Table 2. Terms used to describe diagnostic test characteristics

Information regarding test accuracy helps indicate screening, diagnosis, predisposition, monitoring, prognosis, and drug effectiveness are set out in Table 3:

Screening: Which patients have an asymptomatic disease?
Diagnosis: Which patients have a symptomatic disease?
Predisposition: Which patients could develop the disease?
Monitoring: • Is the disease controlled? • How advanced is the disease? • Has the disease recurred?
Prognosis: Will the disease progress over time?
Is a drug effective?

Table 3. Information regarding test accuracy

10.4.1. The gold standard for diagnostic tests

Comparing the index test results with a reference standard for diagnosing the same target condition in the same participants quantifies the process.

The reference standard could be a gold standard that refers to an experimental model that has been thoroughly tested and is a reliable method. It is often the method accepted and used as the current best available test. However, a gold standard may not be used occasionally because it is expensive or invasive, or patients do not consent to it. In addition, clinicians may decide not to use the gold test for some patients for medical reasons.

10.4.2. Test population

The population of interest must be clearly defined. It would be incorrect to appraise a diagnostic test using a population that does not represent the target population, such as using a population derived from a university student population to appraise a test in care-home patients. The ideal sample for a test accuracy study is a consecutive or randomly selected series of patients in whom the target condition is suspected or the target population for screening studies.

The index test is the new test under evaluation for its accuracy.

The reference standard is the standard against which the index test is compared. It is usually the best test currently available but may not necessarily be used routinely in practice.

The test accuracy is predicated on a one-sided comparison of the index test results and the reference standard. The reference standard is essential to validate the test study's accuracy as there is the assumption that it has a 100 per cent accuracy. This assumption is rarely correct and represents a fundamental flaw in the test. Any inconsistency is presumed to result from errors in the index test. Therefore, the reference standard's selection is critical to the validity of a test accuracy study, and the definition of the diagnostic threshold forms part of that reference standard. A composite reference standard, considered a better indicator of actual disease status, may be used in cases where there is no consensus on the best reference test.

10.4. Designing a diagnostic accuracy study

Table 4 lists aspects to consider when designing a diagnostic accuracy study:

The protocol	The protocol details every step of the study. The problem at this stage should be clearly stated.
Selection of participants for the target population	The target population determines the criteria for including participants in the study. The population is essential in deciding on an appropriate study-setting.
Reference standard	The reference standard should diagnose the same target condition as the index test. The choice of a reference standard (gold or non-gold) determines the methods used when evaluating the index test.

Sample size	An adequate sample size is critical in making inferences from the statistical analysis.
Selection of accuracy	A decision should be made at the protocol stage as to which accuracy measures are to be estimated. This decision will be determined by the test's response (binary or continuous).
Eliminate possible bias	Multiple forms of bias may exist. Therefore, anticipating how to avoid or minimise bias is essential.
Validation of results	Validation ensures an understanding of the reproducibility, strengths, and limitations of the study.

Table 4. Aspects to consider when designing a diagnostic accuracy study

Table 5 sets out a checklist of methodological aspects that should be addressed when designing a diagnostic accuracy study:

Was there a clearly defined population of interest?
For a test accuracy study, the ideal study sample is a consecutive or randomly selected series of patients in whom the target condition is suspected, or for screening studies, the target population.
Was the reference standard applied regardless of the diagnostic test result?
Was an independent and blind comparison with the gold standard of diagnosis?
Did the participants undertake both the new test and the reference test within a short period? Ideally, both tests should be done simultaneously to avoid biases caused by potential alterations in patients' disease status.
Applicability
<ul><li>Are the intended patients similar to the target population?</li><li>Is it possible to integrate the index test into a clinical setting?</li><li>Who will conduct the index test in a clinical setting, and who will interpret the results?</li><li>Is the test affordable?</li></ul>

Table 5. Diagnostic accuracy studies—methodological aspects checklist

10.6. Test accuracy

Test accuracy compares the disease/condition (target condition) estimated by a test of interest (Index test) and the best estimate of the actual disease stated by the reference standard. It is indisputable that most tests result in errors, even if properly carried out.

A false positive is an error in which a test result incorrectly indicates a disease (the result is positive when there is no disease present).

A false negative is an error in which a test result incorrectly indicates no presence of a disease (the result is negative when the disease is present).

New test characteristics can be computed with values obtained for sensitivity and specificity, the positive predictive value, the negative predictive value, the likelihood ratios, pre-test probability and odds, post-test probability and odds receiver operating curve.[4]

Each of these values should be calculated see Table 6.

Patient number:	1	2	3	4	5	6	7	8	9	10	>>>>>>
Reference results:	P	P	P	N	P	N	N	P	P	N	>>>>>>
Index (new test) results.	P	N	P	N	P	P	N	P	N	P	>>>>>>>
	TP	FN	TP	TN	TP	FP	TN	TP	FN	FP	>>>>>>

Number of TP = 4
Number of FP = 2
Number of TN = 2
Number of FN = 2
Total TP+FP+TN+FN = 10

Table 6. Calculation of true positive (TP), true negative (TN), false positive, (FP) and false negative (FN) values

The reference test is always considered to be 100 per cent accurate, although it may not be in reality. The index test results are compared against the reference test results.

The four possible outcomes of cross-classification are represented in a diagnostic 2x2 contingency table, such as the one presented in Table 7:

		Reference standard	
		Positive	Negative
Index test	Positive	TP	FP
	Negative	FN	TN

Table 7. 2x2 table of the results of diagnostic tests

Table 8 explains the terms which relate to test accuracy:

Test characteristic	Explanation	Formula
Sensitivity (true –positive rate)	Is the proportion of subjects with the disorder by the reference test who give a positive result by the Index (new) test	TP/ TP+FN
Specificity (true-negative rate)	The proportion of patients without the disorder and who give a negative test	TN/TN+FP
Positive prediction value (PPV)	The proportion of patients with a positive test who do have the disease	TP/ TP+FP

Negative prediction value (NPV)	The proportion of subjects with a negative test who do not have the disease	TN/TN+FN
The likelihood ratio for a positive test result (LR+)	How much more likely is a positive test to be found in a person with the disease compared to one without the disease	sensitivity/ 1- specificity
The likelihood ratio for a negative test result (LR-)	How much more likely is a negative test to be found in a person with the disease compared to one without the disease	1- sensitivity / specificity
False-positive rate	It is an error resulting from the incorrect indication of a disease's presence, i.e. the result is positive when, in reality, the patient is disease-free.	FP/FP+TN
False-negative rate	Is an error resulting from the incorrect indication that the patient does not have the disease, i.e. the result is negative when, in reality, the patient has the disease?	FN/TP+FN
Accuracy of a test	The proportion of the subjects with the correct result	TP+TN/ TP+FP+FN+TN

Table 8. Explanation of terms relating to test accuracy

10.7. Helpful aide-memoirs for sensitivity specificity and predictive values.

SpPin—when a highly **sp**ecific test is used, a **p**ositive test result tends to rule **in** the disorder.

SnNout—when a highly **s**e**n**sitive test is used, a **n**egative test result tends to rule **out** the disorder.

10.7.1. An explanation of positive predictive value and negative predictive value

PPV = positive predictive value: The proportion of those who test positive with the index test who have the disease

NPV = negative predictive value: The proportion of those who test negative with the index test who do not have the disease

Predictive values depend on the prevalence of the disorder.

Prevalence is the proportion of a particular population affected by a medical condition or disease at a specific time. An increase in the prevalence of a disease in a population will increase the positive predictive value. Conversely, the negative predictive value will decrease.

The likelihood ratio is often more useful than predictive values and can be calculated from sensitivity and specificity numbers. The likelihood ratio remains constant even when the prevalence of the disorder changes. (cf. predictive values).

The likelihood ratio indicates the number of times that patients with a disease are likely to have a particular test result than patients without the disease. Table 9 shows the effect of prevalence on the positive predictive value (PPV).

Prevalence %	PPV %	Sensitivity	Specificity
0.1	1.8	90	95
1	15.4	90	95
5	48.6	90	95
50	94.7	90	95

Table 9. The effect of prevalence on the positive predictive value (PPV)

10.8. The receiver operating characteristic (ROC) curve

A ROC curve is a performance measurement for classification problems at various threshold settings. ROC is a probability curve. The area under the curve characterises the degree or measure of separability. In this section, the following points are discussed.

- An explanation of the ROC curve;
- Defining terms used in a ROC curve;
- The probability threshold that gives the best performance; and
- Relation between sensitivity, specificity, FPR, and threshold.

10.8.1. An explanation of the ROC curve

10.8.1.1. The probability threshold

In medicine, a binary classification problem is knowing the accuracy of the result of a test concerning whether a patient has or has not got a disease. This question requires that a threshold be chosen to convert this probability into an actual prediction. The threshold should be chosen with care. In medically-related situations, a frequent and important consideration is whether a patient has a disease when he is disease-free. The 0.5 probability level is the commonly used threshold: when the probability is more significant than 0.5, the prediction is a 1, i.e. the patient has the disease, or a 0, i.e. the patient does not have the disease.

The probability threshold can be varied depending on the study: this produces different sets of 1s and 0s, and consequently, a different set of predictions.

The area under the ROC curve (AUC), with standard error and 95 per cent confidence interval, can be interpreted as follows:

- the average value of sensitivity for all possible values of specificity;
- the average value of specificity for all possible values of sensitivity;
- The probability that a randomly selected individual from the positive group has a test result indicating greater suspicion than a randomly chosen individual from the negative group.

When the variable under study cannot distinguish between the two groups (there is no difference between the two distributions), the area will be equal to 0.5 (the ROC curve will coincide with the diagonal). When there is a perfect separation of the two groups' values—there is no overlapping of the distributions—the area under the ROC curve equals 1 (the ROC curve will reach the upper left corner of the plot).

The 95 per cent confidence interval is the interval in which the true (population) area under the ROC curve lies with 95 per cent confidence.

10.8.1.2. *P*-value

The *p*-value is the probability that the observed sample Area under the ROC curve is found when the true (population) area under the ROC curve is 0.5 (null hypothesis: area = 0.5). If p is low ($p < 0.05$), then it can be concluded that the area under the ROC curve is significantly different from 0.5 and that, therefore, there is evidence that the laboratory test does have an ability to distinguish between the two groups.

10.8.2. Defining terms used in a ROC curve and the area under the curve (AUC)

The following metrics can be extracted from a ROC curve. The model's precision is calculated using the true row of the predicted labels (Table 10). It indicates how good the model is when making a Positive prediction of the number of patients actually having the disease out of all the patients that the algorithm predicts sick. In Table 10, the precision (positive prediction value) is TP/TP+FP:

		True	False
Predicted labels	Positive	TP	FP
	Negative	FN	TN
		Actual labels	

Table 10. Calculating metrics from predicted labels

Precision is an essential element in avoiding mistakes of true predictions (i.e. in the patients who are predicted as having the disease).

Sensitivity (true-positive rate) TP/TP+FN is calculated using the true column of the actual or real labels. It indicates how many people who are sick are being identified as such. Thus, it is a measure of the percentage of correctly classified true data.

The model's specificity is calculated using the False column of the actual or real labels. Thus, it tells how many of the actual healthy patients are recorded as being without the disease.

Specificity (true-negative rate) TN/TN+FP

It is important in identifying the patients that do not have the disease.

10.8.3. The probability threshold that gives the best performance

Having defined the metrics that can be used, the probability threshold that gives the best performance is given using the ROC curve. It represents how sensitivity and specificity vary with a change in the probability threshold.

Increasing the sensitivity of a test is generally done to the detriment of Specificity and vice versa. However, it is acknowledged that it is preferable for a screening test for a particular condition to be more sensitive than specific. This means that only a small number of patients go undiagnosed, and it is considered acceptable that a certain number of healthy subjects are declared to have that condition.

In a single, succinct format, a ROC curve encapsulates all of the confusion matrices that would be obtained as the threshold varies from 0 to 1.

10.8.4. A standard ROC curve

A standard ROC curve is shown in Figure 2:

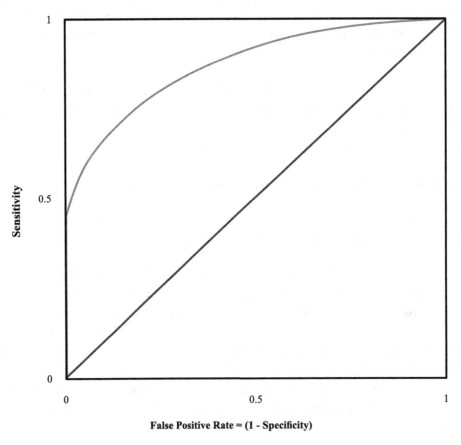

False Positive Rate = (1 - Specificity)

Top curve: a standard ROC curve
Diagonal Line: ROC plot for a random model or classifier

Figure 2. A standard ROC curve with ROC plot for a random model

Sensitivity is recorded on the y axis and measures how accurately people with a disease are identified.

The false positive rate (FPR) or 1- specificity, measures how accurate the real negatives are being recorded. The smaller the FPR, the more accurate the identification of the real negative in the data.

The ROC curve calculates the sensitivity and the false positive rate for several thresholds and plots them against each other.

The representation of the ROC plot for a random model is frequently incorporated in ROC curves to give a rapid comparison of how well the current model is doing. The further the ROC curve of the data under consideration is distanced from the curve of the random model, the better the distance from point A to point B should be, i.e. Ideally, the curve should pass as close as possible to the top-left corner of the diagram.

10.8.5. Explanation of different points of a ROC curve

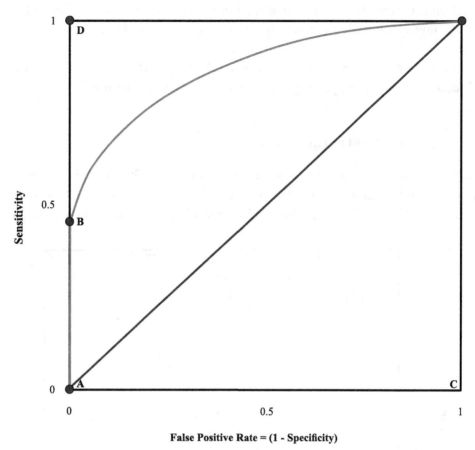

False Positive Rate = (1 - Specificity)

Point A = True positive & nil false negatives; Point B = some true positives & nil false negatives; Point C = only true positives (no false negative) & only false positives (no true negatives); Point D = only true positive and true negatives; Diagonal line = ROC plot for a random model or classifier

Figure 3. The positions of different points of importance, in relation to a ROC plot for a random model or classifier, in interpreting a ROC curve

Point A specifies a probability threshold of 1. At this point, the curve produces no true positives and no false positives. This means that in-dependently of the probability, every sample gets classified as false, which is an acceptable threshold to set as the constructed model only makes false predictions. Note that point A is located on the dotted line, which represents a purely random classifier.

Point B is at a threshold value where some true positive values are acquired, and samples with a high probability of being positive get correctly classified as such. There are no false positives at this point.

Point C is set at the threshold value of 0. Thus, everything is getting labelled as true (cf. point A). If the threshold is set here, the model only creates true predictions.

Point D is the optimal performance point; only true positives and true negatives are recorded; every prediction is correct. Of course, the ideal aim is to get as close as possible to that top left corner, but it is hugely idealistic and unlikely that a ROC curve would reach this point.

Pragmatically, the aim is to identify a point between B and C in the curve that fulfils success on the 0s and success on the 1s and picking the threshold related to that point.

10.8.6. The Area under the ROC curve (AUC)

The area under the ROC curve (AUC is a measurement from values of 0.5 (random model or classifier) to 1 (perfect classifier). It signifies how well the model classifies the true and false data points. The greater the AUC results in the ROC approaching the desired top-left corner.

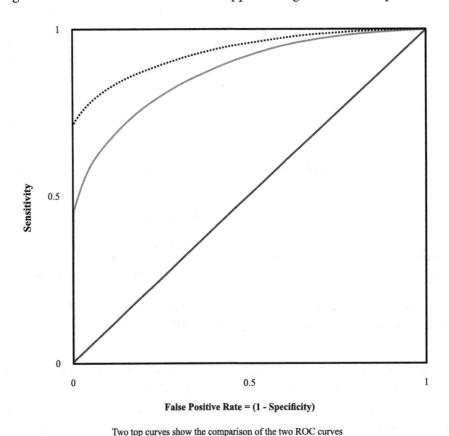

False Positive Rate = (1 - Specificity)

Two top curves show the comparison of the two ROC curves
Diagonal Line: ROC plot for a random model or classifier

**Figure 4. Comparison of two ROC curves in relation to a
ROC plot for a Random Model or Classifier**

Figure 4 shows two different ROC curves in relation to a ROC plot for a random model or classifier. The blue line represents the ROC is better than the model whose ROC is represented by the orange line, as it has more area under it (area between the blue line and the left, bottom and right limits of the graph). Conclusion: the more area under our ROC curve, the better the model is.

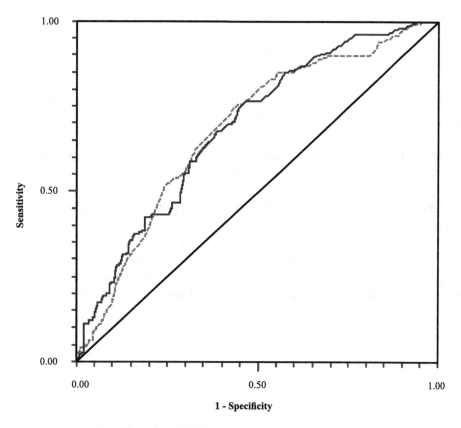

Dotted line = Age; Solid line = ESR; Straight line = Reference line

Figure 5. ROC curves of age and erythrocyte sedimentation rate in cancer against a ROC plot for a random model or classifier

Figure 5 illustrates an example of a ROC curve of age and erythrocyte sedimentation rate in cancer. For age, the area under the curve is 0.684, and for erythrocyte sedimentation rate = 0.690. It can be seen how the curves are closer to the random model reference line (area = 0.5) than to the upper left corner, the point of maximum accuracy of the test. As most diagnostic tests are far from perfect, often, a single test is insufficient. For this reason, clinicians use multiple diagnostic tests administered either in parallel or in series. [5.]

10.9. Summary

The test accuracy compares the disease state estimated by a test of interest, the index test, and the best estimate of the actual disease state provided by the reference standard.

Interpretation of numerical test accuracy metrics requires consideration of the number and consequences of test errors. To decide which dimension of test accuracy is more important in a testing situation, the consequence of being an index test positive or an index test negative needs to be considered.

References

1   Eckert S.E., Goldstein G.R., Koka S. How to evaluate a diagnostic test. *Journal of Prosthetic Dentistry*, 2000; 83: 386-391.

2   Bossuyt P.M, Reitsma J.B, Linnet K., Moons K.G. Beyond diagnostic accuracy: the clinical utility of diagnostic tests. *Clinical Chemistry.* 2012; 58(12):1636–1643

3   Bossuyt P.M.I. L.; Craig J.; Glasziou P. Comparative accuracy: assessing new tests against existing diagnostic pathways. *British Medical Journal.* 2006; 332(7549):1089–1092.

4   Alan D.G,. Bland J.M. Diagnostic tests 1: Sensitivity and Specificity. *British Medical Journal.* 1994; 308 (6943):1552.

5   Baicus C., Ionescu R., Tanasescu C. Does this patient have cancer? The assessment of Age, anaemia, and erythrocyte sedimentation rate in cancer as a cause of weight loss. A retrospective study based on a secondary care university hospital in Romania. *European Journal of Internal Medicine,* 2006; 17:28-31.

Chapter 11. Designing Studies Part 8—Prognosis, Diagnosis, Risk, and Prognostic Study Methods

Santini A.

11.1. Overview

This chapter will address the following:

- Prognosis versus diagnosis;
- Prognostic versus predictive;
- Prognostic versus risk;
- The best design for a prognostic study;
- Expressing results;
- Prognosis;
- Diagnosis;
- Risk; and
- Prognostic study methodology.

11.2. Introduction

Prognostic research involves describing the natural history and clinical course of health conditions by

- Investigating variables associated with health outcomes;
- Estimating an individual's probability of developing different outcomes;
- Investigating the clinical application of prediction models; and
- Investigating determining factors of recovery that can be used in the development of means to progress patient outcomes.

11.3. Terminology

11.3.1. Prognosis versus diagnosis

The terms prognosis and diagnosis are often confused.

Prognosis is a key principle of medical practice. A prognostic factor is a patient characteristic that identifies subgroups of untreated patients having different outcomes.

The term prognostic factors is typically understood to indicate a factor that affects outcome independently of treatment

After the commencement of a disease, the prognosis predicts the course the disease will follow. A diagnosis identifies and names a disease or problem. Knowledge of the prospective course of a disease or illness is fundamental to treating patients with confidence or any measure of success. In addition, specific patient characteristics often give the impression of correctly predicting the outcome of a disease; they need not necessarily cause the outcomes but are so strongly related. These characteristics are called prognostic factors.

In practice, doctors predict an illness's progression in a particular patient, not the course of an illness per se. No two patients with the same diagnosis are identical; each subject's age, sex, disease stage, or genetics, for example, may significantly influence a prognosis and the course the patient's disease will take.

Prognosis in medicine is also used to forecast the future of healthy individuals, such as determining the prognosis of neonates, prenatal tests to evaluate the risk of a pregnant woman giving birth to a Down syndrome baby, and cardiovascular risk profiles to predict heart disease. Types of prognostic factors are listed in Table 1:

Demographics: sex, age.
Behavioural: Obesity, smoking, alcohol consumption.
Disease-specific: Type or location of a tumour, stage of the tumour.
Co-morbidities: Associated conditions with the disease under study.

Table 1 Types of prognostic factors

11.3.2. Prognostic versus predictive

A predictive factor is a patient characteristic that identifies subgroups of treated patients having different outcomes. For example, a prognostic biomarker provides information about the patient's overall cancer outcome, regardless of therapy, whilst a predictive biomarker gives information about the effect of a specific therapeutic intervention. Predictive biomarkers identify patients more prone to encounter an advantageous or disadvantageous effect consequential to medical treatment than similar individuals; they identify subgroups of treated patients having different outcomes. They need not, of necessity, trigger the outcomes of a disease but are so strongly related that they can be used as predictors of the disease's development.

11.3.3. Prognostic and predictive biomarkers

Biomarkers can be are both prognostic and predictive. Prognostic biomarkers are used to categorise patients liable to have a particular outcome. They are commonly identified from observational studies. Recognition of predictive biomarkers requires an appraisal of a treatment modality against a control in patients with and without the biomarker. Prognostic and predictive biomarkers are usually not singularised when data is acquired only from a cohort of patients who have obtained a specific therapy.

11.3.4. Prognostic versus risk

Risk and prognosis describe different outcomes, such as the onset of disease versus a range of disease consequences. Furthermore, risk factors are present before a disease or ailment has arisen (e.g. smoking behaviour, age, gender, or have developed subsequently, e.g. tumour size, alteration in high white cell count). Thus, characteristics related to an increased risk of acquiring a disease are not inevitably identical to those that signpost a worse prognosis or outcome. Prognostic factors can, however, also exist before the commencement of the disease.

11.4. Prognostic Studies

A prognostic study's main objective is to determine the probability of the specified outcome with different combinations of predictors in a well-defined population. Prognostic research describes the natural history and clinical course of health conditions and makes available evidence about disease burden. It is also a method to investigate variables associated with health outcomes of interest. The likelihood of different outcomes occurring can be expressed in a survival curve and may be positive or adverse events.

Prognostic studies of time-to-event data are frequently reported in the literature. These aim to create and authenticate multivariable prognostic models which can be used to forecast survival. Unfortunately, most are retrospective studies in which sample size, before analysis, has not been taken into account.[2] An inappropriate sample size may generate results that may be dubious and questionable.

The standard prognostic study is a cohort study in which a group of people with a particular condition or set of characteristics is followed over time. At the start of a defined period, prognostic studies examine the predictability of a patient's likelihood of developing a disease or experiencing a medical event. The range of factors that may influence outcomes and the expected outcomes such as death or associated complications or changes in circumstances such as pain, or quality of life, as a disease progression are investigated and measured. Such studies lead to identifying prognostic biomarkers, i.e. characteristics that help identify or categorise people likely to have detailed impending outcomes. They include measures such as the body mass index or pathological, biochemical, molecular, or genetic evaluations.

A new prognostic test's accuracy is evaluated by comparing the new or index test with an already established reference test. The reference test for a prognostic test is the observed proportion of the population who develop what is being predicted.

Investigators can use the data acquired in prognostic studies to resolve questions about the associations between risk factors and disease outcomes. For example, smokers and non-smokers can be recognised and enrolled at starting point of the research, and their subsequent incidence of developing heart disease can be weighed up and appraised.

11.5. Study sample and sample size

The sample size is an essential issue for all clinical studies; A barrier to designing good quality prognostic studies, whether prospective or retrospective, is ensuring that enough patients are included in order that the study has the required precision of results. However, little research has been performed specifically regarding the sample size requirements of multivariable prognostic studies.

The study sample includes people at risk of developing the outcome of interest, defined by the presence of a particular condition, such as an illness, undergoing surgery, or being pregnant. Thus, it should represent the population of interest concerning all essential characteristics. To minimise or exclude bias, it must be carefully chosen to represent the population of interest concerning key characteristics and have a sufficiently large number of appropriate patients. There are no clear-cut means of calculating appropriate sample size, though at least several hundred outcome events are preferable. Overestimating the model's predictive performance is in jeopardy when the number of predictors is considerably more significant than the number of outcome measures.

The multivariable character of prognostic research makes it difficult to estimate the required sample size. There are no straightforward methods for this. When the number of predictors is much larger than the number of outcome events, there is a risk of overestimating the model's predictive performance.

The main sample size guidance used by researchers developing prognostic survival models is the events per variable calculation with a lower limit of ten events per variable for each studied candidate predictor.[1, 2] Though a more contemporary report concluded that this number could be lower in certain situations.[3]

11.6. The research question

As with all research studies, prognostic test studies should begin with a written protocol that sets the study in context and rationale. (See chapter 12 on writing a protocol.) The protocol then details how these issues are dealt with during the proposed study. Modifying the original question may occur as the research question is honed; this is a valid outcome.

11.6.1. How to arrive at a research question?

The research question has two purposes:

- To establish where and what kind of research should be undertaken and
- To stipulate the specific objectives of the research study.

To achieve these, a written protocol should be fully developed before commencing the study. It must detail the proposed prognostic test and what is being predicted, how the study is to be organised, what it assesses and evaluates, how specimens, if any, are acquired, dealt with, and stored for testing and how the test results are to be interpreted and used. Also to be included are issues concerning comparator standard prognostic tests or assessments for predicting the same outcome; time-dependent probabilities (time-to-event curves) of what is being predicted; what follow-up time does the prognostic test cover as the number of patients who show evidence of the outcome increases with time, and consequently change prognostic tests' performance characteristics; at what stage in the natural history of outcome development is the prognostic test to be used?; and, importantly, who will use the prognostic test and is it cost-effective?[4]

11.7. Study design

11.7.1. The best design for a prognostic study

The desirable way to study prognosis is in a prospective study, which enables optimal measurement of predictors and outcome. In addition, longer follow-up times can be achieved if the study uses previously created cohorts; the downside is that flawed data may be obtained.

Prognostic retrospective studies are more frequently reported in the published literature. In the main, to randomise patients to different prognostic factors is considered unethical or impracticable; it follows that the standard prognostic study is frequently a cohort study in which one or more groups or cohorts of individuals, who have a disease but have not yet suffered adverse events, are followed up, and the number of outcome events over time is charted.

A case-control study of prognosis may also be undertaken, but the estimated absolute risks are not routinely calculated because cases and controls are often sampled from a source population of unknown size. Moreover, since investigators can choose the ratio of cases and controls, the absolute outcome risks can be manipulated.

A case-control study of prognosis may also be undertaken in which a cohort of patients who have already experienced the outcome event(s) is compared to a control cohort of patients who have not shown signs of the event(s). An estimation of the proportion of individuals in each group with a particular prognostic factor is then calculated.

This type of study design is predisposed to bias, and the absolute risk cannot be assessed. For example, a cohort study is concerned with disease frequency in exposed and non-exposed individuals, whereas a case-control study is about the occurrence and amount of exposure in patients with a specific disease (cases) and patients without the disease (controls).

Data from randomised trials of treatment can also be used to study prognosis. When the treatment is ineffective (relative risk = 1.0), the intervention and comparison group can simply be combined to study baseline prognosis. The groups can be combined if the treatment is effective, but the treatment variable should be included as a separate predictor in the multivariable model. Here treatments are investigated for their independent predictive effect and not their therapeutic or preventive effects. However, prognostic models obtained from randomised trial data may have restricted generalisability because of strict eligibility criteria for the study, low recruitment levels, or large numbers refusing consent.

Table 2 outlines the essentials of cohort studies, and Table 3 outlines the disadvantages of prospective cohort studies in prognostic research:

A cohort study is considered to be the definitive prognostic study. Cohort studies are a type of longitudinal study in which research participants are followed over some time.
Participants who have a common characteristic, e.g. occupation or demographic similarity, and are similar in many ways but differ by a particular characteristic, e.g. middle-aged males who regularly chew betel nut are compared to similar ethnic middle-aged males who do not regularly chew betel. Both cohorts are followed up over time and compared for specific outcome measures such as oral and oesophagus cancer.
The researcher recruits participants when they do not have the outcome of interest. The incidence of the outcome of interest among exposed and unexposed or less exposed participants is then assessed.
No control group is involved in cohort studies. They differ from clinical trials in that no intervention, treaent, or exposure is given to participants.
The intervention in a cohort study is a naturally occurring phenomenon cf. a randomised control trial where the intervention is investigator controlled. Subjects are considered disease-free of the outcome of interest at the beginning of a cohort study.
Cohort studies help investigate rare exposures because their exposure status selects subjects.
Cohort studies concern the life histories of populations' subdivisions and the individuals who represent these subdivisions.

Table 2. The essentials of cohort studies in prognostic research

Large numbers of subjects often require to be studied for a long time.
They are not suitable for diseases with a long latency.
They are inappropriate for the study of rare diseases.
Differential loss to follow-up can introduce bias.
They can be expensive and time-consuming.

Table 3. Disadvantages of prospective cohort studies

Choosing the appropriate study design is crucial in an epidemiological investigation as each type of study design has distinctive strengths and weaknesses.

All sources of bias and confounding must be considered, and steps taken to minimise or eradicate them. In addition, consideration should be given to ethical issues. For example, death or recovery are frequently used estimates in prognosis studies; however, all aspects of a disease, such as pain, incapacity, or debility should also be recorded in detail.

11.8. Study period

The study should begin at a defined point of time in the disease course. All patients must be followed up for long enough so that essential outcomes have occurred.

11.8.1. Bias

To ensure that the sample is unbiased, the study population should include all those with a disease in a defined population (e.g. all patients on a disease register). All participating patients should be followed up from the same defined point in the disease course to guarantee a good prognosis assessment.

Table 4 lists the key factors to be considered in order to minimise bias in prognostic studies:

Minimising bias in prognostic studies
Is the sample size adequate to minimise or exclude bias to the results?
Were the prognostic factors of interest adequately measured in the study participants sufficient to limit potential bias?
Was the outcome of interest adequately measured in participants enough to limit potential bias?
Were potential confounders suitably accounted for to prevent bias concerning the prognostic factor of interest?

Table 4. Key factors to be considered in order to minimise bias in prognostic studies.

11.8.2. Appraising a prognostic study

Table 5 lists the factors to be considered when appraising a prognostic study:

Was there a representative and a well-defined patient sample at a similar point in the disease course?
Was follow-up sufficiently long and complete?
Were objective and unbiased outcome criteria used?
How significant is the likelihood of the outcome events occurring in a specified time?

Were the study patients similar to my own?
Are the results helpful in reassuring or counselling patients?

Table 5. Appraising a prognostic study.

11.8.3. Advantages and disadvantages of prognostic studies

The advantages and disadvantages of prognostic studies are listed in Table 6:

The results can facilitate clinical decision-making, for example, by providing the information necessary to select appropriate treatment.
A more accurate prediction of disease outcomes facilitates patient education and counselling.
Prognostic studies may also allow subgroups of patients to be defined at risk of specific disease outcomes, leading to improved study designs and clinical trials analysis through risk stratification.
Disadvantages of prognostic studies
The results may not be generalisable to local settings, limiting the validity of the study.

Table 6. Advantages and disadvantages of prognostic studies[5, 6, 7]

A checklist for prognostic studies can be found in Table 7:

Does the study sample represent the population of interest concerning critical characteristics?
Is the sample size adequate to minimise or exclude bias to the results?
Were patients enrolled at the same stage in the progression of the disease?
Was the loss to follow-up unrelated to critical characteristics?
Were the prognostic factors of interest adequately measured in the study participants sufficient to limit potential bias?
Was there an adjustment for important prognostic factors?
Was follow-up complete and over an adequate period?
Was the outcome of interest adequately measured in participants enough to limit potential bias?
Were potential confounders suitably accounted for to prevent bias concerning the prognostic factor of interest?
Was the objective outcome criteria assessment blind?
Was the statistical analysis appropriate for the study design?
Generalisability: Are your patients similar to the patients in the study?

Table 7. Checklist for prognostic studies

11.8.4. Judging the quality of individual studies of prognostic tests

Table 8 sets out questions to ask when judging the quality of individual studies of prognostic tests:

1. Was the study designed to evaluate the new prognostic test, or was it a secondary analysis of data collected for other purposes?
2. Were the subjects somehow referred or selected for testing? What was the testing scenario?
3. Was the clinical population clearly described, including the sampling plan, inclusion and exclusion criteria, subject participation, and the spectrum of test results? For example, did the sample represent patients that would be tested in clinical practice?
4. Did everyone in the samples have a common starting point for follow-up concerning the outcome of interest, including any treatments that could affect the predicted outcome?

5. Were the prognostic tests clearly described and conducted using a standardised, reliable, and valid method?
   a. Was the test used and interpreted the same way by all sites/studies, including any indeterminate test results?
   b. Were the test results ascertained without knowledge of the outcome?
   c. Were investigators blinded to the test results?
   d. How were previously established prognostic indicators or other prognostic assessments included in the study and analyses?

6. Was the outcome being predicted clearly defined and ascertained using a standardised, reliable, and valid method?
   a. How complete was the follow-up of subjects, and were losses to follow-up related to the test results or the predicted outcome?
   b. Was the duration of follow-up adequate?

7. Were the prognostic groups predefined based on clinically meaningful decision thresholds for predicted outcome probabilities?
8. Were the results externally validated using an independent sample or internally validated via bootstrap or cross-validation methods?
9. Were any previously established prognostic indicators or prediction models used as comparators to the sample data in the same manner as the potential new prognostic test?
10. Were outcome predictions adjusted for any other factors? Which ones? How?

Table 8. Questions for judging the quality of individual studies of prognostic tests

11.9. Predictors

Prognostic studies may study the natural course or baseline prognosis of patients with a condition or disease using cohorts of patients before the receive any treatment. Alternatively, predictors of prognosis for patients who have received treatments can be investigated. Predictors can be acquired from patients' demographics, clinical histories, medical examinations and tests, disease traits, and prior treatment.

Predictors should be unambiguously and distinctively defined, consistent, and reproducible to enable generalisability from studies to clinical practice. To this end, predictors should be determined and appraised in ways that can be used and are related to practice.

The predictive effect of treatments is small compared with other critical prognostic variables such as age, sex, and disease stage. As indications for treatment and administration are often not standardised in observational studies, this could result in bias.

Predictors should correspond with their intended purpose and intention (for example, a predictor of use in clarifying a patient's prognosis at the time of diagnosis is of little merit as an indicator of disease progression after the start of treatment.[8]

11.10. Outcome

Prognostic studies should concentrate on outcome measures that are pertinent and applicable to patients' needs. Surrogate or intermediate measures, such as hospital stay or physiological measurements, are less helpful if they lack a solid causal relation to a patient's pertinent outcomes. In addition, the study period and the methods of measurement of outcome measures should be clearly defined.

11.11. Interpreting results

11.11.1. Multivariable methodology

Many prognostic studies take account of a single predictor. However, an estimated prognosis is seldom adequately achieved by a single predictor or variable due to dynamics such as the differences in patients' health state and diseases treatment modalities. A multivariable methodology should be considered both at the prognostic study design stage and later when data are analysed. They are generally referred to as prognostic models, prediction models, prediction rules, or risk scores. They allow a permutation of predictor values to estimate an absolute risk or probability of an individual's outcome. An added advantage is that a comparison can be made between specific predictors or characteristics that may be more costly to measure than inexpensive or easily measured predictors.[9, 10, 11, 12, 13]

The foremost use of prognostic models in informing patients about the risk of developing a disease or giving information regarding their illness's future progression. Prediction models are intended to help doctors make decisions by providing more objective estimates of probability and other relevant clinical information by improving the understanding of the factors of the progression and consequence of patients with a specific disease.

Additionally, they aid in the doctor-patient relationship concerning choices of the type and extent, if any, of additional treatment. Prognostic models are also used to compare performance differences between hospitals and select appropriate patients for therapeutic research.[14, 15]

11.11.2. Survival analysis

Survival analysis studies the time between entry into a study and a suitable occurrence of an event. Initially, such analyses were performed to information on time to death in fatal conditions, but they can be applied to many other outcomes and mortality.

Survival analysis is usually applied to data from longitudinal cohort studies. There are, however, problems when analysing data relating to the time between one event and another:

All times to the event occurring will differ, but it is unlikely that these times will be normally distributed. The subjects might not all have entered the study simultaneously, so there are unequal observation periods.

Some patients might not reach the endpoint by the end of the study. For example, if the event is recovery within twelve months, some patients might not have recovered in the twelve-month study period. Patients can leave a study early, not experience the event, or be lost to follow-up. The data for these individuals are referred to as censored.

Both censored observations and unequal observation periods make determining the mean survival times difficult because we do not have all the survival times. As a result, the curve is used to calculate the median survival time.

11.11.3. Median survival time

Median survival time is the time from the start of the study that coincides with a 50 per cent probability of survival—that is, the time taken for 50 per cent of the subjects not to have had the event. This value is associated with a p-value and 95 per cent confidence intervals.

11.11.4. Kaplan-Meier survival analysis

The Kaplan-Meier estimator plot is a series of declining horizontal steps that approach the actual survival function for that population with a large enough sample size. On the plot, small vertical tick-marks state individual patients whose survival times have been right-censored.

The Kaplan-Meier estimate is one of the best options to measure the fraction of subjects living for a certain amount of time after treatment. In clinical or community trials, an intervention's effect is assessed by measuring the number of subjects who survived over time after that intervention. The time starting from a defined point to the occurrence of a given event (such as death) is called a survival time and group data analysis as survival analysis. This can be affected by subjects under study that are uncooperative and refuse to remain in the study, or when some of the subjects may not experience the event of death before the end of the study, although they would have experienced or died if observation continued, or the investigators lose touch with them midway in the study.

These situations are described as censored observations. The Kaplan-Meier estimate is the simplest way of computing survival over time despite all these difficulties associated with subjects or situations. The survival curve can be created assuming various situations. It involves computing probabilities of event occurrence at a certain point of time and multiplying these successive probabilities by any earlier computed probabilities to get the final estimate. This can be calculated for two groups of subjects and also their statistical difference in the survivals. This can be used in Ayurveda research when comparing two drugs and looking for the survival of subjects.

The Kaplan-Meier survival analysis looks at event rates over the study period rather than at a specific time point. It is used to determine survival probabilities and proportions of individuals surviving, enabling a cumulative survival probability estimation. The data are presented in life tables and survival curves.

The data are first ranked in ascending order over time in life tables. Next, the survival curve is plotted by calculating the proportion of patients who remain alive in the study each time an event occurs, taking into account censored observations. The survival curve will not change at the time of censoring but only when the next event occurs.

Censored patients are assumed to have the same survival prospects as those who continue in the study.

Time is plotted on the *x*-axis, and the proportion of people without the outcome (survivors) of each time point are plotted on the *y* axis. Thus, a cumulative curve is achieved, with steps at each time an event occurs. Small vertical ticks on the curve indicate the times at which patients are censored.

A survival curve can be used to calculate several parameters:

- The median survival time, which is the time taken until 50 per cent of the population survives;
- The survival time, which is the time taken for a certain proportion of the population to survive; and
- The survival probability is the probability, at a given time point, that an individual will not have developed at the endpoint event.

A survival curve can also be used to compare the difference in the proportions surviving in two groups and their confidence intervals, such as when comparing a control population with an experimental population.

Features of the Kaplan-Meier estimator are summarised in Table 9:Further information on this topic can be found in chapter 17.

1. The Kaplan-Meier curve is an estimator used to estimate the survival function. It is the visual representation of this function that shows an event's probability at a respective time interval.
2. In overall survival curves, the event of interest is death from any cause. This provides a broad, general sense of the mortality of the groups. In disease-free survival curves, the event of interest is the relapse of a disease rather than death.
3. A patient is scored as censored if he or she did not suffer the outcome of interest. In survival analysis, patients who do not have an "event" during a specified period are said to have censored observation.
4. Censoring is present when information on time to outcome event is not available for all study participants. For example, a participant is censored when information on time to event is unavailable due to loss to follow-up or non-occurrence of the outcome event before the trial ends.
5. In cancer studies, most survival analyses use the following methods: • Kaplan-Meier plots to visualise survival curves; • Log-rank test to compare the survival curves of two or more groups; and • Cox proportional hazards regression to describe the effect of variables on survival.
6. Several methods have been described to deal with the problem of informative censoring. These include imputation techniques for missing data, sensitivity analyses to mimic best- and worst-case scenarios, and use of the dropout event as a study endpoint.

Table 9. Kaplan-Meier summary

11.11.5. Log-rank test

The log-rank test is a hypothesis test to compare two samples' survival distributions. It is a nonparametric test and appropriate to use when the data are right-skewed and censored.

11.11.5.1. Comparison of log-rank test with Kaplan-Meier and other tests

The Kaplan-Meier test provides a method for estimating the survival curve; the log-rank test provides a statistical comparison of two groups; the Cox's proportional hazards model allows additional covariates to be included.

The log-rank test tests the null hypothesis of no difference in survival between two or more independent groups. The test compares the entire survival experience between groups and can be thought of as a test of whether the survival curves are identical (overlapping) or not. It is used to test the null hypothesis that there is no difference between the populations in the probability of an event at any time point. The analysis is based on the times of events.

The log-rank test is a better method as it takes the entire follow-up period into account. In addition, it is a significance test and helps decide whether or not to accept the null hypothesis that there is no difference in the probability of survival in the different groups. However, it does not indicate the size of the difference between the groups, unlike the hazard ratio.

The log-rank test is so-called because the data are first ranked and then compared with observations and expected outcome rates in each group, similar to a chi-squared test. The log-rank test does not consider other variables.

11.12. Cox proportional hazards regression

The hazard rate is the probability of an endpoint event in a time interval divided by the time interval duration. The hazard rate can be interpreted as the instantaneous probability of an endpoint event in a study if the time interval is short. The hazard rate might not be constant during the study.

A *p*-value and confidence intervals complement the hazard ratio. It is assumed that the hazard ratio remains constant throughout the study. If the hazard ratio is one, the two arms have an equal hazard rate.

If the hazard ratio is > 1, the experimental arm has an increased hazard.

If the hazard ratio is < 1, the experimental arm has a reduced hazard.

Although the hazard ratio interpretation is similar to relative risk and the odds ratio, the terms are not synonymous. The hazard ratio compares the experimental and control groups throughout the study duration, unlike the relative risk and odds ratio, which only compare the proportion of subjects that achieved each group's outcome at the end of the study.

It is not possible to calculate the hazard ratio from a 2x2 contingency table.

Cox proportional hazards regression is used to produce the hazard ratio.

It is the multivariate extension of the log-rank test.

It is used to assess the effect of treatment on survival or other time-related events and adjusts other variables' effects.

Additional reading

Riley RD, Hayden JA, Steyerberg EW, Moons KGM, Abrams K, Kyzas PA, et al. (2013) Prognosis Research Strategy (PROGRESS) 2: Prognostic Factor Research. PLoS Med 10(2): e1001380. https://doi.org/10.1371/journal.pmed.1001380

Transparent Reporting of a multivariable prediction model for Individual Prognosis or Diagnosis (TRIPOD) Statement. https://www.tripod-statement.org/resources/

References

1   Laupacis A., Sekar N., Stiell I.G. Clinical prediction rules. A review and suggested modifications of methodological standards. *Journal of American Medical Association* 1997;277:488-494.

2   Concato J., Peduzzi P., Holford T.R, Feinstein A. R. Importance of events per independent variable in proportional hazards analysis. I. Background, goals, and general strategy. *Journal of Clinical Epidemiology* 1995;48:1495–1501.

3   Vittinghoff E., McCulloch C..E. Relaxing the rule of ten events per variable in logistic and Cox regression. *American Journal of Epidemiology* 2007;165:710–718.

4   Riva JJ, BA, Malik KMP, BSc, Burnie JS, BSc, Endicott AR, Busse JW. What is your research question? An introduction to the PICOT format for clinicians. *The Journal of the Canadian Chiropractic Association* 2012; 56(3): 167–171.

5   Laupacis A, Wells G, Richardson S, et al. Users guides to the medical literature. V. How to use an article about prognosis. *Journal of the American Medical Association* 1994; 272:234–237

6   Fletcher R, Fletcher S. Clinical epidemiology: the essentials (5ᵗʰ ed.), Lippincott Williams & Wilkins, 2013.

7   Mak K, Kum CK. How to Appraise a Prognostic Study. *World* Journal of *Surgery* 2005; 29: 567–569.

8   Walraven vC, Davis D, Forster AJ, Wells GA. Time-dependent bias was common in survival analyses published in leading clinical journals. *Journal* of *Clinical Epidemiology* 2004;57:672-682.

9   Murray DW, Carr AJ, C Bulstrode C. Survival analysis of Joint Replacements. *The Journal of Bone & Joint Surgery(UK)* 1993;75-B: 697-704.

10 Riley RD, Abrams KR, Sutton AJ, Lambert PC, Jones DR, Heney D, et al. Reporting of prognostic markers: current problems and development of guidelines for evidence-based practice in the future. *British Journal of Cancer* 2003;88:1191-1198.

11 Concato J. Challenges in prognostic analysis. *Cancer* 2001;91:1607-1614.

12 Reilly BM, Evans AT. Translating clinical research into clinical practice: impact of using prediction rules to make decisions. *Annals of Internal Medicine* 2006;144:201-209.

13 Moons KG, Alan DG, Vergouwe Y, Royston P. Prognosis and prognostic research: Application and impact of prognostic models in clinical practice. *British Journal of Medicine* 2009:338:b606.

14 Knaus WA, Wagner DP, Draper EA, Zimmerman JE, Bergner M, Bastos PG, et al. The APACHE III prognostic system. Risk prediction of hospital mortality for critically ill hospitalised adults. *Chest*1991;100:1619-1636.

15 Le Gall JR, Lemeshow S, Saulnier F. A new simplified acute physiology score (SAPS II) based on a European/North American multicenter study. *Journal of the American Medical Association* 1993;270:2957-2963.

Chapter 12. Writing a Protocol

Eaton K.A.

12.1. Overview

This chapter will address the fifth of the ten stages in a research project suggested in the introduction to this book.

Chapters 4 to 11 have described how to design (plan) a research study. The next stage is to justify the necessity and feasibility of the proposed study and write a detailed plan in a research protocol. This chapter outlines the structure and topics that should be covered when writing a research protocol and is divided into the following sections:

What is a protocol, and why is a written protocol necessary?

The topics which should be covered in a protocol and its layout

Suggested further reading

12.2. What is a protocol, and why is a written protocol necessary?

A research protocol is a detailed plan of a proposed project that provides written evidence of the need for the proposed study and its feasibility. It is a key stage and should demonstrate that the proposers have, as far as possible, considered all relevant points before starting the project.

Research ethics committees, research and development committees and funding bodies will only consider an application if accompanied by a protocol. It allows any individual or organisation the opportunity to make a judgment about the scientific, financial, and ethical aspects of a proposed study. It also supplements any application forms that have been submitted and can be used as a resource to provide answers to questions arising from the application form(s). The protocol also provides its authors with a reference point during a study. It can, and should, constantly be referred to, to check that all project stages are being performed consistently in a scientific manner, within budget, and on schedule.

Some organisations, such as universities, the National Institute for Health Research, the European Commission, and the Medical Research Council issue-specific guidelines on the contents of a protocol. Before writing, it is wise to check if the organisation that the protocol is to be submitted to has such guidelines, and if it does, follow them.

150

Time spent designing and writing a protocol is time well spent and will benefit the subsequent stages of the project. Help and advice should be sought before writing it. A wide range of opinions should be canvassed, from statisticians, ethics committee chairpersons, and clinical colleagues.

A protocol should include justification of the need for the project and a detailed plan that sets out for the investigation. It should specify

- what is to be investigated;
- where and when the research will take place;
- procedures and methods to be used;
- a proposed timetable; and
- resources required (technical, scientific, ethical, and financial).

12.2.1. The topics which should be covered in a protocol and its layout

The following topics that should be covered (this list is based on one originally produced by the Leeds Teaching Hospitals NHS Trust Research and Development Department)[1].

1. Title;
2. Administrative details and a summary;
3. Introduction;
4. Aim;
5. Statement of the problem;
6. Methods;
7. Data security;
8. Analysis of data;
9. Proposed schedule;
10. Facilities required;
11. Budget;
12. Further considerations; and
13. References.

Remember that no two protocols are precisely the same, and their layout should be planned accordingly. In addition, there are variations to the format suggested in this chapter, such as those recommended by the NHS Health Research Authority and the National Institute for Health Research. As previously mentioned, readers are advised to visit the websites of these organisations if they wish to obtain funding from them and write the relevant protocols following these organisations' guidelines. The URLs for the two websites are listed at the end of this chapter.

12.2.2. Title

The title should explain the project. It will usually be longer than the title used if any papers arising from the research are published. In addition, the names of the principal investigators and others involved in the study should be included, together with their affiliations, contact details, and roles in the study. Failure to include these details at this stage has occasionally led to disputes in the past.

Example

A study of complete denture hygiene procedures employed by non-institutionalised, old age pensioner patients of six general dental practices in the North of Scotland.

In addition to the title, the front page should record a protocol number, version (draft) number, and the date when the protocol was written or last revised (the version number and date must be updated as and when amendments are made), as it is not uncommon for several drafts of a protocol to be written.

12.2.3. Administrative details and a summary

The following administrative details and a summary should follow the title page:

- A contents page, which details relevant sections and sub-sections and lists page numbers;
- A page(s) with a list of names and affiliations of the researchers with spaces for them to sign and date their signatures. The postal and e-mail addresses and telephone numbers for members of the research team should also be included, together with their roles in the project, such as chief investigator (CI), principal investigator (PI), and statistical advisor. Further details which describe the functions of PIs, CIs and all those involved in a research project can be found in the NHS Health Research Authority's UK policy framework for health and social care research (2020); and
- A summary of the main study issues should include the title, aims, design, experimental or other scheduled treatment, the sample, and the endpoint. In addition, a flowchart of the schedule can be added.

12.2.3. Introduction

This should explain why the study is necessary, refer briefly to previous work relating to the problem and put the proposed research in the context of what has gone before. It should also provide evidence that a literature search has been performed and refer to significant and relevant studies. Finally, its concluding sentence should link to the next section of the protocol the aim.

Thus, the literature indicates that previous studies in Scotland have only investigated the complete denture cleaning habits of the institutionalised elderly, not those living at home.

12.2.4. Aim

The study's aim(s) and objectives should be set out clearly. Essentially, the aim is the overall goal to be achieved, and objectives are steps to achieve the aim. The aim should be specific to the population to be studied and not give the impression that its results can be generalised to a broader population.

For example: Aim: To investigate the complete denture hygiene procedures employed by non-institutionalised old aged pensioners who attend a sample of general dental practices in the North of Scotland.

Objectives: To assess the use of chemical denture cleaners in the study group. To assess whether there are variations related to gender and age.

12.2.5. Statement of the problem

This statement should provide a summary of precisely what the project is trying to achieve. It should give a more detailed background to the problem than the brief scenario sketched out in the introduction and end with a question.

For example, Fife et al. (2017) found that institutionalised elderly patients frequently could not clean their complete dentures adequately. The proposed study will address whether or not this finding is also true for the non-institutionalised elderly.

12.2.6. Methods

Having established what the project aims to achieve, the remaining sections should explain how it is proposed to carry out the necessary work. The methods section should

- detail exactly which procedures are to be used;
- show that the proposals are possible and practical;
- identify potential problems and suggest solutions to them;
- detail the proposed methods for data gathering and data processing; and
- address the issues of patient consent, data security and ethics approval.

Each study will have its particular characteristics. However, virtually all will have a 'study population', and details of this population and how it is to be scientifically sampled must be explained. Laboratory methods should be described if they are used, as should proposals for the use of questionnaires. Before writing a protocol, it is wise to discuss recommendations for population sampling, data collection, and analysis with a statistician so that they can be justified in the protocol.

In particular, the following points should be considered:

- The population to be sampled with details of inclusion and exclusion criteria;
- How confidentiality and anonymity for individual subjects will be maintained;
- An explanation of how the sample size will be calculated, the power of the sample and how subjects will be recruited. The topic of power calculation is covered in the chapter on questionnaires;
- Randomisation should include the technique used to randomly select subjects and, when appropriate, allocate them to study groups. It should also describe any other factors that were considered and used and any other factors considered during the process. If the study is double-blind, the procedure to ensure that this happens and reasons for breaking the blinding (e.g. not withholding a new lifesaving procedure or drug) should be given;
- Informed written consent should detail the process used to obtain it, together with information on how informed written consent will be accepted from minors or adults who cannot provide it. Patients or other participants in a study should be given a verbal explanation of the nature of the study, including any potential risks, and they should also be given an information leaflet or letter. Suppose they are asked to complete a questionnaire, either in hard copy or online. In that case, there must be a box at the beginning of the questionnaire for them to tick to indicate that they agree to participate, understanding that the information they provide will be treated as confidential and that they will not be identified in any publication or other communication which may arise from the study. Patient/participant information leaflets, consent forms and questionnaires must be attached to the protocol as appendices.
- Study procedure, a section that describes how the study will be conducted. If patients are required to make visits during the study, it should detail what will happen at each visit, including all examinations and tests;
- Study drug supply gives details of how drugs will be supplied, packaged, stored securely and labelled;
- Concurrent medication/treatment specifies any medication(s) that should not be taken during the study;
- Questionnaires should be piloted before their distribution unless they have been successfully used in previous studies. Details of the piloting should be included in the protocol, and a copy of the questionnaire should accompany the protocol as an annex or appendix. See Chapter 9 for further details of questionnaires.

12.2.7. Example of the first part of the methods section of a protocol

A preliminary check of patient records and dental laboratory bills has indicated that during the last year, a total of one hundred edentulous patients aged older than 65 years were seen in the six practices which have agreed to take part in this study. A power calculation has indicated that for a 95 per cent confidence level and a 0.05 confidence interval, at least 235 individuals who meet the inclusion criteria for the study must be recruited. After the start date for the study, all patients who meet the inclusion criteria will be invited to wish to take part. The study will run until at least 235 have been recruited and have completed the questionnaire. The nature of the study will be verbally explained to potential participants, who will be given a patient information sheet). If they agree to take part, participants will be given a written informed consent form to sign

The patients will be asked about their denture cleaning habits using a questionnaire This questionnaire has been piloted on a sample of twenty volunteers. The patients' names will not appear on the questionnaires. Instead, each questionnaire will be given a unique study number and, when completed, stored in a locked filing cabinet.

NHS ethics approval for the study will be sought via the Integrated Research Application System (IRAS). IRAS is described in more detail in Chapter 13, about ethics. It is a single system for applying for the permissions and approvals for health and social care community care research in the United Kingdom.

The methods section should then describe how the resulting data that will be analysed, the timetable, facilities required, budget and dissemination of results, as will now be detailed.

12.2.8. Security of data

Details of methods used to keep data security must be included. They may consist of encrypted USBs, locked filing cabinets with keys held only by specified individuals, and password-protected computers. There should also be an explanation of how the study will meet the General Data Protection Regulations (2018).

12.2.9. Analysis of data

The description of the proposed analysis of data must be written in the context of advice sought from a statistician before writing a protocol. In addition, it should detail the methods to be employed in analysing, interpreting and presenting the data. Chapter 16- Analysing Data explains this aspect in further detail.

12.2.10. Proposed schedule

This should set out a timetable for the project and include details of the proposed start and finish dates and the expected hours involved.

12.2.11. Facilities required

Apart from those available in workplaces, other facilities may well be required. All should be listed, including the need for additional workspace, equipment, technical help, advisers, computing facilities, and transport.

12.2.12. Budget

It is essential to be aware of the costs before commencing any project, whether self-funded or partly or wholly funded by a private organisation or public body. The budget should be realistic and include the costs of

- salaries and wages;
- purchase or hire of equipment;
- consumables and transport;
- time taken by all investigators (including administrative and practice staff);
- telephone calls and photocopying; and
- dissemination of the results.

If external funding is sought, the budget will have to be justified. If no external funding is sought or is not forthcoming, those taking part in a study should be aware of its costs. For example, if a university department is leading the project, it will almost certainly charge a university overhead to cover the cost of the use of its premises and equipment. Typically, this may be between 30 and 100 per cent of the total budget. See Chapter 14 – Obtaining Funding for further details of how to structure budgets for research studies.

12.3. Further considerations

Research governance requires that all research be entirely justifiable and that all those involved, including the researchers, are safeguarded.

Approval from an ethics committee will be required if humans or animals are involved in any way. In addition, during the study, if it becomes apparent that it is necessary to amend the protocol in any way, permission to do so must be sought from the ethics committee which approved the study.

All research-active NHS care organisations are required to have local implementation plans. This ensures that any research funded by or involving the NHS, its patients and its employees (including contractors, such as general dental practitioners) is conducted within the UK Policy Framework for Health and Social Care (2017[2]).

It is recommended that an informal approach should be made to the chairperson or secretary of the relevant research ethics committee at an early stage. Furthermore, as mentioned earlier, the ethics committee will request a copy of the protocol and require a detailed submission, which may have to be presented in a prescribed format. This may or may not influence the style in which a protocol is written.

General managers of NHS trusts, primary care trusts, and health boards should be able to give details of the names and telephone numbers of ethics committees chairpersons on request.

The plans for the dissemination of results once the study has been completed should be outlined. Typically, this will involve presentations at research meetings and publications in scientific journals (see chapter 18 – Writing up and Disseminating the Results).

Check that, where appropriate, the protocol addresses the following issues:

- Assessment of efficiency;
- Assessment of safety;
- Subject withdrawal;
- Deviations from the protocol;
- Data recording;
- Statistical considerations;
- Data and document confidentiality;
- Quality control/assurance; and
- Ethical considerations.

Finally, give the draft protocol to someone who has had had no involvement in or knowledge of its development and ask them if they feel that they could undertake the study using it as their blueprint.

Suggested Further Reading

O'Brien K, Wright J. How to write a protocol. *Journal of Orthodontics* 2002; 29: 58–61.

NHS Health Research Authority (2018) Protocol Section in HRA Planning and Improving Research. www.hra.nhs.uk/planning-and-improving-research/

National Institute for Health Research (2020) Advice on Protocols in Clinical Trials Toolkit www.ct-toolkit.av.uk/routemap/protocol-development, accessed on 23 January 2021

Acknowledgement

The author wishes to thank the Director of Leeds Teaching Hospitals NHS Trust Research and Development Department for permitting the reproduction of sections of Writing a Research Protocol Guidance Notes for Researchers in section 2 of this paper.

Ario Santini, Kenneth A Eaton

References

1　The Leeds Teaching Hospitals NHS Trust Research and Development Department.

　Writing a Research Protocol Guidance Notes for Researchers. 200? Accessed from www.leedsteachinghospitals.co/sites/research_and_development/successful.php#Protocol Accessed on 12 December 2010.

2　NHS Health Research Authority. UK policy framework for health and social care research 2020. Accessed from www.hra.nhs.uk/planning-and-improving-research/ on 21 December 2020.

Chapter 13. Research Ethics and Obtaining Ethics Approval

Eaton K.A, Palmer N.R.

13.1. Overview

The previous chapter outlined how to write a protocol. The next stage, stage 6, has two elements: obtaining ethics approval and obtaining funding. Each is the topic for a separate chapter. As described earlier, evidence-based practice is the gold standard of healthcare and has been described as a scientific milestone of the last century.[1] Developed initially as evidence-based medicine in 1991, the concept has been adopted by other disciplines and professions to encompass most health fields.[2] However, the highest standard of evidence must be used to inform health decision making, so the primary research on which this evidence is based must be ethical and scientifically sound.

This chapter will set out the primary ethical considerations for researchers to design and conduct ethical research, including procedures for governance and review. However, although legal and regulatory issues will be discussed, this chapter does not constitute legal advice, and researchers should always seek appropriate guidance on legal issues where necessary.

This chapter is divided into the following sections:

- Definition of ethics in biomedical research;
- The development of codes of practice;
- Applying ethical practice to clinical research;
- Publication ethics;
- Governance arrangements for health-related research in the United Kingdom, general guidance;
- Additional considerations; and
- Summary

13.1.1. A note on terminology

The authors of this chapter have chosen the word *participant* to describe individuals taking part in a research project, prefixed by *potential* when referring to those who have been invited to participate but have not yet provided their consent. In health-related studies and clinical trials, these may be patients, or they may be healthy volunteers. The word *subjects* can also be used to describe those taking part in research, but participant is often preferred as it is less impersonal.

13.2. Definition of ethics in biomedical research

Ethics are rules of conduct. All those involved in research are ethically bound to respect human life and people's autonomy.

Good research practice demands that researchers

- respect the rights of participants in their studies;
- listen to and share information with them; and
- treat them courteously and caringly.

The rules that apply to research are similar to those that apply to day-to-day clinical practice. They are a set of principles or a code of behaviour to protect patients from unreasonable actions by clinicians.[3, 4] Over the years, biomedical researchers have agreed nationally and internationally to accepted standards. In 1964, the World Medical Association Declaration of Helsinki[5] underscored twelve fundamental principles for human biomedical research, revised on nine occasions.

The issue of research in developing countries was taken up by the Council for the International Organization of Medical Sciences (CIOMS), which, in collaboration with the World Health Organization, proposed guidelines for international research. The guidelines were further amended in 1993 as the International Ethical Guidelines for Biomedical Research Involving Human Participants.[6] In addition, a common framework for observational studies in medical research was proposed in 2009.[8]

The Medical Research Council and the Royal College of Physicians have also published guidance in the United Kingdom, as has the Health Research Authority.

Ethical principles must also be applied to safeguard researchers and the environment from harm and ensure that any research project does not waste resources, financial or other. In addition, universities and other organisations involved in research ensure that the research they support is conducted and reported ethically to avoid the potential for reputational damage.

Research with human subjects has been described as exemplifying "the perennial conflict between the good of the individual and the good of society"[7] and research ethics has evolved to provide a framework for attempting to resolve this dilemma, and in so doing, to maintain public trust in research.

13.3. The development of codes of practice

Discussion of research ethics came to the fore in the middle of the twentieth century, mainly in response to specific historical events involving serious abuse and exploitation of human subjects.[8] This section will demonstrate how the codes have evolved and will highlight incidents of research misconduct and its implications.

13.3.1. Nuremberg Code

The revelations of unethical human experimentation carried out under the Nazi regime that emerged from the Nuremberg Trials at the end of World War II led to the Nuremberg Code in 1949.[9] Accepted as the first internationally recognised ethical standard for research with human subjects,[10] the Code lists voluntary consent as essential. Other principles included in the Code stipulate that the research must be well designed and should benefit society. In addition, risks to subjects should be minimised, and researchers should be suitably trained for the research activities they undertake.

13.3.2. Declaration of Helsinki

Some weaknesses in the Nuremberg Code were identified in its application, and these were addressed in the Declaration of Helsinki, which the World Medical Association adopted in 1964. The Declaration has been revised nine times, most recently in 2013.[5] The focus on voluntary consent in the Nuremberg Code implied that research involving subjects lacking the capacity to consent would be unethical. In recognition of the injustice of excluding subjects from research from which they, or others like them, could benefit, the Declaration of Helsinki introduced guidelines for ethically obtaining consent for incompetent subjects such as children, or those with cognitive impairments. The Declaration also introduced the use of control groups in clinical research.

From its first edition, the Declaration has prioritised the best interests of the subjects involved in research, and this focus continues in the current version, which states: "While the primary purpose of medical research is to generate new knowledge, this goal can never take precedence over the rights and interests of individual research subjects."[5]

13.4. Continuing bad research practice

During the 1960s, research institutions in the United Kingdom and the United States began to develop procedures for reviewing research proposals in line with the principles set out in these published codes of practice.[11] However, despite establishing these oversight mechanisms, cases of unethical research practices continued to come to light through the actions of whistleblowers. For example, during the 1960s, clinicians Maurice Pappworth in the United Kingdom and Henry Beecher in the United States published details of many cases of unethical medical experimentation. Pappworth published his concerns in the British press about research that he claimed had risked patients' lives and had been carried out purely to advance the careers of those involved.[12] Beecher identified ethical failures in research that had been supported by leading institutions and published in prominent journals, indicating that unethical research was not confined to Nazi experimenters.[13]

Both Pappworth and Beecher suffered criticism by the medical establishment, although their actions, and broader evidence of the prevalence of unethical research, prompted a reassessment of research oversight.

The origins of the United Kingdom's national network of National Health Service (NHS) research ethics committees (RECs) arose from a report published by the Royal College of Physicians in 1967.[11] In the United States, legislation governing research involving human subjects was passed in 1974, which led to the creation of the National Commission for the Protection of Human Subjects of Biomedical and Behavioural Research.[14] In 1979, the National Commission published the Belmont Report,[15] which set out an ethical framework for research involving human subjects.[7]

13.4.1. The Belmont Report

The Belmont Report was mainly developed as a response to the publication of details of research scandals that had occurred since the establishment of the Nuremberg Code and the Declaration of Helsinki, including historical cases that had come to light for the first time and that threatened to undermine public trust in the research enterprise[7] seriously.

The approach to ethical regulation taken by the Belmont Report was to set out three principles for ethical research involving human subjects while acknowledging that these principles may sometimes conflict and should be applied according to the particular details of each case.[15]

The principles established by the Belmont Report are: respect for persons (which places a focus on informed consent from research subjects and includes additional protections for those who cannot consent); beneficence (which requires maximisation of the benefits of research, and minimisation of the risks); and justice (which requires a fair distribution of benefits and burdens of research).

The Belmont Report has become one of the most influential documents concerning the ethics of research involving humans.[7] It has formed the basis of research ethics review models in several countries, including the United States and the United Kingdom.

13.4.2. Beauchamp and Childress and the four principles approach

Two of the most influential figures in biomedical ethics are Tom Beauchamp and James Childress, who developed the four principles theory in 1979.[16] Incorporating a number of established theories of ethics, such as consequentialism and deontology, the four principles approach constituted a "framework of four broad moral principles: respect for autonomy, non-maleficence, beneficence, and justice."[16] The four principles theory builds on and develops the principles set out in the Belmont Report, specifying "respect for autonomy" rather than Belmont's "respect for persons," and including "non-maleficence" alongside "beneficence," which, in the Belmont Report, includes both positive and negative consequences.[17]

13.5. Research misconduct and its implications

Despite the establishment and operation of ethical and legal standards for research involving human subjects, details of scandals continue to come to light.

13.5.1. Wakefield and MMR

A paper published in the Lancet in 1998 claimed a link between the measles, mumps and rubella vaccine (MMR) and autism in children.[18] The lead author was Andrew Wakefield, a British gastroenterologist. Despite weaknesses in the study, such as a small sample size and uncontrolled design, the paper and its claims were widely publicised.[19]

Other studies discrediting the claims were published soon afterwards.[20] Then, in 2004, an investigation by the Sunday *Times* uncovered evidence that Wakefield had received financial support from a law firm that was suing vaccine manufacturers before embarking on the study. Most of the children involved in the study were named in the legal case.[7]

In 2010 Wakefield was found guilty of dishonesty and irresponsibility by the General Medical Council (GMC), the UK regulator, which held that he "abused his position, subjected children to intrusive procedures such as lumbar puncture and colonoscopy that were not clinically indicated, carried out research which flouted the conditions of ethics committee approval and brought the medical profession into disrepute."[21] *The Lancet* retracted the paper after this decision,[19] and Wakefield was struck off the medical register by the General Medical Council, which found him guilty of serious professional misconduct, later that year.[22]

However, Wakefield's fraudulent research had so damaged public trust in the MMR vaccine that during the mid-2000s, coverage in the United Kingdom fell to around 80 per cent, when it should be at 95 per cent for population protection, and this inevitably led to measles outbreaks.[23] Coverage has continued to be poor, with the World Health Organisation reporting tens of thousands of measles cases in Europe which have inevitably led to some deaths.[22]

13.5.2. Paolo Macchiarini and tracheal transplants

A more recent case of research misconduct involved Paolo Macchiarini, a surgeon with an international profile. In 2008, along with several colleagues, he carried out an operation in Spain on a woman with breathing problems to transplant a trachea (windpipe) from a deceased donor that had been seeded with the recipient's stem cells.[24] *The Lancet* reported this innovative surgery as a success, and in 2010 Macchiarini was recruited by the Karolinska Institute in Sweden as both a guest professor and a lead surgeon at the Karolinska University Hospital.[25] Macchiarini went on to carry out other transplants, using artificial tracheas built from plastic polymer seeded with patients' cells.[26]

However, after post-surgery complications and deaths of patients who had received the transplant, questions were raised by clinicians involved in their after-care and academics who had co-authored several papers on the procedures, and a number of investigations were launched.[27]

After conflicting outcomes in several investigations that have subsequently been recognised as flawed, Macchiarini and seven of his co-researchers were found guilty of scientific misconduct and dismissed by the Karolinska Institute in 2018.[26] He was also subsequently convicted of forging documents and abuse of office in Italy in 2019.[28]

It was found that Macchiarini had overstated the success of the artificial trachea technique, had provided inaccurate or misleading descriptions of the condition of patients when papers on the method were published, was primarily responsible for the publication of incorrect or incomplete data, had failed to get proper authorisation from a research ethics committee to carry out the surgical procedures, and had failed to secure informed consent from the patients.[27] In 2015, of the original eight patients who received transplanted organs, only two were documented as surviving, and they had both had their artificial trachea removed.[25] It has been claimed that in all, twenty artificial trachea operations were carried out by Macchiarini in various countries across the world, and only three of the twenty patients are still alive.[28]

While the principal actor in this case is Paolo Macchiarini,[25] it has been observed that research misconduct is rarely the fault of one "bad apple" or narcissistic individual alone. Wider contextual issues, such as competition and market forces, often contribute to the pressures that can lead to bad practices, alongside inadequate responses from organisations in investigating high profile cases with the potential to be reputationally damaging.[25]

13.6. Applying ethical practice to clinical research

It is, of course, important to remember that the majority of research is carried out ethically, by honest and dedicated researchers, in the public good. However, the central ethical challenge of all research involving humans is to avoid exploitation, particularly in the case of clinical research, which requires that human subjects are placed at risk of harm for the benefit of others.[29] Thus, the primary purpose of research ethics is to ensure that human subjects are protected in this endeavour. One of the ways this is achieved is by assessing research on ethical grounds before it is undertaken, or "prior ethical review."[11]

13.6.1. Aim of clinical research

The aim of clinical research is the generation of new knowledge. This contrasts with the aim of clinical therapy, which is the treatment of a specific patient. However, the distinction is not always clear cut in that

- Patients may benefit from participation in a research project by receiving "new" types of treatment;
- Future patients may benefit from the data collected during clinical research.

A further blurring occurs in that the Declaration of Helsinki requires all participants to be given a detailed explanation of precisely what is involved before enrolling in a research project.[5] To do this, researchers will invariably produce a detailed checklist of points to cover during such an explanation. Thus, it can be argued that potential recruits for clinical research projects may often be better informed and protected than those undergoing routine clinical treatment.

13.6.2. Providing information to participating patients

When a detailed explanation of what is involved is given to a potential recruit for a research study, the following points should be covered:

- The reasons for conducting the study;
- An explanation of the study design;
- The methods of identification of the participants;
- A list of possible benefits and potential risks;
- The process of obtaining informed consent; and
- Privacy and confidentiality.

13.6.3. Reasons for conducting the study

In clinical studies, it is a prerequisite that the project is ethically as well as scientifically defensible. In ethical terms, research is justifiable and praiseworthy, as long as it causes no significant harm to participants. Justification must be based on the premise that research is permissible only when it produces beneficial results and limits or prevents harm.

13.7. Study design

A further prerequisite of clinical research is that the project is scientifically sound. A scientifically sound project fulfils two ethical requirements:

- It is not wasteful of resources, including funds, participants' time, or laboratory space; and
- Its design reduces the risk of harm or injury to the participants involved.

It follows from this that no clinical research should proceed without first drawing up a protocol and having it peer-reviewed by a research ethics committee.

Prior ethical review of research involves assessing elements of the methodology concerning research ethics principles, broadly based on those set out in the Belmont Report. Therefore, these elements should be a central consideration in the design of research, so researchers should make sure that they are addressed from the earliest stages of research planning.

One approach that can help researchers focus on research ethics is studying a research ethics review application form while designing the research protocol. Incorporating the headings from the document can help to ensure that all relevant ethical issues are covered. For example, the NHS research ethics application form is the online Integrated Research Application System (IRAS) form for health-related research, which also includes question-specific guidance, incorporates all the relevant policies.

13.7.1. Identification and recruitment of participants

Arrangements for identifying potential participants, and recruiting them in to the research, should be clear. Where participants with a particular health condition are sought, only those with an appropriate legal basis, such as a member of their care team, can access medical notes on behalf of the researcher.

Careful consideration should be given to choosing the person who makes the first approach to potential participants to ensure that there can be no perception of coercion. For example, this could be the case where there is a power imbalance between the recruiter and the potential participant, who may, wrongly, assume he or she will receive adverse treatment should the potential participant refuse to become involved in the research.

Recruitment material should avoid overstating benefits and should not include improper inducement or statements that could be coercive.

Two problems arise from the identification and recruitment of participants:

- Vulnerable patients must be protected from being coerced into a study, and
- Denying entry, for any reason, to persons who may benefit from the research.

Participants should be selected for reasons directly related to the problem being studied. For example, it is ethically wrong to select participants because they are easily accessible or can be manipulated or if their position is compromised.

The Hopewood House[30] and Vipeholm studies[31] carried out before the Declaration of Helsinki are two examples involving unethical dental research. They used vulnerable subjects who were given no alternative but to participate.

People can be vulnerable to the influence that others may have on them or to economic exploitation. Therefore, they should not be paid at a level that could be viewed as coercive to participate in studies, but they can be reimbursed for any expenses that they may incur.

13.8. Risks and benefits overview

It is the responsibility of the researcher to assess the risks and benefits of a study at the outset, in clinical research. This is part of the justification for conducting the research and must be available and disclosed as part of the informed consent process. However, the way the risks are presented can have a significant bearing on the way they are perceived, interpreted and accepted.

Research ethics committees and peer review groups may lack the expertise to assess risk and benefit. If they do, then in confidence, they can seek second opinions. Furthermore, participants and investigators may differ in their assessment of the adverse consequences of clinical research.

The conceptual terms harm and risk are ill-defined in all relevant codes and guidelines. Risk is the probability and magnitude of future harm. Feinberg (1984)[32] defined harm as psychological, social or economic damage and physical damage. A participant may be "harmed" when their interests have been set back or compromised.

Researchers cannot be expected to identify all threats to the interests of participants. Still, they are expected to make it a duty to determine the likelihood and severity of known risks.

13.8.1. Risks

As established in ethical codes of practice, and contained within the concepts of beneficence and non-maleficence from the Belmont Report and Beauchamp and Childress's four principles approach, for research to be ethical, the wellbeing of participants must be safeguarded. Risks must be minimised and reasonable concerning the expected benefits of the study. The risks or burdens and the benefits of being involved in the research must be summarised and assessed, including a discussion of the probabilities and the consequences of harm. Risks must be minimised and mitigated, and efforts to protect participants evidenced.

Risks related to research participation may include[33]

- Medical risks, such as death, disability, injury, toxicity, nausea, shortness of breath, or adverse drug reactions;
- Psychological risks, such as pain, discomfort, distress, anxiety, remorse, shame;
- Social risks, such as discrimination, stigma, bias, identity theft;
- Financial risks, such as having to cover the costs of medical bills, or loss of earnings; and
- Legal risks, such as liability for child support as a result of paternity discovered during genetic testing.

The research proposal should include all the information needed by the research ethics committee to assess the risks inherent in the research and the measures taken by the researcher to mitigate the risks. The criteria used will depend on the nature and aims of the study and the participant population, and the types of tests and interventions that are planned. Some measures used to minimise risk include[7]

- Conducting a review of the published literature related to the research to better understand the potential risks;
- Checking for known medication allergies, for studies involving administration of drugs, by obtaining a medical history from the participant;
- Excluding research participants from the study who may be at increased risk due to factors, such as medical condition, age, pregnancy status, or other factors;
- Ensuring participants are monitored while they are in the study and receive appropriate follow-up after its completion;
- Ensuring any unanticipated problems and adverse events are reported to the REC, the institution, and the Sponsor promptly, and to other relevant authorities in line with legislative requirements;
- Providing support, such as making counselling services available for participants who experience distress, for research in which participants are asked about stressful events they have experienced, such as trauma, physical or sexual abuse;
- Ensuring that investigators and staff have appropriate levels of training, knowledge, and experience for all types of research, in order to conduct the study safely and effectively; and
- Ensuring measures to protect privacy and confidentiality are implemented for all types of research.

Different types of research will involve different risks, for example, research that takes place in another country from that in which the study is managed; research involving children; research taking place in developing world countries. Therefore, careful consideration of specific risks relating to these different research contexts is needed to assure research ethics committees that they will be appropriately mitigated.

Any risks to researchers themselves should also be assessed and minimised. These can range from exposure to dangerous chemicals, pathogens, or toxic substances, to risks of emotional distress when dealing with sensitive or upsetting issues in the context of research. Researchers should be suitably trained if required to undertake exposure-prone procedures, and consideration should be given to the provision of access to debriefing, support networks, or professional counselling for researchers who face distressing issues in the course of carrying out their research activities.[34]

13.8.2. Benefits

While the risks and benefits of specific research studies are seldom known with certainty in advance, as part of a research ethics review, the foreseeable risks and inconveniences of a research project, once they have been mitigated, are weighed against anticipated benefits. Benefits could be to the individual participants themselves, in the form of closer supervision, improved knowledge about their disease or condition, or access to improved healthcare.[35] Or the benefits may relate to other present and future patients, with no direct benefits to the study participants. Even when participants will not benefit directly from their participation, it has been shown that they can benefit indirectly from altruistic motivations, such as a sense of connection to society, to science, or their community or the institution hosting the research.[36] Some research participants have reported that the desire to help others was instrumental in their decision to participate. Others reported a therapeutic effect from the opportunity to share their story with the researchers.[37]

Anticipated benefits should be listed in participant information documentation alongside the possible risks to help potential participants decide whether or not to participate. However, they should not be overstated or framed in a way that could constitute improper inducement.

13.9. Informed consent

Informed consent is the most important principle in ethical research. It implies that the potential participant is given all the relevant information, in a form that they can understand, before they decide whether or not to participate in a study. The process involves an ongoing dialogue between the researcher and the participant to allow full access to all relevant information regarding the project before completing and signing a form. In addition, there must be severe doubts that a participant is being respected, protected from harm, and fairly treated without informed consent.

Participants can only give informed consent if they have

- Been given all relevant information in a form that they can understand;
- Been free from any coercion or improper inducement;
- Have the mental capacity to decide to participate or not; and
- Actively agreed to participate.

The researcher should give the participant an information sheet containing the following points before obtaining their written consent:

- The reasons for the study;
- The research techniques to be used;
- The reason the participant is being invited to participate;
- The benefits and consequences of the study for both the participant and society;
- The anticipated risks, discomfort and inconvenience;
- The time commitment;
- The intent, if any, to conduct a follow-up study;
- The intent to retain data and what is to be done with the data in the future;
- The extent and manner in which confidentiality is to be maintained;
- Any rules regarding termination of the study and withdrawal of the participant; and
- The right of the participant to withdraw from the study without penalty or denial of other treatments.

Incorporating "respect for persons" and "respect for autonomy" from the Belmont Report and Beauchamp and Childress's four principles approach, the concept of informed consent is important for promoting trust between research participants and researchers[7] and is central to the conduct of ethical research. Consent has been described as a form of mutual agreement between researchers and participants, setting out their intentions to behave in particular ways.[38] The requirement for participants to provide consent to their involvement in research is established in common law and is set out as a legal requirement for clinical trials.[5]

To be able to provide informed consent to participate in a research study, participants must be provided with appropriate information about the research to be able to understand the personal implications of involvement. In healthcare research this information is usually provided to participants in a participant information sheet (PIS) that explains the study.

It is essential to apply a proportionate approach to seeking consent. The procedures used and the information provided should be appropriate to the nature and complexity of the research, the associated ethical issues, and the balance of risks and benefits inherent in the study. Overly lengthy and complex procedures and information can risk overwhelming a potential participant.

For consent to be valid, it must[39]

- Be given freely, with no undue influence;
- Be by a person who is competent to do so, with the necessary mental capacity; and
- Be someone who has been adequately informed.

Anyone asked to give his or her consent to take part in a research project should

- Be neither deceived nor coerced (and can judge that he or she is not deceived or coerced);
- Not be overwhelmed with information but able to control the amount of information received; and
- Have the opportunity to withdraw consent previously given.

One way to avoid producing PIS documents that are overly lengthy and confusing to potential participants is to take a layered or tiered approach. This involves providing initial summary information that potential participants can use to decide whether they are interested in taking part in the research. This initial summary should include details on how to access more comprehensive information about the study, provided in a user-friendly format, and presented in one or more additional layers.[40] In addition, consideration should be given to the types of media used to provide the information. For example, videos, animations, audio, or brochures can complement, or even replace, the more traditional form of text-based PIS on paper, dependent on the needs and requirements of the participant population.

The provision of information on its own is not sufficient to assume understanding. Often, the verbal explanation provided by the researcher at the point of seeking consent, accompanied by interactive questioning, does most to support understanding.

Potential participants must be provided with sufficient time to fully consider whether or not they wish to take part in the research. The amount of time provided should be proportionate to the complexity of the study and the level of risk that participants will face. In addition, they should have the opportunity to ask questions of the researcher and others, if necessary, before they come to a decision.

13.9.1. Capacity to consent

When seeking consent, researchers must be able to assess the capacity of potential participants to understand the information provided and be able to decide for themselves whether or not they wish to participate. Where necessary, they should seek the advice and assistance of a professional who has experience in assessing capacity.

When assessing capacity, the researcher must be sure that the potential participant is able to

- understand the purpose and nature of the research;
- understand what the study involves, its benefits (or lack of benefits), risks and burdens;
- understand the alternatives to taking part;
- retain the information for long enough to make an effective decision;
- make a free choice; and
- be capable of making this particular decision at the time it needs to be made.

Research projects where it is intended to recruit adults aged over 16 who lack capacity fall within the Mental Capacity Act 2005 (MCA). The MCA requires that the research is reviewed and approved by an NHS REC, defined in the Act as the "appropriate body", before it is initiated. The requirements for approval are set out in Section 31 of the Act:

- The research must be linked to an impairing condition that affects the person who lacks capacity or the treatment of that condition; and
- There are reasonable grounds for believing that the research would be less effective if only people with capacity are involved; and
- Arrangements are in place to consult carers and to follow the other requirements of the Act (Mental Capacity Act Code of Practice 2007);
- The research must have some chance of benefitting the person who lacks capacity. The benefit must be in proportion to any burden caused by taking part, or
- The research aims to provide knowledge about the cause of, or treatment or care of people with the same impairing condition or a similar condition.

The Act includes the requirement that the researcher consults with specified people to determine whether the person who lacks capacity should be included in the research. It also stipulates that any objections a person who lacks capacity makes during the study must be respected. The MCA applies in England and Wales. Similar legislation applies in the devolved nations: the Adults with Incapacity (Scotland) Act 2000 in Scotland, and the Mental Capacity Act (NI) 2016 in Northern Ireland.

13.9.2. Privacy and confidentiality

Privacy is a characteristic of limited accessibility to a person. Confidentiality refers to the status of the information about a person and the management of this information. In all clinical research studies, information is gathered which may be termed confidential. In the context of dental research, patients must be protected against undue access to their privacy. Consideration must always be given to their right to be excluded from the study without penalty, in other words, to be left alone.

Participant anonymity can often be maintained by identifying participants solely by numbers rather than by name. However, in dental epidemiological studies, where patient records are used in many instances, access restriction or confidentiality must always be considered when formulating a protocol.

Each Health Board in Scotland and Trust in England/Wales/Northern Ireland has a Caldicott Guardian(s).[41] The use or transfer of patient-identifiable information, except for routine clinical care, requires approval. In addition, researchers are required to comply with common law confidentiality, the Data Protection Act 2018, and the UK General Data Protection Regulation (UK GDPR).

While often discussed in tandem, privacy and confidentiality are separate concepts. Privacy refers to the prevention of unwanted intrusion into an individual's private space or information. Confidentiality refers to the implementation of safeguards to protect personal data.

Information and data from individuals and patients are essential for health-related research. To ensure their continued participation in the research enterprise, researchers must maintain the public's trust by taking all necessary measures to protect privacy and confidentiality[42]. Breaches to confidentiality, in addition to the harms caused to the individuals to whom the data refer, can lead to reputational damage to researchers and their institutions.[7]

Measures that researchers can use to protect privacy and confidentiality in health research include

- Securing appropriate consent for access to identifiable information to identify potential participants;
- Limiting access to identifiable data to members of the research team;
- Ensuring research team members have had appropriate training on privacy and confidentiality;
- De-identifying, where possible, personal data as soon as possible; and
- Maintaining appropriate technological measures to safeguard identifiable data, such as password protection and encryption.

Participant information sheets must include full details about the methods used to collect research data and the associated measures to protect privacy, as well as details of how confidentiality will be safeguarded during data analysis and storage. However, while researchers have an ethical and a legal (in line with data protection legislation) obligation to protect data confidentiality, there may be circumstances where a researcher is obliged to breach confidentiality, and participants must also be made aware of this via participant information documentation. This could be, for example, if the researcher learns of a risk of harm to the participant, or a third party, that they are obliged to report to the relevant authorities. It would be usual to discuss this with the participant before deciding on a course of action. There may also be a statutory requirement for a researcher to breach confidentiality in certain circumstances (in compliance with prevention of terrorism legislation, or if evidence of child abuse or neglect is uncovered, for example), and if this is foreseen as a possibility, a plan to manage this eventuality should be formulated in advance.[43]

Advances in health-related research can lead to additional risks to privacy and confidentiality that researchers and research ethics committees must address. Wearable technology, electronic health records and data linkage, and advances in genetic analysis can all lead to risks to participants that were unforeseen when the early codes of ethics were drafted.[42] Researchers should work with data protection experts at their institutions to ensure they can take account of the implications of these advances and developments and employ all appropriate technical measures to safeguard participant data.

13.10. Publication ethics—publication and dissemination of findings

Ensuring that the research results are disseminated to research participants and other groups or communities with interest is good practice and can maximise the benefits of the study.[44] A lay summary of the study findings provides recognition for participants' contribution and can help maintain trust in the research enterprise. Information on publication and dissemination arrangements should be included in the participant information (see https://www.hra.nhs.uk/planning-and-improving-research/best-practice/publication-and-dissemination-research-findings/).

There are numerous types of unethical behaviour relating to the publication of scholarly literature. They include falsification of results, plagiarism and simultaneous submission of a manuscript to more than one journal. The Committee on Publication Ethics (COPE) investigates any cases of breaches of publication ethics, which are reported to it. Its members are editors, publishers and institutions. It has issued guidelines and recommends that all journals and publishers follow core practices[45] and publish guidelines and instructions for authors.

The core practices that journals should follow include

- A clearly described system for dealing with allegations of misconduct by authors;
- Policies on authorship and contribution;
- A system for complaints and appeals;
- Policies on conflict of interests;
- Policies on data sharing and reproducibility;

- Providing ethical oversight;
- Policies on intellectual policy, journal management and the peer review process; and
- A system for post-publication discussions and corrections.

The International Committee of Medical Journal Editors (ICMJE) has also issued Recommendations for the Conduct, Reporting, Editing, and Publication of Scholarly Work in Medical Journals (2019),[46] including and reiterate COPE's core practices. These recommendations will be considered in Chapter 18 on writing up and dissemination.

13.11. Governance arrangements for health-related research in the United Kingdom

13.11.1. Health Research Authority

The body with responsibility for providing approvals and opinions on health-related research studies in the United Kingdom is the Health Research Authority (HRA).[1] It oversees the assessment of governance and legal compliance and research ethics review for research involving the NHS and Health and Social Care. Researchers submit applications for review via the online Integrated Research Application System (IRAS) which provides a single system for applying for the permissions and approvals required.[2] The IRAS system incorporates comprehensive information, including question-specific guidance, to assist researchers with compiling their submissions. The HRA has a number of e-learning modules that are available to researchers.[3]

HRA approval applies to all project-based research taking place in the NHS in England and Wales. Studies with sites in Northern Ireland, Scotland or Wales are supported through existing UK-wide compatibility systems. In addition, each country accepts relevant centralised assurances from national coordinating functions to avoid duplication. For studies that have NHS sites in Northern Ireland or Scotland, the HRA will share information with participating nations. The relevant R&D coordinating function will provide advice on the procedures to set up sites in their country. For studies that are led from Northern Ireland or Scotland but have English and/or Welsh NHS sites, the R&D coordinating function in the lead nation will share information with the HRA to enable HRA Approval for English and Welsh sites. Further guidance on seeking HSC R&D Permission in Northern Ireland can be found on the HSC website.[4] Further guidance on seeking NHS R&D permission in Scotland can be found on the NHS Research Scotland Permission Coordinating Centre website.[5]

13.11.2. United Kingdom policy framework and sponsorship

United Kingdom health and social care research is governed by the UK Policy Framework for Health and Social Care Research,[47] which sets out principles of good practice and responsibilities for the individuals and institutions involved in health-related research. The Framework stipulates that all research in the NHS or Health and Social Care organisations, involving patients, their tissues, or identifiable data, or their relatives or carers, must have a sponsor. This is defined as "the individual, organisation or partnership that takes on overall responsibility for proportionate, adequate arrangements to set up, run and report a research project."[47] The Sponsor must authorise the IRAS form before submission, so researchers must establish which organisation will take on this role during the planning phase of their project. For researchers based within an NHS trust, it is usual for this organisation to sponsor. For university students, the university will usually agree to act as a sponsor. Universities will also usually provide sponsorship for their academic staff conducting funded non-commercial research. For commercial studies, it is generally the commercial organisation, or their legal representative, that will take on the role of Sponsor.

13.12. Stages in seeking approvals for research in health and social care

13.12.1. "Is it research?"

The first step for researchers seeking approval from the HRA is to determine whether their study classifies as "research" as defined by the UK Policy Framework for Health and Social Care Research (2017).[4]. Research is defined as "the attempt to derive generalisable or transferable new knowledge to answer or refine relevant questions with scientifically sound methods" (p 5). The HRA, in collaboration with the Medical Research Council, has designed a decision tool to help researchers with this task.[6] Studies classified as "audit" or "service evaluation" should comply with local NHS approval arrangements instead of following the HRA Approval procedures.

13.12.2. Integrated Research Application System (IRAS) form

The initial step in completing the IRAS form involves filling in several filter questions; the answers will define the sections that appear in the rest of the form to create the "full dataset." Next, the researcher must study the guidance to ensure the correct options are selected in the filter so that the project follows the right path for approval.

Health and social care research involving staff only, with no involvement of patients of their identifiable data, will generally require the governance and legal checks carried out through HRA Approval. However, research involving NHS or adult Social Care patients, their relatives or carers, or their identifiable tissue or data will also need to be reviewed by an NHS Research Ethics Committee (REC). NHS REC review is also required under the legislation covering people who lack the capacity to consent (Mental Capacity Act 2005), research involving human tissue samples (Human Tissue Act 2004), and a range of other health-related research.[7] The requirement for REC review is identified by the correct completion of the filter questions. Projects that do not qualify for research ethics review by an NHS REC should comply with the lead researcher's institution's relevant research ethics review requirements. For example, research supported by a university will require a research ethics review via university structures.

13.12.3. Supporting documentation

The HRA provides guidance and templates for the supporting documentation that must be submitted with the IRAS application. The main documents include

- A research protocol: a complete description of the research study that provides a set of instructions for its conduct;[8]
- A participant information sheet: user-friendly information to inform potential participants of the details of a study and what participation will involve;[9]
- A consent form: document to record informed consent decision;[10]
- Investigator(s)' CVs.[11]

13.12.4. General guidance

The points to consider in any proposal submitted to a REC will depend on the nature of the study in question. However, many have been explained in the chapter on writing a protocol.

Researchers are often critical of the Research Ethics Committee (REC) process by which their projects are approved, complaining that it is too complex, trying, and sometimes unreasonable. RECs are looking for evidence that researchers are sensitive to ethical issues, particularly to participants' interests, and that information given to potential participants explains the trial fully and truthfully. Researchers can improve their chances of success at an ethical review by preparing a suitable protocol and, in particular, by paying attention to the wording of participant information leaflets.

The following sub-sections give general guidance on issues that frequently result in an unfavourable report by an REC.

13.12.5. Patient care

The care and protection of participants is a key area of concern for RECs. A proposal should demonstrate that:

- Careful consideration has been given to the risks, inconveniences and discomforts to which participants might be exposed.
- Complete disclosures of these have been given to participants.
- Measures had been put in place to avoid any risks and to support participants where possible.

13.12.6. Informed consent

RECs frequently levy criticism at the use of language in the participant information leaflets/letters.

- Use simple language, write in lay terms, and avoid technical terms.
- Ensure that any written material given to participants is accessible.
- Demonstrate that inappropriate participant expectations have not been created and that trials have not been presented too enthusiastically.

13.12.7. Scientific issues

RECs see scientific issues as having ethical dimensions. They will look for

- A scientifically sound design (note, an unclear research question destroys the validity of research and may lead to an unethical study);
- Clearly defined subjects, interventions, and outcome measurements;
- A study that has sufficient power to test the hypothesis;
- Participants who are chosen without bias; and
- Exclusion and inclusion criteria that are correctly and fully described.

Applicants must recognise the degree to which their proposed research is likely to attract scientific scrutiny from RECs and prepare their applications so that the scientific design, rationale, and methods are robustly and clearly explained.

In perusing their remit, RECs check that the proposed methodology, scientific design and conduct of a study are appropriate and practical. They will consider

- Scientific issues including flaws in the rationale of methods;
- Sampling;
- Research question;
- Instruments or measures; and
- Approach to analysis and power calculation

13.12.8. Publication of results

The Declaration of Helsinki expands its guidance to publishing results (Article 16), stating that information regarding any study should be publicly available. Ethical publications extend to publication of the results and consideration of any potential conflict of interest. For these reasons, RECs will expect to receive reports on the completion of projects they gave ethics approval for. Researchers should seek publication only in refereed journals so that their peers review their work before publication. It is scientifically unethical to publish the same report, in slightly different formats, in several journals.

13.12.9. Patents and copyrights

Some clinical research can lead to investigators seeking patents or obtaining copyrights. If this occurs, the ethical constraint is that such patents and copyrights must not be used to restrict research or the treatment of patients.

13.12.10. Fraud

It is unlikely that any clinician undertaking research for the first time would knowingly set out to commit fraud. However, fraud can include the misappropriation or misuse of research funds and the falsification or fabrication of results, which may result in harm to patients from unsafe treatment. Plagiarism of results can also be construed as fraud.

13.13. Additional considerations

13.13.1. Justice

The emphasis so far has been on protecting research participants. While research participants must not be subjected to undue influence and exploitation, it is essential to ensure that no one is unfairly excluded from participation in research. This concept is framed as "justice" within the Belmont Report and Beauchamp and Childress's four principles approach.

Historically, ethics codes have emphasised that individuals and groups considered vulnerable should not routinely be involved in research. This category has included children, people who lack capacity, pregnant women, and prisoners. However, there is evidence that the health of these populations has been adversely affected by excluding them from research involvement.[7] This has ranged from a lack of research into the areas that affect them most, for example, for people with intellectual and developmental disabilities,[48] to a lack of data on the safety and efficacy of medicines used in children.[49]

The principle of justice requires that all decisions on inclusion and exclusion must be justified. Thus, while vulnerable populations must be protected from harm relating to research involvement, they should not be unfairly excluded from research from which they, or others like them, could benefit.

13.13.2. Public and patient involvement

An essential element in the design and development of high-quality research is public involvement.[12] INVOLVE, the national advisory group that supports public involvement in NHS, public health, and social care research, has produced guidance for researchers on involving the public in designing and developing their projects.[50] It sets out the benefits of public involvement as

- Making research more relevant;
- Helping define what is acceptable to participants;
- Improving the process of informed consent;
- Improving the experience of participating in research; and
- Improving the communication of findings to participants and the wider public.

Seeking the input of people who have lived experience of a condition or service, as a patient or carer, can improve the quality and relevance of research, contributing to producing research studies that respect the dignity, rights, safety, and wellbeing of participants. In addition, confirmation that a study directly addresses the concerns of those it seeks to involve, and ultimately, to benefit, can help secure a favourable opinion from a research ethics committee.

13.14. Summary

This chapter has set out the key elements of ethical research to provide researchers with guidance to design projects that uphold the highest ethical standards. Consideration of the aspects described, including the development of good quality and user-friendly information for potential participants, suitable consent procedures, and appropriate plans to disseminate the findings, will improve prospects of success in securing a favourable opinion from a research ethics committee.

The key ethical points to consider in clinical research projects are

- Does it have scientific merit?
- Is it justified?
- How will informed consent be obtained?
- Do the benefits outweigh the risks?
- How will the participants be selected?
- How will the privacy and confidentiality of the participants be protected?

References

1   Dickersin K, Straus SE, Bero LA. Evidence-based medicine: Increasing, not dictating, choice. *British Medical Journal*. 2007; 334: s10.

     See: https://www.hra.nhs.uk/approvals-amendments/ (viewed 31.03.21)

2   Trinder L. (ed.) *Evidence-Based Practice: A Critical Appraisal*. Oxford: Blackwell; 2000

     See: https://www.myresearchproject.org.uk/ (viewed 31.03.21)

3   Beauchamp TL, Childress J. *The Principles of Biomedical Ethics*. 5th edition. New York, NY: Oxford University Press; 2001

4   Woff L. Ethics of research on human biological materials. *Nature Biotechnology.* 2008;26: 29-30.

See: https://research.hscni.net/approval-research-hsc (viewed 06.04.21)

5   World Medical Association (1964). *Declaration of Helsinki: Ethical Principles for Medical Research Involving Human Subjects* (2013 revision), available at: https://www.wma.net/policies-post/wma-declaration-of-helsinki-ethical-principles-for-medical-research-involving-human-subjects/ (Accessed on 1 April 2021).

See: https://www.nhsresearchscotland.org.uk/services/permissions-co-ordinating-centre/permissions (viewed 06.04.21)

6   Council for International Organizations of Medical Sciences. *International ethical guidelines for biomedical research involving human subjects.* Geneva Council for International Organization of Medical Sciences; 1993.

See: http://www.hra-decisiontools.org.uk/research/ (viewed 31.03.21)

7   Resnik DB. *The Ethics of Research with Human Subjects: Protecting People, Advancing Science, Promoting Trust.* Switzerland: Springer; 2018

See Governance Arrangements for Research Ethics Committees https://www.hra.nhs.uk/planning-and-improving-research/policies-standards-legislation/governance-arrangement-research-ethics-committees/ (viewed 31.03.21)

8   Wertheimer A. *Rethinking the Ethics of Clinical Research—Widening the Lens.* Oxford: Oxford University Press; 2011

See: https://www.hra.nhs.uk/planning-and-improving-research/research-planning/protocol/ (viewed 01.04.21)

9   Nuremberg Code Trials of war criminals before the Nuremberg military tribunals under Control Council Law No.10,1949, l.2:181-182, Washington DC: US Government Printing Office.

See: http://www.hra-decisiontools.org.uk/consent/ (viewed 01.04.21)

10   Capron AM. Human Experimentation. In Veatch, R.M. (ed.), *Medical Ethics.* Boston: Jones and Bartlett; 1989. pp125-172.

See: http://www.hra-decisiontools.org.uk/consent/ (viewed 01.04.21)

11   Hedgecoe, A. Scandals, ethics, and regulatory change in biomedical research. *Science, Technology and Human Values.* 2017;42: 577-599.

See: https://www.hra.nhs.uk/planning-and-improving-research/research-planning/prepare-study-documentation/ (viewed 01.04.21)

12   Harkness, J., Lederer, SE., Wikler D., Laying the ethical foundations for clinical research. *Bulletin of World Health Organisation.* 2001;79: 65-372.

See: https://www.hra.nhs.uk/planning-and-improving-research/best-practice/public-involvement/ (viewed 01.04.21)

13 Jones DS, Grady C, Lederer SE. Ethics and clinical research—The 50th anniversary of Beecher's bombshell. *New England Journal of Medicine*. 2016; 374:2393-2398.

14 Shamoo; AE, Resnik, DB. *Responsible Conduct of Research*. Third Edition. Oxford: Oxford University Press; 2015

15 National Commission for the Protection of Human Subjects of Biomedical or Behavioural Research, *The Belmont Report: Ethical principles and guidelines for the protection of human subjects of research*,1979, Washington DC: Department of Health, Education, and Welfare

16 Beauchamp T, Childress J. Principles of Biomedical Ethics: Marking its fortieth anniversary. *American Journal of Bioethics*. 2019;19 (11): 9-12.

17 Veatch; RM. Reconciling lists of principles in bioethics. *Journal of Medicine and Philosophy*. 2020;45: 540-559.

18 Wakefield AJ., Murch SH, Anthony A, Linnell J, Casson DM, Malik M, Berelowitz M, Dhillon AP, Thomson MA, Harvey P, Valentine A, Davies SE, Walker-Smith JA. **RETRACTED**: Ileal-lymphoid-nodular hyperplasia, non-specific colitis, and pervasive developmental disorder in children," *The Lancet*, 1998;351: 9103: 637–641.

19 Rao TS, Andrade C. The MMR vaccine and autism: Sensation, refutation, retraction, and fraud. *Indian Journal of Psychiatry*. 2011; 53: 95-96.

20 Flaherty DK. The vaccine-autism connection: A public health crisis caused by unethical medical practices and fraudulent science. *Annals of Pharmacy*. 2011;45: 1302-1304.

21 Dyer C. Wakefield was dishonest and irresponsible over MMR research, says GMC. *British Medical Journal*. 2010;340:c593

22 Kmietowicz Z. Measles: Europe sees record number of cases and 37 deaths so far this year. *British Medical Journal*. 2018; 362:k3596

23 Omer S. The discredited doctor hailed by the anti-vaccine movement. *Nature*. 2020;586: 668-669.

24 Macchiarini P, Jungebluth P, Go T, Asnaghi MA, Rees LE, Cogan TA, Dodson A, Martorell J, Bellini S, Parnigotto PP, Dickinson SC. Clinical transplantation of a tissue-engineered airway. *The Lancet*, 2008; 372, .9655:2023-2030.

25 Berggren C, Karabag SF. Scientific misconduct at an elite medical institute: The role of competing institutional logics and fragmented control. *Research Policy,* 2019; 48: 428-443.

26 Hawkes N. Macchiarini case: Seven researchers are guilty of scientific misconduct, rules Karolinska's president. *British Medical Journal*. 2018; 361:k2816.

27 Vogel G. Report finds misconduct by surgeon. *Science*. 2015; 6238: 954-955.

28 Day M. Disgraced tracheal transplant surgeon is handed 16-month prison sentence in Italy. *British Medical Journal*. 2019;367:l6676

29 Emanuel EJ, Wendler D, Grady C. An ethical framework for biomedical research. in Emanuel EJ, Grady C, Crouch RA, Lie RK, Miller FG, Wendler D. (ed.), *The Oxford Textbook of Clinical Research Ethics*, 2008, Oxford: Oxford University Press, pp123-135

30 Harris R. Biology of the children of Hopewood House, Bowral, Australia. IV. Observations of dental caries experience over five years. *Journal of Dental Research* 1963;42:1387-1399.

31 Gustafsson BE. The Vipeholm dental caries study. *Acta Odontologica Scandinavia*. 1954;11:232-264.

32 Feinberg J. *Harm to others*. New York: Oxford University Press, 1984.

33 Levine RJ. *Ethics and Regulation of Clinical Research*: Second Edition. Newhaven: Yale University Press; 1988

34 Butler AE, Copnell B, Hall H. Researching people who are bereaved: Managing risks to participants and researchers, *Nursing Ethics*. 2019;26: 224-234.

35 Rennie S, Day S, Mathews A, Gilbertson A, Luseno WK, Tucker JD, Henderson GE. The role of inclusion benefits in ethics committee assessment of research studies. *Ethics and Human Research*. 2019;41: 13-22.

36 Carerra JS, Brown P, Brody JG, Morello-Frosch R. Research altruism as motivation for participation in community-centred environmental health research. *Social Science and Medicine*. 2018;196: 175-181.

37 Lakeman R, McAndrew S, MacGabhann L, Warne, T. That was helpful…no one has talked to me about that before: Research participation as a therapeutic activity. *International Journal of Mental Health Nursing*. 2013;2:76-84.

38 Faden RR, Beauchamp TL. *A History and Theory of Informed Consent*. New York, Oxford: Oxford University Press; 1988

39 O'Neill, O. Some limits of informed consent. *Journal of Medical Ethics*. 2003;29: 4-7.

40 Antoniou EE, Draper H, Reed K, Burtis A, Southwood TR, Zeegers MP. An empirical study on the preferred size of the participant information sheet in research. *Journal of Medical Ethics*. 2011; 37: 557–562.

41 Department of Health. Caldicott Guardian Manual 2010, accessed 11 December 2020. www.dh.gov.uk.publications.

42 Lowrance WW. *Privacy, Confidentiality and Health Research*. Cambridge: Cambridge University Press; 2012.

43 Blightman K, Griffiths SE, Danbury C. Patient confidentiality: When can a breach be justified? *Continuing Education in Anaesthesia Critical Care and Pain*, 2014; 14: 52–56.

44 Long CR, Stewart MK, McElfish PA. Health research participants are not receiving research results: A collaborative solution is needed. *Trials*. 2017;18:1-4.

45   Committee on Publications Ethics (2017) Core Practices, accessed 1 April 2021. www.publicationsethics.org.

46   International Committee of Medical Journal Editors (2019). Recommendations for the Conduct, Reporting, Editing, and Publication of Scholarly Work in Medical Journals, updated December 2019. Accessed 2 April 2021. www.icmje.org.

47   Health Research Authority. UK Policy Framework for Health and Social Care Research. London: HRA; 2017

48   Chu LF, Utengen A, Kadry B, Kucharski SE, Campos H, Crockett J, Dawson N, Clauson KA. Nothing about us without us—Patient partnership in medical conferences. *British Medical Journal.* 2016;354:l3883

49   Wong I, Sweis D, Cope J, Florence A. Paediatric medicines research in the UK. *Drug Safety.* 2003;26: 529-537.

50   Health Research Authority/INVOLVE. *Public involvement in research: Impact on ethical research.* Southampton: INVOLVE; 2016.

Chapter 14. Obtaining Funding

EATON K.A, REED D.

14.1. Overview

This chapter is divided into the following sections:

- Introduction;
- Possible sources of funding;
- How to improve chances of obtaining funding; and
- Suggested further reading.

14.2. Introduction

First-time researchers and those studying for masters and doctorate degrees need funding during their research training, as there are fees to pay for postgraduate degrees and living costs to be met. Studies cost thousands or millions of pounds to run. This chapter will suggest where to look for funds for research training and funding studies and how to improve the chances of obtaining such funding.

Applying for funding can be frustrating and time-consuming, and even the best full-time researchers have funding applications rejected. It may be the intention to seek funds for either the full cost of a study or only part of it. When funding is being sought, some thought should be given to the relevance of the research concerning the interests of the funding authority since some funding sources are relatively specific in what research they will or will not support.

It is therefore essential to read and apply any guidance which the funding body may have produced. If any points are unclear, it is acceptable to make an informal approach to the organisation concerned and seek further guidance, before submitting a protocol, as this may avoid much wasted time and effort.

For clinical studies, it is essential to demonstrate that patients were consulted when the proposed project was designed and stress the benefits to patients expected to result from the proposed study.

14.3. Possible sources for research funding

14.3.1. For research training

One consequence of the increased emphasis on evidence-based practice is that there is a need for practitioners to critically appraise the research which underpins the evidence. To do this, as described in Chapter 2, they need to assess the validity of the research objectively. In future, undergraduate courses must provide appropriate training to enable this to happen. Some may wish not only to have an understanding of research processes but to perform some research themselves. There are growing opportunities for training to acquire the necessary skills during fellowship, masters, doctoral, and postdoctoral studies.

Funding for this training may come from the UK Government through grants from seven research councils, such as the Engineering Physical Sciences Research Council (EPSRC) and the Medical Research Council (MRC) and the National Institute for Health Research (NIHR). In addition, since 2017, the Government has been encouraging continuous learning via apprenticeships, which range from level 2 to level 7 (master's level) (with level 8 [doctoral level]) also part of the long-term aspiration. Many apprenticeships at level 7 present opportunities for participants to develop research skills and conduct small work/practice-based projects during their apprenticeship.

Some universities, both in the United Kingdom and overseas, offer scholarships to research students. However, opportunities vary greatly, and it is best to search individual university websites.

Employers, both in the public and private sector, may also fund studies for master's and doctoral degrees either wholly or partially. They may also offer interest-free loans repayable over time to fund their employees' studies. Examples include the UK Armed Forces, which have paid all fees and continued to pay salaries of service personnel whilst they study for approved postgraduate degrees and some schools in Medway, Kent, which have reimbursed 50 per cent of the fees for part-time MSc degrees for their teachers once the teachers have completed an MSc programme.

Charitable foundations, such as Leverhulme (www.leverhulme.ac.uk), Nuffield (www.nuffieldfoundation/org), and the Wellcome Trust (www.wellcome.ac.uk) fund research studies and fellowships for doctoral and postdoctoral students working on projects they have funded.

Several small charitable bodies can provide research students with small grants (www.findamasters.com/funding/guidance/charities.aspx). Many restrict such grants to members of their group—for example, the Clan Forsyth Society, which only considers applications from its clan members (www.clanforsyth.com).

Small grants may be available to help with the costs of attending conferences to present their research findings. For example, the National Conference of University Professors (NCUP) offers travel grants (www.ncup.org).

Some dental bodies corporates are starting to show a research interest, especially if it might improve their efficiency or help raise their public profile.

Thus there is a wide range of possibilities for obtaining funding to pay the costs of research training in part or totally.

14.3.2. National Institute for Health Research (NIHR)

The NIHR has several schemes to enable all healthcare workers, including dentists and other dental team members working in both primary and secondary care, to obtain research training (www.nihr.ac.uk).

Two are of particular relevance to dentists and dental care professionals who wish to pursue full- or part-time careers as clinical academics. They are the pre-doctoral clinical academic fellowship scheme and the doctoral fellowship scheme. The clinical academic training fellowships enable healthcare workers in bother primary and secondary care, who have little formal research experience, to undertake research training, master's degrees and then submit applications for doctoral fellowships. To ensure that they do not lose income during their training, the NIHR pays their salary costs (including their employer's National Insurance and pension contributions) whilst they train, and they can request to continue to work one day per week in their practice. The doctoral fellowships offer the same benefits but over a more extended period (the time taken to complete a doctorate). They also pay laboratory costs and any fees. The authors of this chapter are aware of general medical practitioners and at least one general dental practitioner and one dental hygienist who have obtained doctorates through the NIHR's doctoral fellowship scheme. Competition for NIHR fellowships takes place annually (www.academy-awards@nihr.ac.uk).

Apart from funding research training, the NIHR also funds a wide range of healthcare research on various topics. Current topics can be viewed at the NIHR's website (www.nihr.ac.uk).

14.3.3. Apprenticeships

Currently, several different types of apprenticeships might be of interest to dental professionals wishing to extend their research skills and conduct a small research project as part of an apprenticeship. In November 2021, examples included a senior leader apprenticeship for those who may be interested in developing skills and research related to business and administration; or an advanced clinical practitioner apprenticeship (for those wishing to focus on training and research related to clinical practice); or a clinical scientist apprenticeship for dental professionals who might wish to perform practice-based research within their workplace. It is worth keeping an eye on the government apprenticeship website[1] as new apprenticeships are being developed continuously.

Some higher education institutions offer premium-rate programmes, such as a master's in business administration (MBA), which can be part-funded by the apprenticeship levy and topped-up with part additional payment to meet the commercial rate required by the training provider.

Thus, apprenticeships can offer an excellent route for developing research skills and an opportunity to conduct a practice-based study funded through the apprenticeship levy.

Details on how to take advantage of apprenticeship opportunities can be obtained from local apprenticeship-training providers, who will advise on the application process to those interested and their employer. For lists of apprenticeships and training providers, see the government apprenticeship website,[1] which can be searched by postcode to identify training providers for all levels of apprenticeship. The arrangements for apprenticeship schemes in Scotland, Wales and Northern Ireland differ from those in England. Details can be found at https://www.apprenticeships.scot/, https://gov.wales.apprenticeships, and https:// indirect.gov.uk/campaigns/apprenticeships. Further details can be found in Appendix 3.

14.3.4. Research funding from international organisations

It is unlikely that individuals who are new to research will seek funds for projects instead of research training from large international organisations. However, they may be junior researchers within a large international research project funded by bodies like the Bill and Melinda Gates Foundation (www.gatesfoundation.org) or the European Commission (www.europa.eu/info/research-and-innovation/funding/funding-opportunities_eu).

14.3.5. Small research grants from UK organisations

It is far more likely that new researchers may seek funds for small research projects from local or national organisations. For oral health research, these include:

14.3.5.1. The British Society for Oral and Dental Research (BSODR)

The BSODR (formerly The British Society for Dental Research) is dedicated to enhancing and promoting high-quality research to improve oral health in the United Kingdom (www.bsodr.org). The BSODR also constitutes the British division of the International Association for Dental Research (IADR), the global body responsible for promoting oral health research worldwide.

14.3.5.2. The Faculty of Dental Surgery (FDS) of the Royal College of Surgeons of England

In collaboration with the relevant specialist societies, the FDS annually offer fellowships and pump-priming grants of up to £10,000 for research in orthodontics, oral surgery, oral medicine, gerontology, paediatric dentistry and anaesthetics in dentistry to its members. It also funds and promotes research in other aspects of oral care (www.rcseng.ac.uk/dental-faculties/fds).

14.3.5.3. Dental manufacturers

Dental manufacturers may be a source for covering the costs of materials or equipment only or may, in addition, provide capital funding. However, if dental manufacturers provide funds, care should be taken in establishing the ownership of the research findings and any limitations on publication.

14.3.6. The internet

Most universities have a website where research funding opportunities may be listed. For example, the website of the University of Newcastle School of Dental Sciences (www.ncl.ac.uk/dental)

14.4. How to improve chances of obtaining funding

14.4.1. Overview

There are two types of grant applications.

- Those made in response to a call for applications by a funding organisation (funder-initiated applications); and
- Those made de novo by the researcher(s) (investigator-initiated applications).

In both cases, meticulous planning is essential for success. Before submitting either type of grant application, it is necessary to establish

- Exact details of the topics for which funding is sought;
- The correct application procedure (which forms to use, time limits for applications, and other details);
- The amount of money which could be available; and
- Who to contact at the funding organisation concerned for informal advice.

As a preliminary to making an unsolicited application, it is important to establish whom to approach and, perhaps more importantly, how to approach them. Two key questions which should be asked, and for which expert advice will inevitably be necessary if these questions are to be answered satisfactorily are

- Why should the organisation wish to fund the planned research?
- How can the organisation be convinced that the project can be carried out successfully?

14.4.2. Expert advice and alliances

A proven track record of demonstrable expertise and success in the relevant research areas is of great importance when applying for large research grants. Unfortunately, in the United Kingdom, very few healthcare workers in primary care and very few general dental practitioners (GDPs) and dental care professionals have such track records in research.

The most successful applicants for grants for investigator-initiated research into emergency medicine have been those who had appropriate research expertise and experience, knew the scientific field concerned in detail, identified a timely research question, and consulted the funding organisation for detailed discussions before submitting applications.[2]

Although the research question is often defined in advance for funder-initiated research, in other respects, the same basic success criteria apply to this type of project.

Experience has shown that it is almost essential for new researchers wishing to obtain research funds to form alliances with, and obtain expert advice from, established researchers (typically from university departments or industry) if they are to be successful.

Relatively small awards are made to GDPs with little or no previous research experience. However, there is invariably considerable competition for these awards, and applicants are well-advised to obtain help from experienced researchers with their application forms and protocols.

Success in winning such awards, followed by successful completion of the project and a resulting publication, does help to establish a track record, as does the possession of a research degree such as a PhD or other doctorate.

Above all else, expert advice is important in defining the total cost of a proposed programme of research. Considerable difficulties may arise if a project is only partly completed and the available funds have been spent. Both under- and overpricing of an application may result in rejection.

14.4.3. Writing the application

The application is a research protocol structured to the particular specifications and requirements of the funder. The application should cover

- The aims and objectives of the project;
- The methods to be employed;
- The proposed timetable of work;
- Full details of the resources required, including a schedule of payment; and
- Details of how any funds awarded will be managed.

The onus is to demonstrate to the funder(s) that the applicant(s) can conduct the proposed project effectively. This involves not only having a good idea but presenting it clearly and concisely to whoever has been appointed to assess the application.

14.4.4. Features of a well-written application

14.4.4.1. Content

If application forms are provided, they will almost certainly cover the headings described in Chapter 12 (writing a protocol). In addition, it will provide sections for the senior investigator(s) to set out a brief CV and details of previous work and publications relevant to the application. The latter are frequently of crucial importance as the best indication of future success is past success.[2]

Those who assess research grant applications look for experience in previous projects relevant to the proposed project and a good publication record. These are deemed to demonstrate productivity and expertise. Also, they look for sufficient detail in the methods section to demonstrate how the research problem will be tackled. A short report of a successful pilot study is also beneficial for the funding body.

A North American review of successful research grant awards[3] suggested that they had the following attributes.

- Achievable specific aims;
- A testable hypothesis;
- Preliminary data to support the hypothesis;
- A relevant research plan and experimental design;
- Appropriate resources;
- Addressed a significant issue/question;
- A clear explanation of validation and quality control processes; and
- An explanation of how any findings would affect clinical practice or public health.

14.4.4.2. Physical appearance of the application

A well laid-out, well-written application enhances the chances of success and demonstrates a thorough approach to the assessors. Only include relevant information and write in a concise style, using plain, grammatically correct English. It is a good idea to download or photocopy the application forms and make draft copies to avoid corrections on the final form.

14.5. Final checks

Check that the application

- Identifies the appropriate granting body or agency to contact for your proposal (this is of paramount importance as each body usually has its particular sphere of activity);
- Describes succinctly the goal of the proposed research and how its aim(s) will be achieved;
- Identifies the problem that the research is intended to address, details what is known about the problem in the scientific literature and highlights the perceived gaps or limitations;
- States precisely what it will have achieved if the project succeeds, and the likely effect of a successful research project;
- Describes, if possible, how the research is likely to contribute to patient care and patient benefit;
- Details experimental design and describes how it will answer the set questions;
- States clearly that the applicants are aware of any potential limitations in their approach and, if possible, proposes an alternative approach if the first approach fails (unless this is done, the reviewers may identify them and reject the proposal);
- Gives examples of any previous personal works that suggest that the proposed study will succeed;
- Describes the study's design briefly, how the sample size will be calculated, and, if applicable, what randomisation procedure will be used;
- Describes how it is planned to recruit research subjects and what criteria you will be set for including or excluding particular individuals;
- Describes how informed consent will be obtained and which authorities have given ethics approval for the research; and
- States clearly how the collaborators in the study will strengthen the proposal.

Suggested further reading

A search of the Internet will reveal many sources of advice on writing grant applications, including the United States National Institute of Health. Bethesda, MD 20892, USA Advice on preparing research grant applications. At http://www.grants.gov/web/grants/team-grants.hl

References

1 UK Government, Apprenticeship Training Courses 2021, accessed 14 November 2021. https://findapprenticeshiptraining.apprenticeships.education.gov.uk/Courses.

2 Simons-Morton DG. Funding Avenues for Research in Emergency Medicine at the National Institutes of Health and the National Heart, Lung and Blood Institute. *Academic. Emergency Medicine*, 1996;3:202-204.

3 Bain RL, Nyberg LM. Funding for urolithiasis research: progress and strategies for future NIH support. *Journal of Endourology*,. 1995;9:299-300.

Chapter 15. Piloting the Methods and Project Management

SUVAN J.

15.1. Overview

This chapter addresses the seventh stage of a research project. Once the study protocol has been written, which provides the blueprint for a project, and funding plus ethics approval have been obtained, the next stage is to pilot (test) the project methods then conduct (implement) and manage the study.[1] Increased emphasis on the importance of evidence-based practice and the role of research evidence in clinical guidelines has brought enhanced awareness of quality aspects of clinical research conduct. Study management facilitates adherence to the protocol, regulations or research governance to ensure participant safety and robust results are achieved in an efficient manner.[2]

The chapter is divided into the following sections:

- Introduction;
- Piloting the methodology;
- Logistical elements of project management;
- Regulatory aspects of project management;
- Summary; and
- Further resources

15.2. Introduction

This chapter expands the reader's understanding of research operations, that is, the preparation and deployment of the project in a manner directed toward accomplishment of the research objectives. The principles are the same regardless of the size or location of the project, whether a general practice or the facilities of a large international pharmaceutical company. Even the best-designed study may go drastically wrong if poorly implemented, rendering the collected data meaningless. This often occurs due to seemingly small mistakes, even in a single but critical step in the conduct of the study methodologies embedded within the protocol. Piloting the study methods followed by attentive and continual management are crucial for the success of any study. The underlying concept of robust study conduct lies in the aim to minimise bias, working at all times to ensure that results are as valid as possible.[3]

In addition, any study involving humans or samples collected from humans (for example, studies in a pathology laboratory) must be conducted in a manner compliant with the regulations governing clinical research.[4, 5] Finally, as discussed in the chapter on ethics approval, codes of ethical behaviour are designed to protect study participants and individuals who might eventually benefit from the treatment being investigated.[6] Thus, elements of project management facilitate scientific features while other elements focus on participant protection and regulatory compliance.[5, 7]

The subsequent sections of this paper will outline and explain simple procedures or practical steps proven to minimise bias during a study implementation, whilst also facilitating participant protection and resource use. These aspects lie within the two key operational aspects of clinical research conduct referred to as methodology piloting and project management.

15.3. Piloting the methods

Establishing a framework for clinical study implementation begins by piloting all protocol steps and the associated methods to confirm the feasibility and consistency of the defined operational procedures. Piloting should incorporate elements of training, calibration, clinical visits and study schedule, systems to obtain appropriate study supplies, recruitment procedures, as well any support activities by external collaborators be they administrative, technical, clinical, or laboratory in nature.[8] Although a robust, well-designed protocol seems overtly clear when written, research projects are conducted by individuals, not machines. Furthermore, implementation of a detailed protocol may give rise to unexpected issues, many of which can be highlighted during piloting. Keep in mind, the most well-deliberated plan may overlook some highly unexpected or undesirable surprises. The following sections highlight procedures that should be followed to help minimise the need for amendments which can be laborious and time consuming following study commencement.

15.4. Training

Accuracy in clinical research data collection is paramount for robust results.[9] Therefore, all individuals involved in or interfacing with the project should be thoroughly familiar with their defined study tasks or methodologies beyond the extent of knowing how to perform them correctly. The target is that the task is so practiced that it not only can be performed correctly but is difficult to be performed incorrectly. In addition, the consistency of each individual and between individuals is vital. For example, in some epidemiological studies, researchers responsible for gathering data should be trained to the same consistent standard, and any potential researcher who is an outlier in terms of observations or consistency should be excluded. Therefore, it follows that all persons responsible for carrying out a given task should be trained to the same gold standard, during simultaneous training, when possible. This small step avoids variation (and thus bias) in explanations or the understanding of key elements of potentially technique sensitive measurements or procedures.

15.4.1. Calibration

Many procedures incorporated in research projects are already well known to clinicians. Healthcare professionals often have pre-existing routines, habits, or approaches in performing what are normally thought of as standard techniques. However, a study protocol may require small modifications to a standard procedure, or a change in sequence of procedures compared to standard clinical practice. Calibration is a part of piloting methodologies serving to confirm the planned procedures are highly repeatable.[9,10] It often assists to "reprogram" researchers to perform common tasks in a highly consistent manner. It is a form of training aimed at a performance level that ensures the data gathered are within a predefined limit of error (repeatability) when repeating the same task multiple times. Repeatability refers to the level at which a single individual can repeat the same task in a consistent manner minimising variation, particularly important when collecting data based upon clinician measurements or assessments. This is referred to as calibrating against oneself or intra-examiner repeatability.

Calibration may also target minimising differences in the performance of procedures between two or more designated individuals known as inter-examiner calibration.[10] Examiner calibration is performed to train examiners in standardised techniques and quantify the inter-examiner variation. The measure of variability obtained during calibration can later be accounted for during analysis and interpretation of the study data. Calibration may also refer to agreement during duplicate performance of any study intervention. For example, how interview questions are asked in obtaining qualitative data, the consistency with which use of a study product is explained to participants at the time of product dispensing, or the technique used for a medical procedure. Perhaps a good example of a technique sensitive procedure is recording of blood pressure as variation can occur due relatively small differences such as cuff positioning, participant position, or whether the participant is speaking or quiet during the measurement. Ensuring each clinician performs it in precisely the same manner is essential to internal validity of the results.

15.4.2. Schedules

All aspects of scheduling and visit or procedure timing should also be piloted before a study commences to facilitate definition of time required for each task or procedure included as a part of each unique study visit. Accurate definition of "time per task" serves to facilitate overall predictions of time required per participant/visit and defines overall associated clinic and administrative time. Piloting timing of each step may allow study coordinators to see imbalances or bottlenecks in the flow of a study appointment. This can be particularly important in scenarios where a participant is seen by multiple researchers during a study visit. For example, one researcher may assess a condition using one index or measurement tool and a second researcher assessing another aspect thereafter. In the context of the overall project, efficient use of time is a critical element of study implementation as each study has set costs/funding that require maximisation of resource use to meet defined budgets. Particularly in practice settings, consideration must be given to study implementation to minimise influence on regular practice activities.

15.4.3. Supplies

Piloting of the project is a confirming step for anticipated supply requirements both in terms of supply specifications and quantities. All products used in a study should be identical, including instruments, materials, and pharmacological or over-the-counter (OTC) agents. For example, different brands of medical instruments may have minor differences in graduations or calibrations that could introduce variability of measurements. Biological products such as regenerative membranes or patient self-care products should be supplied from the same production lot for all study participants. This may need to allow for the shelf life of a product or medication, hence the need for accurate estimates of time for study recruitment and time needed to complete all study visits. An example to demonstrate this might be saliva sample tubes available in various shapes and sizes with some more suitable for storage and others suited for sample collection. When one tries to spit into such a collection tube, it is realised how important the design of the tube can be to the amount of saliva collected. In a study assessing a biofluid, bio-substance, such as bacterial biofilm or a biomarker, the detection level of the assessment technique, dye, or assay might also affect the ease and consistency of assessments performed, and therefore results.

15.4.4. Recruitment

Recruitment strategy is one of the most important aspects of any study and has been shown to be improved by piloting prior to study commencement.[10, 11] Recruitment spans from the first approach to inform a potential participant of a project, to explain the study, and then follow up to confirm their interest to participate and obtaining written informed consent. A participant is only considered recruited once they have signed the consent form. Bottlenecks or unanticipated challenges in any of these steps can affect overall recruitment rates substantially.[12] If difficulties are encountered at one stage, the entire study may be delayed, which can increase costs, due to extra staffing or facility costs associated with the extended time needed to complete the study visits for all participants.

The delicate manner that the study objectives or procedures are explained may significantly influence the willingness of potential participants to consider participation. Explanations provided by staff involved in recruitment need to be consistent and honour patient autonomy in line with regulatory requirements.[13] If it is feasible and within regulatory guidance, an opt out approach enables greater numbers to be recruited compared to an opt in approach. In this approach, participants may tentatively be included and proceed to the next step of scheduling with the condition that they initiate contact to withdraw after consideration of study information provided, then the tentative appointment will be cancelled. Approaches and systems such as this should be tried and defined based on experiences encountered during piloting. In any explanation, there can be the glass half full approach or the glass half empty message. The challenge is to discern how the patient would see the glass half full when considering study participation. This can be quite different to a clinician's view of the benefits of study participation.

Piloting is an opportunity to explore patient views. It is advised to get feedback from potential study participants as to the adequacy of information and the manner of presentation, or even the feasibility of the study visits or procedures. It is noteworthy that many potential participants are most concerned about the novel element of the research; is it the intervention or the methods of measurement. Many studies do not include a novel intervention but instead might be investigating the effect of a known intervention on an unexplored outcome. It is worthwhile to clarify this to alleviate concerns when interventions or products are not investigative. On the other hand, it is important to highlight if indeed the intervention is novel as full transparency of information is part of good clinical practice (GDP) consent guidance.[7]

15.4.5. Support requirements

Some steps in research study conduct rely on external collaboration or support. Identified partnerships should also be tested prior to study commencement to ensure services to be provided are commensurate with the study protocol and are deliverable in line with protocol requirements. For example, a dental study investigating the effects of different impression materials on the characteristics of dental restoration crown margins would depend upon partnership with dental technicians and a dental laboratory. In such a case, it might be desirable to have all the work done by one clinician and one technician to minimise variability. This approach might have implications for laboratory production time especially as the scheduling and return of constructed restorations would be dependent on availability of that one person. Ensuring a backup individual is trained should the designated laboratory technician be unable to carry out the task is part of piloting and preparing the system. Piloting of external partnerships can be even more important than those internal to the study setting as the study principal investigator would likely have minimal control of factors that may affect the activities of external collaborators working as part of the research team.

15.5. Logistical elements of project management

For ease of discussion, project management is presented in two sections: the first focuses on logistical elements, the second on those defined by regulatory guidelines. However, it should be noted that these two aspects overlap and are interdependent rather than mutually exclusive. For example, logistics promote study conduct to minimise bias while maximising efficiency in every step. Regulatory guidance highlights that a study conducted in a disorganised, inefficient manner with inadequate attention to consistency is an unethical study and puts participants at risk.[6] Hence, operational details of either logistical aspects or research regulations and governance facilitate both of these two facets of study implementation. Project management is ultimately the responsibility of the principal investigator. However, this is normally delegated to a study coordinator for day-to-day implementation supplemented by regular study update meetings. It is a distinct research role as it requires substantial allocated time due to the need for comprehensive and continual focus on detail.[14]

15.5.1. Project initiation

The first step in managing a research project is the organisation of the study commencement which occurs through a study initiation meeting. The initiation meeting is held with all study team members present including the principal investigator and the statistician. It should be held before piloting study methodologies (referred to earlier) and confirms final agreement and understanding by all study team members on every aspect of the study protocol and its implementation. It informs each member of study activities that are within their individual role or responsibility. Roles are confirmed and defined to the final level of detail. The meeting agenda is determined by the protocol with the normal format being to go step by step through each page of the protocol clarifying methods, roles, supplies, and other factors that characterise each step. A typical study initiation meeting requires a minimum of three hours depending on the size of the complexity of the protocol and the size of the research team. Imagine it to be an enactment of the study visits, hence is often referred to as a dry run of the study. It may involve role playing, to provide examples of study recruitment conversations, during which a clinician explains facets of study participation to an individual unaware of the project details. Elements of the piloting or training mentioned earlier may be combined with study initiation hence sometimes may require as much as one or more days. The meeting is led by the study coordinator and principal investigator with other key roles leading pertinent sections. For example, the study examiner might coordinate discussions of study assessments with treatment clinicians leading discussions of study treatments.

Beyond defining roles and tasks, the study initiation meeting is a time to define and set practical systems in place that will orchestrate consistent and smooth running of the study. Without defined systems linking together as a chain or sequence of gears, the risk for bottlenecks or problems in the study are high. Furthermore, any break in the chain can put the quality of the data at risk.

15.5.2. Participant recruitment

Following study initiation, the subsequent project management focus is study recruitment. The techniques employed should allow for eventual calculation of the recruitment rate (ratio of those enrolled compared to potential participants approached). Logs should be kept, recording participants deemed suitable for inclusion in the study. This can be used to direct distribution of study participant information leaflets and invitations to participate. A record of study information distribution should be kept including date sent or provided. As participants agree to or decline participation, this is noted in the log together with the reason if participation is declined. As mentioned, the number of participants recruited divided by the number approached provides the recruitment rate, an element critical to study resource allocation and flow. For example, if one out of every five individuals approached agrees to participate versus one out of every ten approached, the effect on recruiting time is far more significant and the resources to distribute information are higher. In addition, use of recruitment logs allows researchers to discern if difficulties in recruitment are related to too few suitable participants or too few suitable individuals agreeing to participate. This is important as the potential solution would be different in each case.

Furthermore, scientific publication requires reporting of recruitment rate and reasons for non-participation to facilitate consideration of potential selection bias at the time of study recruitment.

15.5.3. Participant flow and retention

Once participants are enrolled in the study, the demands of management increase as it is vital to ensure all study procedures, visits, or aspects such as the return of questionnaires, occur within time frames defined in the study protocol. It is essential to retain as many study participants as possible to the end of the study to minimise bias associated with loss-to-follow-up. Various computer programs facilitate tracking of study visits from simple Excel spreadsheets to complex databases, designed specifically for this purpose. It is essential that the date of every visit is logged, allowing easy identification of missed visits or visits taking place outside accepted time windows defined in the protocol. In studies with extended follow-up or numerous participants, this works to prevent participants from "falling between the cracks" if they miss a visit. When a study appointment is cancelled, it should normally be rescheduled as soon as possible as it is easy to forget a patient who has left a message on a voicemail system. Participants attending at timepoint that deviate from those defined in the protocol or drop-outs may result in significant bias in the study results, particularly if too many the participants lost during follow-up were part of the same group within the study, for example in a test or control group or if the loss results in insufficient numbers to reach the protocol defined study sample size.

15.6. Project monitoring and quality assurance

The Oxford Advanced Learners online dictionary defines monitoring as "to watch and check something over a period of time in order to see how it develops, so that you can make any necessary changes."[15]

In the context of clinical research, it is precisely the same. Monitoring is carried out throughout a study in the same manner as an ongoing audit of all aspects to ensure study compliance with both the protocol and regulatory guidelines.[4, 11] Monitoring includes observing each task including all clinical and laboratory procedures and administrative tasks to verify consistency with the initial training or systems agreed upon during study initiation. It can be easy for clinicians to drift back to previous clinical habits over time, therefore constant follow-up serves to remind the study team of details previously agreed.

Without ongoing monitoring, small critical changes can be overlooked. For example, imagine a scenario related to the saliva samples mentioned earlier. During the study initiation, it is agreed that saliva should be placed immediately into a -20°Celsius freezer in an area in the back of the clinical practice some distance from the clinic area. Some weeks after the study commencement, a member of the study team normally responsible for storing the sample after collection notes that there is a 4°C refrigerator closer to the clinic area. For pragmatic reasons, the thought emerges to collect all samples from the morning session in the 4°C refrigerator before taking them all to the -20°C in a batch at midday to avoid losing time walking back and forth to the -20°C freezer during the clinical visits. A simple timesaving step evokes a disaster for the samples as it is forgotten that substantial biological information is lost from saliva with each minute that passes prior to freezing. Such an error can occur so easily without notice and can occur due to attempts to improve an alternate aspect of the study, in this case clinical efficiency. In the scenario cited, regular monitoring of study activity and tasks picked up the change allowing quick reversion to the original plan.

Constant communication within the study team is essential and an efficient way to monitor all activity.[16] Depending on project complexity, size, duration, the weekly occurrence of study visits, and the study team size, study meetings may be held weekly, biweekly, or monthly. Less frequently than monthly is not advised as small errors can have significant effect on the study data if not discovered early. Evaluation and discussion of each step with potential to impact on study data or study efficiency at regular intervals allows the study team to capitalise on aspects working well and alter those that could be improved. Efficiency in all aspects of the study implementation is vital, hence the need for ongoing assessment of operational aspects.

Monitoring of study data collection forms and study files is another essential part of study monitoring and can also highlight areas where study conduct as gradually digressed away from the study protocol. This may be performed internally by members of the study team or alternatively by a person external to the team. In many studies funded by an industrial sponsor, the sponsor will be responsible to monitor source documents and study data collection forms plus procedures of the study.

15.6.1. Contingency plans

Contingency plans are part of any successful project management. In the same manner that specifically defined project plans must be in place before a study begins, a good contingency plan is required to cope with the unexpected. This is most pertinent regarding the study personnel and their defined roles, in particular those that have a particular responsibility such as a calibrated study examiner. As discussed previously, some may be very specifically trained, therefore a plan should be in place for cover should they be unable to carry out their defined role.

15.7. Regulatory elements of project management

Reverting to research governance, project management carries with it many requirements defined by regulatory bodies. Although sometimes time consuming and often criticised for their effect on timeliness of study conduct, regulations are essential for protection of study participants, researchers and ultimately improving the quality of all aspects of study management. For example, regulatory guidance requires documentation of all study activities to a level that would enable the project to be re-enacted, much like a theatre play, should any issue arise around a treatment or product at the time it is implemented on a broader scale. In addition, it defines the systems that should be in place to ensure accurate data protection and archiving of all information related to the study.

15.7.1. Study initiation

Regulatory requirements at the time of study initiation include full documentation of all steps that have been taken to ensure appropriate training of members of the study team. These form the contents of the study initiation report. In addition, the primary study file, sometimes referred as the investigator file, is started at this point. It contains a copy of all documents such as the protocol, participant information sheet, consent form, communication with ethics committees, sample data collection forms, equipment specifications, delegation logs, recruitment logs, and study product details. It also includes sample signatures of all individuals who may sign study forms, curricula vitae and professional registration details of researchers.

15.7.2. Study duration

Throughout the duration of the study regulatory elements of study management are focused on communication with the ethics committee with attention to two main facets related to participant safety. The first is the requirements for reporting adverse events experienced by participants during the study. Documentation of adverse events in the study forms is compulsory, including assessment of the nature of the event, the seriousness and possible relation to the study. In the rare event of a severe event, particular attention must be given to adverse events that result in hospitalisation. All hospitalisations must be reported to the principal investigator within twenty-four hours and to the ethics committee within a defined limit of time, typically fifteen days maximum, in addition to the usual procedures following incidents within a clinic or practice. Repeat occurrence of a similar adverse event may require a study to be stopped to protect participants. Therefore, this is a vital step of study management and documentation. It is important to know regulatory guidance on adverse events for the jurisdiction where the study is taking place.

The second important regulatory aspect is communication with the ethics committee regarding any required changes to the protocol during the study. It is not unusual that alterations to a study protocol are identified during the study. This can be for logistical reasons, such as to improve study recruitment or, sometimes due to new scientific knowledge that has come available since study initiation. Amendments are only allowed after submission and approval by the original ethics committee that has approved the project before it started. It will usually involve altering participant information leaflets and consent forms which in turn requires the reconsenting of active study participants with the updated version of the consent form. This formal process for any alterations to the initial protocol facilitates consistency in study procedures.

15.7.3. Study closure

Similarly, as there are defined regulatory procedures to study initiation and monitoring during active recruitment and follow-up, there are also defined steps at the end of a study. For example, the end date is usually defined as the last participant last study visit, however after this, time is allocated to data preparation for analysis and final reporting of results to ethics committees, study sponsors and participants in some cases. In addition, research governance defines the required time for study documents need to be kept or archived and techniques for destroying study samples or documentation following the defined archive period. In general, about one third of the overall study duration is attributed to study initiation, about one third to active recruitment and follow-up and one third for data management and study closure tasks. Based on this, the overall study duration can be defined by calculating the time needed for study visits then adding equal time prior to commencement of study visits and following completion to allow for study preparation and closure tasks.

15.8. Summary

Irrespective of the research study setting, i.e., a primary dental care practice, a teaching hospital or a laboratory, attention to minimising bias is situated at the heart of robust study results. Piloting methodologies and project management emerge as invaluable parts of performing research. A well-constructed blueprint (protocol) is essential but only as good as the implementation to achieve valid results. Piloting of methodologies and project management demand equal, if not more, time and effort as construction of the plan. Therefore, a well-defined strategy and sufficient resources should be set a priori to ensure adequate operational aspects are not overlooked.

Further resources

Pocock, S. J. 2013,. *Clinical trials; a practical approach.* Chichester West Sussex: Wiley, 2013.

Association of Clinical Research Professionals https://acrpnet.org/.

National Institute for Health Research Clinical Trials Toolkit, https://www.ct-toolkit.ac.uk/.

Department of Health (DH). Research Governance Framework for Health and Social Care London: DH; 2005, http://www.dh.gov.uk/en/publications.

National Institute of Health Research Clinical Research Guide https://www.nihr.ac.uk/documents/clinical-trials-guide/20595.Giannobile, W., Burt, B., Genco, R. (Editors), 2010, *Clinical Research in Oral Health*, Wiley-Blackwell; 2010.

References

1 Eaton KA, Santini A. An Introduction to Research for Primary Dental Care Clinicians: Part 3: Stage 5. Writing a Protocol. *Primary Dental Care.* 2011(2):91–94.

2 UK MRC. Good Research Practice 2021, https://mrc.ukri.org/research/policies-and-guidance-for-researchers/good-research-practice/.

3 Farrell B, Kenyon S, Shakur H. Managing clinical trials. Trials. 2010;11(1):1-6.

4 NHS-HRA. UK Policy Framework for Health and Social Care Research: NHS Health Research Authority 2020, available from: https://www.hra.nhs.uk/planning-and-improving-research/policies-standards-legislation/uk-policy-framework-health-social-care-research/.

5 Rickham P. Human experimentation. Code of ethics of the world medical association. Declaration of Helsinki. *British Medical Journal.* 1964;2(5402):177-183.

6 Santini A, Eaton KA. An Introduction to Research for Primary Dental Care Clinicians: Part 4: Stage 6a. Obtaining Ethical Approval. *Primary Dental Care.* 2011(3):127-132.

7 Barth I, Krafft H, Weber G, Keller-Stanislawski B, Cichutek K. Good clinical practice in the European Union. *Human Gene Therapy.* 2008;19(5):441-442.

8 Giannobile WV, Burt BA, Genco RJ. Clinical research in oral health: John Wiley & Sons; 2009.

9 Polson AM. The research team, calibration, and quality assurance in clinical trials in periodontics. *Annals of Periodontology.* 1997;2(1):75-82.

10 Pocock SJ. Clinical trials: a practical approach: John Wiley & Sons; 2013.

11 Prescott R, Counsell C, Gillespie W, Grant A, Russell I, Kiauka S, et al. Factors that limit the quality, number and progress of randomised controlled trials: a review. *Health Technology Assessment.* 1999;3:1-143.

12 Mapstone J, Elbourne D, Roberts I. Strategies to improve recruient to research studies (Cochrane Methodology Review). The Cochrane Library. 2004(1).

13 Wade J, Donovan JL, Lane JA, Neal DE, Hamdy FC. It's not just what you say, it's also how you say it: opening the 'black box' of informed consent appoinents in randomised controlled trials. *Social Science & Medicine.* 2009;68(11):2018-2028.

14 Farrell B. Efficient management of randomised controlled trials: nature or nurture. *British Medical Journal.* 1998;317(7167):1236-1239.

15 Turnbull J, Lea D, Parkinson D, Phillips P, Francis B, Webb S, et al. Oxford advanced learner's dictionary. International Student's Edition. 2010.

16 Bertram S, Graham D, Kurland M, Pace W, Madison S, Yawn BP. Communication is the key to success in pragmatic clinical trials in practice-based research networks (PBRNs). *The Journal of the American Board of Family Medicine.* 2013;26(5):571-578.

Chapter 16. Collecting and Collating Data

SANTINI A., HOWE M-S.

16.1. Overview

This chapter describes how to collect and collate data, which is stage 8 in a research study. After an introduction, the chapter covers

- Data collection;
- Data management systems;
- Data validation;
- The use of pre-existing records;
- Data confidentiality; and
- Training data collectors.

16.2. Introduction

Data collection is the systematic procedure in which measurements and observations are collected during a research study. The collected data are subsequently analysed, and conclusions are made regarding the study.[1] Table 1 below sets out an overview of data collection and analysis.

Before collecting data, it is imperative to consider the following:

- The aim of the research;
- The type of data to be collected;
- The types of study appropriate to obtain the required data; and
- The methods and procedures to be employed to collect, store, and analyse the data.

Data collection methods should be clarified during the earliest stages of a research study. Details of the type of data and the methods of acquiring and analysing them should be written into the research protocol and related to the study's stated aim. Once collected, they should be stored in a form that allows the analysis of the acquired data.[2]

Data collection	Analyses
• Data are collected in a convenient form; • An account and conclusions are composed around it; • In the account and conclusions, discussions should be kept concise and interesting.	• Analysing results for a case study tends to be based more on opinion or interpretation than statistical methods; • There is no right or wrong answer in a case study; • Though numerical data are helpful, the main objective is to judge trends or processes and not analyse every datum; • Maintain focus by referring to the original reference points.

Table 1. Data collection and analyses

The many types of study and aspects of their design have been covered in earlier chapters of this book.[1] The covered topics include quantitative studies; randomised controlled studies; qualitative studies; systematic reviews; sampling; questionnaires; screening and diagnostic testing; and prognosis, diagnosis, risk, and prognostic study methods.

16.3. Collection of quantitative and qualitative data

As described in previous chapters, research methodology can be separated into two main categories, quantitative research and qualitative research.

Quantitative data is information about quantities, and therefore numbers, and qualitative data is descriptive and deals with observed occurrences, which are not usually measured.

The foremost characteristic of quantitative data is that they are gathered using structured research instruments. The results should be based on larger sample sizes that are representative of the population. The research study can usually be replicated or repeated, given its high reliability.[3, 4]

Table 2 sets out the differences between quantitative and qualitative research studies:

Character	Quantitative Data	Qualitative Data
Definition	Expressed in quantities, values, or numbers	Expressed by quality
Research question	Test theory Validate	Build theory Describe
Nature of Data	Numerical	Descriptive
Measurability	Measurable (such as length, size, weight, and time)	Generally not measured Narratives and descriptive
Research process	Tightly structured Known variables Set methodology	Loosely structured Unknown variables Variable methodology

Collection Method	Using an objective approach. Data collected and analysed by statistics Numerical Sample size calculated, often large Specific measurement instruments	Using a subjective approach. Data acquired by observation. Text, image Sample size not calculated, often small Non-standardised interviews
Data Structure	Structured: establishes the level of occurrence	Unstructured: describes the depth of understanding
Data analysis	Statistical Deductive reasoning	Looking for themes and patterns Inductive reasoning
Reliability	A statistical approach lends weight in terms of authority and reliability	Not so reliable and objective
Data Collection Techniques	Experiments and quantitative surveys	Qualitative surveys.
Outcome presentation	Statistical Numerical Formal	Words Narrative

Table 2. Differences between quantitative and qualitative approaches to research

16.3.1. Qualitative data

Qualitative data are also known as categorical or nonnumerical data.

Examples of qualitative data include

- Gender;
- Marital status;
- Nationality;
- Binary data (when only two possibilities are available for a categorical variable);
- Multi-category data (occurs when there are more than two possible categories).

16.3.2. Quantitative data

Quantitative data are also known as numerical data and are classified as either discrete or continuous.

Discrete data have a finite number of possible values and tend to be comprised of integers (whole numbers).

Continuous data has infinite possibilities. Continuous data values can include decimal places:

Diameter of tumours: 1.50 cm, 2.65 cm

Height of children: 0.92 m, 1.27m, 1.52m

The types of data that may be collected are listed in Table 3:

Quantitative data are presented in numbers and graphs. Statistical methods are used to analyse the acquired data.
Qualitative data are presented in words, phrases or sentences. The researcher then interprets and classifies them.
Primary data are originally sourced data collected firsthand by the researcher for a specific research purpose or project. Examples of primary data: establishing opinions towards health services, determining the health needs of a population or society, determining the job satisfaction of the employees, measuring the service quality provided by employees.
Secondary data are acquired from already existing datasets. They have been collected previously for a specific purpose and documented. As a result, secondary data are speedily accessed, unlike primary data. To create a new dataset, variables for analysis can be selected from one secondary data source or combined from different sources. Examples include hospital record cards, census data, books, websites, and government records.
Cross-sectional data are collected by observing subjects or themes at a single time point or single space point. Their primary limitation is that they cannot describe changes over time or cause and effect relationships in which one variable affects the other.
Categorical variables represent types of data that may be divided into groups. Categorical data are qualitative and cannot be measured numerically. The categorical data are also known as attributes. Examples include race, sex, age group.
Univariate data: A data set consisting of observation on a single characteristic is a univariate data set. When the observations are categorical responses, the data are said to constitute a univariate data set.
Time series data are collected when the same measurements, such as blood pressure, temperature, weight, and populations are recorded over different periods, such as hourly, daily, monthly, and yearly. The data accumulated in this fashion are termed time-series data (e.g. population in a different period).
Ordered data: This refers to data recorded as ordered categories that constitute an ordered data set. They differ from categorical variables only in that there is an explicit ordering of the variables. For example: pain grades ordered data may be low, medium, and high.

Table 3. Types of data

16.3.3. Converting quantitative data to qualitative data

Qualitative data tend to be measured on nominal or ordinal scales. Quantitative data tend to be measured on interval or ratio scales.

Nominal and ordinal data can be analysed with non-parametric statistics. On the other hand, interval and ratio data can be analysed using parametric statistics.

Quantitative data can be converted into categorical data by using cut-off points.

For example, biological measurements or results from rating scales are often converted into disease or no disease. This is because categorical data are easier to tabulate and analyse. However, the conversion means some data are discarded, and it gets harder to detect a statistically significant difference. Also subjects at either side of the cut-off point end up with very different levels of risk.

16.4. Data variables and scales

A typical data classification is made by placing data into one of four measurement scale types: nominal, ordinal, interval, and ratio. Interval and ratio data are designated continuous scale data.

The measurement scale specifies the kinds of mathematical analyses that can be carried out on the acquired data. For example, measurement scales are used when describing the properties of variables.

An appropriate study design or methodology should refer back and apply to the stated aims and objectives of the study and is central, not only for the realisation of the study but also for acquiring satisfactory data. Good data collection follows from the researcher having a grasp of the strengths and weaknesses of different research designs.

Having decided on the type of data to be collected, the next step is to choose the method best suited for the study (Table 4):

Experimental clinical research is mainly a quantitative method.
Surveys, observations, archival research and secondary data collection can be quantitative or qualitative methods.
Interviews and focus groups are predominantly qualitative methods.

Table 4. Choosing a quantitative or qualitative method

16.4.1. Data variables

A variable is when there are two or more values for a characteristic that is under investigation. Variables may be classified into different categories. A continuous variable has an infinite number of possible values; for example, in measuring patients' ages, it would be possible, although unlikely, to record them down to the nearest second. However, discrete variables have a set number of values; for example, the Löe and Silness (1963) Gingival Index[6] has four discrete values—0, 1, 2, and 3—for the assessment of gingival inflammation. Variables in research may also be classified as administrative or research. Administrative variables contain metadata, which describes the content and context of the data and enhance the value of the data stored as it may record, for example, dates, times and personnel involved. Research data are the variables and outcomes from the research activity and comprise the data used for the primary analysis.

16.4.2. Data scales

The different types of data scales are described in this sub-sub-section, and the statistical tests used to assess them are included in Table 4.

16.4.2.1. Nominal

Nominal data is the simplest of the measurement scales where each observation is allocated a description or name. The only inferences that can be made are based on whether the categories are the same or not and the frequency with which categories occur. Consider data showing the preferred types of hat, where the options were beret, beanie, ascot cap, and balmoral cap. The resultant data will only allow a count of the number of times each type of chosen hat or a comparison, based on people's response. For example, the first three people preferred a beret, and the fourth person's preference was different from the first three.

Data scale	Description	Statistical test
Nominal data (Categorical data)	Numbers are used only to identify different categories and have no meaning themselves.	Chi-squared Mode
Ordinal data	Numbers are used to show a sequence or order but do not indicate numerical differences.	Median Percentile
Interval data	Numbers reflect standard and equal units of measurement and the size of differences.	Mean Standard deviation Regression Analysis of variance
Ratio data	Similar to interval data but with a true zero point	Same as Interval data, plus Geometric mean/harmonic mean Coefficient of variation

Table 4. Data scales and statistical tests used to assess them

16.4.2.2. Ordinal

Ordinal data also uses descriptions or labels. However, there is a collation between the labels. e.g. Consider asking twenty people to rate the pain reduction after taking a prescribed analgesic, giving them the choices of no difference, slightly, moderately, significantly. The generated data could be, nine reported no difference; three reported slightly, two reported moderate difference;

and five reported a significant difference. Nominal data also allows relative comparisons to be made (e.g. person a, b, and c experienced slightly less pain but not as much as persons x and y). A summary of the variables can be made based on the median. In the above sample, the median level of pain reduction is "no difference."

Continuous scale data (interval or ratio): In continuous data points where there is a function of series and category. The grade between each number is the same and measurable. Continuous scale data consist of two types of data scales, interval scale and ratio scale.

The only difference between interval and ratio scale data is whether or not the referred scale has an absolute zero.

16.4.2.3. Interval data

Interval data have been assigned a numeric value. This permits the calculation of quantitative differences between values. For example, Edinburgh temperatures measured in degrees centigrade over seven days in February were 9, 8, 8, 7, 6, 8, and 8. From the first day to the fourth day, temperatures fell by two degrees. By the fifth day, the temperature was three degrees lower than the first; the seventh day was two degrees higher than on the fifth day. These calculations cannot be made with ordinal scores, as the numbers represent a category. Another example applies to the assessment of pain. It cannot be specified with any certainty that the quantification of pain reduction difference between no difference and slightly different is equal to the quantification of pain reduction between moderately different and significantly different. Interval data's power is that averages and variances can be computed, which are fundamental to statistical and analysis calculations, such as correlation, linear regression.

16.4.2.4. Ratio data

On a ratio scale, numbers have units of equal size and rank order. The scale has an absolute zero. For example, consider the temperature data above. Ratios cannot be calculated with the Celsius readings For example, it is not very meaningful to state that on a day when the temperature was 9°C, it was 9/6 warmer than on day five when the temperature was 6°C.

Compare this with four athletes completing a training schedule. If the athletes completed twelve, fourteen, seven, nineteen hours of training per week, a valid statement is that we can say that the second athlete completed twice as many hours as the third person. The defining property of ratio scale data is the capability of calculating ratios. Another way of recognising a ratio scale is to determine if the value of 0 on the scale signifies the absence of everything. In this example, zero hours means precisely that an athlete did not complete any training. Compare that with the temperature example. Zero° C does *not* mean there was no temperature.

Table 5 compares interval scale data and ratio scale data:

Interval scale data
When numbers have units that are of equal magnitude as well as rank order on a scale without an absolute zero
Interval data can have an arbitrarily assigned zero. This, however, does not relate to an absence of the measured variable.
Example: temperature in Celsius.
Ratio scale data
When numbers have units that are of equal magnitude as well as rank order on a scale with an absolute zero.
Examples include heart rate, blood pressure, distance.

Table 5. Interval scale data versus ratio scale data

16.5. Data management systems

Data management deals with the entire procedure of what is done with data once they have been collected (see Table 6, below).

It is essential to plan the details of data management from the study's inception and outline it in the study protocol. As explained in Chapter 13, a data manager who is fully responsible for the organisation's storage, security, administration, and data analysis should be appointed.

First-time researchers, who may, for example, be undertaking a small research project as part of an MSc degree, will generally have to be data managers under their supervisors' watchful eye for any data they collect.

A database is a detailed collection of data that stores organised information efficiently and logically. Once an appropriate study has been designed, data are interpreted and reported.

Data, in the framework of databases, denotes the single items that are stored in a database. They can be stored individually or as a set.

Data management describes how data are
<ul><li>Stored, electronically or otherwise;</li><li>Cleaned;</li><li>Manipulated in an appropriate manner; and</li><li>Analysed.</li></ul>

Table 6. Data management

Standardisation of data reduces repetitiveness and facilitates the comparison and analyses of data, as seen in Table 7:

Good database design will
- reduce repetitiveness (such as entering an address or age for a patient multiple times);
- store data in a convenient form for analysis.

Table 7. Good database design and coding conventions

The design of a data management system should cover many issues. Loss of collected data is to be avoided; this would lead to the usually unrealistic necessity of repeating a study or experiment. There are also ethical reasons for safeguarding records, whether these be clinical records or personal details.

Table 8 outlines the main points to be considered:

- Questionnaires should be kept securely in locked cabinets and rooms;
- Identification data should be stored separately;
- The database should be password-protected;
- Adequate database backup procedures should be in place;
- Avoid loss by using backup storage;
- Keep the files and discs separate from the computer; and
- Long-term storage of data should be seven years for observational studies, fifteen years for clinical trials.

Table 8. Points to bear in mind when designing a data management system

16.5.1. Database software

Database software, referred to as a database management system, creates databases.

There are several types of database software, usually classified into six subtypes: analytical database software; data warehouse database software; distributed database software; end-user database software; external database software; and operational database software.

The various functions of database software include

- Data storage;
- Data backup and recovery;
- Data presentation and reporting;
- Multi-user access control;
- Data security management; and
- Database communication.

Care must be taken when entering data into the electronic database. Any inaccuracy in the data entry process will undoubtedly lead to the final data set being inaccurate and inadequate. This is particularly true concerning manually entered data.

The types of database software available and commonly used are given below[4] in Table 9 and types of data entry in Table 10:

- Excel—spreadsheet software useful for simple stats;
- Access—facilitates data entry and tabulation;
- SAS—generally useful for statistical analysis;
- SPSS—incorporates data spreadsheets and robust statistical techniques.

Table 9. Types of database software

Manual entry	Direct entry
• Single entry: one person only enters all the data; • Double-entry: two independent people enter the same forms, and any differences between the two are reconciled. (This is a form of double checking and is more time consuming and expensive.)	• Data collection forms on a computer screen allow direct entry via a web page; • Forms can be fed into a scanner.

Table 10. Types of data entry

16.6. Data validation

Data should also be validated. Validations are quality assurance processes that confirm the data's accuracy during the various phases of the study. Validation should occur before data entry, during data entry and post-data entry.

Table 11 describes data validation methods:

- **Visual review**
Cross-matching data on a questionnaire with source data.

- **Value range checks**
Checking that numbers in the database make sense.
e.g. cholesterol levels should be > 0 and < 20 mmol/L

- **Field type checks**
Checking that text is not entered into numerical fields.

- **Logical**
If an entry is classed as a non-smoker, then cigarettes per day should be 0.

Table 11. Data validation methods

To uphold good data management strategies, data managers should refer to and use the points outlined in Table 12:

- Do not collect data that are already accessible.
- Retain a record of existing sources of data
- Be aware of questionnaire design difficulties.
- Consider and address the expected data inaccuracies.
- Appropriately maintain confidentiality.

Table 12. Data management checklist to support data management strategies

16.7. The use of pre-existing records

An extensive assortment of data is available from pre-existing records, such as hospital admission records and reports. Properly used, these can provide important information. However, they are not without their advantages and disadvantages. Though their use may be time-saving and reduce study expenses and avoid complications associated with de novo data collection, the utmost care should be used to collect such information and use it. Only research data that are necessary to answer the study question should be collected.

Because of the relative ease of accessing the data, researchers should be on their guard against collecting inaccurate or incomplete data. However, not only would this be time-consuming, but it will incur an added expense.

A list of advantages and disadvantages of using existing databases is summarised in Table 13.

Advantages	Disadvantages
Usually specific to a topic e.g. Mortality data ➜ Death Registry • By law, some databases are necessarily complete, such as coroners' reports; • Readily accessible to authorised personnel; • Data have already been collected; • Saves time; and • Reduces expense.	Data may be • incomplete, missing, or not collected; • available as summary statistics only • inaccurate (depending on the vigilance and training of those extracting/entering the data) • not collected for research purposes and biased, e.g. measurement, selection, interviewer biases • of limited accessibility due to confidentiality or business interest, for example Medical records may be subject to • Ambiguity; • Variability in clinician interpretation; • Omission; • Error; • Illegibility; • Selection bias; • Variability in interpretation or handling of missing data; and • Transcription errors.

Table 13. Advantages and disadvantages of using existing databases

16.7. Data confidentiality

Data protection and related data confidentiality refer to the suitable and appropriate use of information about individuals. It pertains to an individual's fundamental right to privacy. It concerns recognising the right of an individual to have control over their own identity and their interactions with others and balancing this with the interests of the populace as a whole. Data protection legislation covers everyone who keeps other people's data. This includes employees, volunteers, service users, members, supporters and donors.

Several institutions, including royal colleges, acknowledge the responsibility of safeguarding personally identifiable data.

Table 14 summarises these principles for data confidentiality, followed by organisations such as the Health and Social Care Information Centre (HSCIC) and the Nuffield Trust:

• Personally identifiable data must be safeguarded by ensuring anonymity or confidentiality under an explicit agreement with the data source's custodian;   • Data collected must be used only for the study designated in the application for ethical approval;   • All personal identifying information from questionnaires and computer files should be removed;   • Link study ID codes with individuals and store them separately from research data; and   • Ensure that no identifiable data is published.

Table 14. Principles for data confidentiality

16.7.1. Caldicott Principles

These principles apply to the use of confidential information and when information is shared and between individuals or organisations for whatever purpose. They affect the collection and use of data from a research study. When a novel or challenging judgment or decision is required, it is advisable to involve a Caldicott Guardian.[6]

See Table 15:

Principle 1: Justify the purpose(s) for using confidential information
Every proposed use or transfer of confidential information should be clearly defined, scrutinised, and documented, with continuing benefits regularly reviewed by an appropriate guardian.
Principle 2: Use confidential information only when it is necessary
Confidential information should not be included unless necessary for the specified purpose(s) for which the information is used or accessed. The need to identify individuals should be considered at each stage of satisfying the purpose(s) and alternatives used where possible.
Principle 3: Use the minimum necessary confidential information
Where the use of confidential information is considered necessary, each item of information must be justified so that only the minimum amount of personal data is included as required for a given function.

Principle 4: Access to confidential information should be on a strictly need-to-know basis
Only those who need access to confidential information should have access to it. Then only to the items they need to see. This may mean introducing access controls or splitting information flows where one flow is used for several purposes.
Principle 5: Everyone with access to confidential information should be aware of their responsibilities
Action should be taken to ensure that all those confidential handling information understand their responsibilities and obligations to respect patient and service users' confidentiality.
Principle 6: Comply with the law
Every use of confidential information must be lawful. All those handling personal information are responsible for ensuring that their use and access to that information comply with legal requirements set out in statute and under the common law.
Principle 7: The duty to share information for individual care is as important as the duty to protect patient confidentiality
Health and social care professionals should have the confidence to share confidential information in patients' best interests and service users within the framework set out by these principles. In addition, they should be supported by the policies of their employers, regulators and professional bodies.
Principle 8: Inform patients and service users about how their confidential information is used.
A protocol by which this can be achieved should be in place.

Table 15. The Caldicott Principles

16.7.2. Information commissioner's office on General Data Protection Regulation (GDPR)

The General Data Protection Regulation (GDPR) was a legal framework that outlined standards for collecting and processing personal information from persons living in the European Union (EU). On leaving the EU in December 2020, the UK GDPR supplanted the EU GDPR. In all particulars, the UK legislation is the same as the EU GDPR, differing only in modifications which makes it work in a UK-only context.

For further information, search the Information Commissioner's Office (ICO) for the webinar "Keep data flow at the end of the UK's transition out of the EU."

16.7.3. What is GDPR compliance?

Under the terms of GDPR, researchers and organisations have to ensure that personal data is gathered legally and under strict conditions. Furthermore, those who collect and manage it are obliged to protect it from misuse and exploitation and respect the rights of data owners. Failure to comply with the regulations can incur penalties for not doing so.

16.8. Health and Social Care Information Centre (HSCIC)

The Health and Social Care Information Centre (HSCIC), which replaced the NHS Information Centre, has the responsibilities set out in Table 16. They are particularly relevant to researchers.

Collecting, analysing, and presenting national health and social care data
Setting up and managing national IT systems for transferring, collecting, and analysing information.
Publishing a code of practice on how personal confidential information of patients should be handled and managed by health and care staff and organisations
Building up a library of "indicators" that can be used to measure the quality of health and care services provided to the public
Providing a register of all the information collected and produced by HSCIC and publishing it while safeguarding individuals' confidential data.

Table 16. The Health and Social Care Information Centre's Responsibilities

The HSCIC website includes a helpful search facility that allows searching by topic, category, geography, and organisational groups (www.hscic.gov.uk/searchcatalogue).

16.8.1. The Nuffield Trust

The Nuffield Trust summarises large amounts of existing data on care through interactive maps, bubble charts, animations and bespoke visualisations that show the interactions individuals (anonymised) have with care services (www.nuffieldtrust.org.uk/data-and-charts).

16.9. Training data collectors

All data collectors involved in a study should be adequately trained in the data collection procedures s specified in the study's protocol. In addition, they should have a clear understanding of the relevant information sources and the protocol involved in any review, adaptation and improvement of data collection forms that will be used.

16.9.1. Calibration

Data collectors should collect data in a standardised and consistent manner as detailed in the research study's protocol. To ensure consistency of data collection, everyone who collects data during a study should undergo calibration training. Following data collector training, the collectors should check their efficiency and the suitability of the data collection form(s) they will be using. Collectors should be blinded to the study hypothesis. In addition, when groups comparisons are made, they should also be blinded to the patient's group assignment.

The components of data collectors' training are listed in Table 17.

Check all phases of the extracting process to confirm • data availability; • appropriateness of the procedures; and • data collector performance.
Arrange regular feedback from the data collectors who may identify • confusing and misleading questions; • unforeseen ambiguities or conflicts; and • inefficiencies in data collection form layout.

Table 17. Components of data collectors' training

16.9.2. Inter-examiner reliability and intra-examiner reliability

In statistics, inter-examiner reliability is the degree of agreement among a study's data collectors. It is an assessment of the homogeneity or consensus in the ratings, scores, and measurements generated by the examiners (data collectors).

Inter-examiner reliability is the degree of agreement in ratings between different examiners. Intra-examiner reliability is the degree of agreement in ratings given by the same person on different occasions. Both are characteristics of test validity.

When there is a disagreement among examiners (raters), either the scale used to make measurements is defective, or the examiners need to be re-trained to make consistent measurements.

Several statistical processes can be used to determine inter-rater reliability. Discussion of these is beyond this chapter's scope, as different statistics are appropriate for different types of measurement. Some options are: the joint probability of agreement; Cohen's kappa and the related Fleiss's kappa; inter-rater correlation; concordance correlation coefficient; and intra-class correlation.

16.10. Summary

Data collection is crucial to a research project, and failure to accurately collect data may lead to the following problems:

- The research hypothesis is not answered correctly;
- The study has problems with validity and is difficult to repeat;
- Incorrect findings may cause harm to participants when applied in a broader setting; and
- Public health policy may be compromised as a result of misleading analyses and conclusions inferred from inaccurate data.

Table 18 provides a final checklist:

• Identify and separate participant/patient identification and research data;
• Print patient ID code on every page;
• Provide special instructions where necessary;
• Use self-coding forms:
       What is the sex of the patient?
       1=Male; 2=Female; 9=Unknown
• Check the completeness of data collection.

Table 18. A final checklist

Recommended further reading and helpful resources

An Introduction to Managing Research Data. Andrew Burnham, University of Leicester, 2013. www2. le.ac.uk/services/research-data/documents/an-introduction-to-managing-research-data-v1-1.

The Census and Survey Processing System (CSPro) is a US Government public domain software package for census and surveys. It can be used by many people, from non-technical staff assistants to senior demographers and programmers. It is used primarily for data entry, editing, tabulation, and dissemination (**www.census.gov/population/international/software**/cspro).

Data Management Plans—a UK Medical Research Council guidance, including a downloadable guide: www.mrc.ac.uk/research/research-policy-ethics/data-sharing/data-management-plans.

The Nuffield Trust summarises considerable quantities of data through interactive maps, bubble charts, animations and bespoke visualisations that show the interactions individuals (anonymised) have with care services. www.nuffieldtrust.org.uk/data-and-charts.

References

1   Johnston T M, An introduction to research for primary dental care clinicians: part 7: stage 8. Collecting data; *Primary Dental Care*, 2012;19 39-43.

2   Dawson A. A Practical Guide to Performance Improvement: Data Collection and Analysis. AORN J. 2019;109(5):621-631.

3   Gentil ML, Cuggia M, et al. Factors influencing the development of primary care data collection projects from electronic health records: a systematic review of the literature. *BMC Medical Informatics Decision Making*. 2017;17(1):139.

4   Gill P, Stewart K, Treasure E, Chadwick B. Methods of data collection in qualitative research: interviews and focus groups. *British Dental Journal.* 2008;204(6):291-295.

5   Raftery J, Roderick P, Stevens A. Potential use of routine databases in health technology assessment. *Health Technology Assessment* 2005;9(20):1-92.

6   Crook MA. The Caldicott report and patient confidentiality. *Journal of Clinical Pathology.* 2003; 56: 426–428.

Chapter 17. Analysing Data

Howe M-S., Richards D.

17.1. Overview

This chapter addresses the ninth stage of a research study.

Once data have been collected and collated, it is necessary to analyse them. If the data have been derived from quantitative research, then statistical testing is usually required.

After the introduction, this chapter covers the following:

- Types of data in quantitative studies;
- Measures of variability;
- Choosing a summary measure;
- Standard error of the mean;
- The 95 per cent confidence interval;
- Tests for statistical probability and the p- value;
- Presenting data;
- Statistical tests;
- Survival data;
- Transforming data;
- Kappa;
- Receiver operating characteristic (ROC) curves;
- Analysing multiple variables;
- Meta-analysis; and
- Bayesian analysis.

17.2. Introduction

There are two scenarios where it is essential to understand the foundations underpinning medical statistics. The first instance is when the researcher is undertaking the initial critical appraisal of the literature following the development of their research question. Just because a paper has used reporting guidelines and been through the peer-review process does not guarantee the accuracy of data analysis or the quality of the conclusions. The second instance is when designing a study protocol to ensure that the data measurement, collection, analysis, and results are robust.[1, 2, 3] To this effect, it is recommended that researchers sign up for a postgraduate course in essential medical statistics, familiarise themselves with a good reference book,[4] and take advice from a specialist medical statistician at the outset of designing a study.

To clarify a couple of terms at the beginning of this chapter: a variable is a value that can vary, and a statistic is any quantity calculated from a set of data.

17.3. Types of data in quantitative research

17.3.1. Quantitative data

Quantitative data are data expressing a certain quantity, amount or range. They are always ordinal, which means they can be arranged in numerical order from smallest to largest and measured numerically as either

Continuous—data that are measured and can take any value (within a range), such as height or time; or

Discreet—data that are counted and can only take specific values, usually counts (integers).

17.3.2. Categorical data

Categorical data occur when the item under investigation falls into a specific separate category or class. This data can be treated as non-ordered or ordinal but not necessarily as interval because the measured differences between a category or class may be subjective. Categorical data can also be continuous (number of individuals falling into a series of categories by age or ethnicity) or dichotomous (binary), such as sex (male/female).

17.3.3. Summarising quantitative data

One of the simplest forms of summarising continuous data is identifying the centre of the data distribution and measuring the data's variability.

17.3.4. Measures of the centre of the data

Mean is the simple average of the data:

$$\text{Mean} = \frac{\sum_{i=0}^{n} x_i}{n}$$

Median is the middle value and is not skewed by a small proportion of extremely large or small values, and therefore provides a better representation of a "typical" value.

Mode is the number that appears most often in a set of numbers.

A simple example to show the effect of the different measures is shown in Table 1:

Data	4, 3, 3, 4, 5, 3, 7, 9, 15, 21, 89
Mean	14.8
Median	5
Mode	3

Table 1. Summarising quantitative data

17.4. Measures of variability

Standard deviation

The standard deviation measures how dispersed the data are and compares the average difference between the mean and each data value. It is often abbreviated to SD or S.

$$\text{Standard deviation} = \left\{ \frac{\sum_{i=1}^{n}(x_i - \bar{x})^2}{n-1} \right\}$$

17.4.1. Range

The difference between the smallest and largest value is the range and is presented as the minimum and maximum.

17.4.2. Interquartile range

The interquartile range (IRQ) describes the middle 50 per cent of values ordered from lowest to highest. The statistical dispersion is equal to the difference between seventy-fifty and twenty-fifth percentiles.

17.5. Choosing a summary measure (quantitative data)

To establish which of the above methods are best suited to initially summarise the data, it is helpful to know how it is distributed (Figure 1).

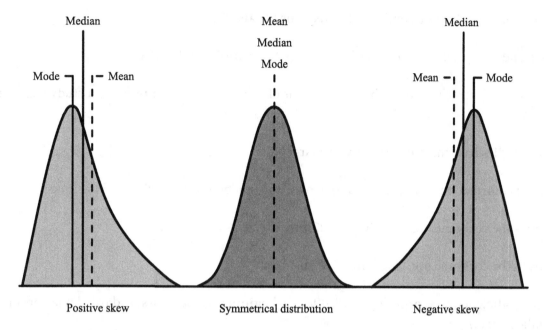

Figure 1. A general relationship of mean and median under differently skewed unimodal distribution

If the data has a symmetrical (normal) distribution, then use the mean and standard deviation.

If the data are skewed, then use the median and interquartile range.

The range (minimum to maximum) can be used in addition to the standard deviation.

17.5.1. Choosing a summary measure (categorical data)

Categorical data are usually summarised in a table showing the frequencies per category with either the overall proportions or percentages.

17.6. The standard error of the mean

The standard error of the mean (SEM) is a statistic representing the standard deviation associated with repeated sampling and recording of the means within a study (sampling distribution). The SEM is sensitive to the number of samples so that as the number increases, the SEM reduces. However, if the number of samples is large, then the sample means follow a normal distribution (central limit theorem).

Standard error of a sample mean (SE) = $\dfrac{SD}{\sqrt{n}}$

There can sometimes be confusion between the SD and SE:

The standard deviation (SD) describes the variation between individuals.

The standard error (SE) describes the amount of uncertainty in the result of a study (repeated sampling).

Small studies have more uncertainty and larger SEs.

Further information can be found in the following Students 4 Best Evidence blog links:

https://s4be.cochrane.org/blog/2014/10/22/simply-mean-average/.

https://s4be.cochrane.org/blog/2016/05/27/median/.

https://s4be.cochrane.org/blog/2018/09/26/a-beginners-guide-to-standard-deviation-and-standard-error/.

17.7. The 95 per cent confidence interval (CI)

Alan et al. (2013) have provided an excellent explanation of the importance of understanding the need to report uncertainty and using confidence intervals: "Statistical analysis of medical studies is based on the key idea that we make observations on a sample of subjects and then draw inferences about the population of all such subjects from which the sample is drawn."[5]

If a researcher could measure every individual in a population, then the mean value of the parameter measured would be exact, and there would be no uncertainty around that value. However, as the sample size reduces, the certainty around the mean lessens, requiring the addition of a confidence interval. A research protocol typically sets a confidence interval at 95 per cent, meaning that there can be 95 per cent confidence that the interval contains the true value.

To construct a confidence interval, it can be assumed that if many independent samples are taken from the population under investigation, there would be normal sampling distribution.

A normal distribution curve is divided into three standard deviations above and below the mean (Figure 2):

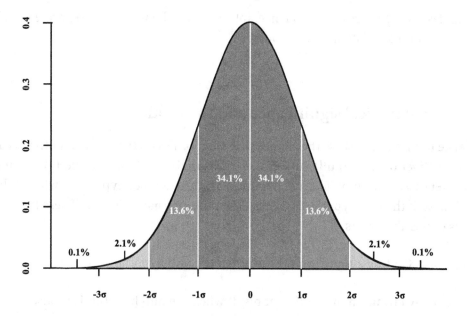

Figure 2. Normal distribution curve with standard deviations

Two (1.96 is more precise) standard deviations on either side on the central value of the normal distribution curve represents just about 95 per cent of the area under the curve.

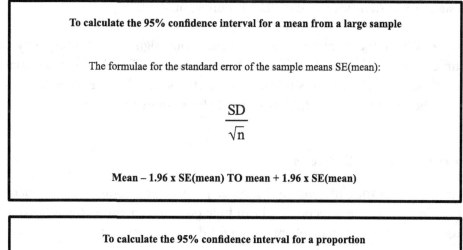

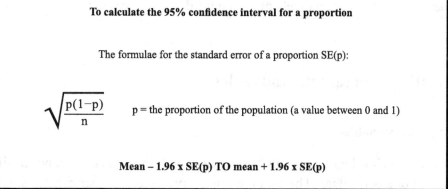

Figure 3. To calculate the 95 per cent confidence interval for a mean

Note: When describing ranges or confidence, intervals use the word *to* to separate the values, as a dash could be confused with a negative value.

17.8. Tests for statistical significance and the *p*-value

A significance test is used to show the chance that a hypothesis is true. The hypothesis can either be true (alternative) or false (null), and this is measured using the *p*-value (probability value written in lower case italics as *p*). The null hypothesis is the reference hypothesis with no difference or association, so if the null hypothesis is false, then the alternative is true. These two states lead to two types of possible errors.

Type 1 (α) error— Getting a significant result when the null hypothesis is true

Type 2 (β) error—Getting a non-significant result when the null hypothesis is false.

17.8.1. *p*-values

Definition: the probability, given that the null hypothesis is true, of obtaining data as extreme or more extreme than that observed. This probability is usually set at 0.05 (5%), so if $p < 0.05$, this is considered statistically significant and $p \geq 0.05$ is non-significant.

Important note: Where there are small sample sizes, a non-significant finding only concludes there is insufficient evidence to find a difference between groups. Therefore, it is essential to assess if there are sufficient samples for the study to be correctly powered. Power is typically set at 80% $(1 - \beta)$, where the chance of a type 2(β) error should be no more than 20 per cent.

17.8.2. One or two-sided (tailed) tests

A two-sided test allows the difference to be either positive or negative. A one-sided test only assesses the difference in one direction and can hide potential harmful effects. Two-sided tests should be used unless there is an excellent reason for doing otherwise.[6]

17.9. Presenting data (graphs and tables)

17.9.1. Categorical variables

A categorical variable's values are the labels associated with those variables, and the distribution is either a count or a percentage. The data are usually presented as a bar chart/histogram or pie chart (Figure 4):

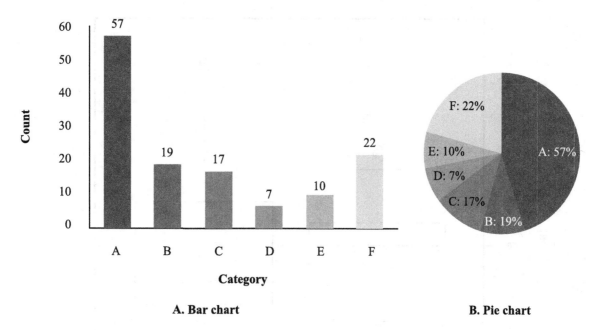

A. Bar chart   **B. Pie chart**

Figure 4. Categorical charts

17.9.2. Quantitative variables

17.9.2.1. Histograms

Quantitative data can also be presented as a histogram. The data are plotted into bins on the x axis. The bins are usually specified as consecutive, non-overlapping intervals of a variable. By looking at the shape of the distribution, one can assess whether the data are skewed or distributed normally (Figure 1).

17.9.2.2. Box and whisker plot

This chart contains six pieces of summary information.

- Median—horizontal line in the box;
- Upper quartile—the top edge of the box;
- Lower quartile—the bottom edge of the box;
- Maximum—top of the whisker;
- Minimum—bottom of the whisker; and
- Outliers—separate circle outside the plot.

A box-whisker plot is handy in presenting and summarising asymmetric/skewed distribution data (Figure 5).

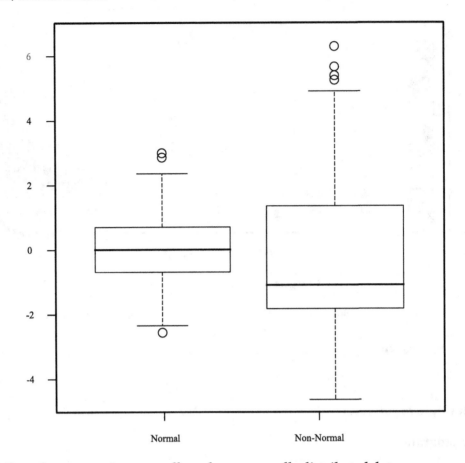

Figure 5. Box plots comparing normally and non-normally distributed data

17.9.3. Tables

Guidelines for data tables

Peacock et al. (2017) have produced an excellent book, *Presenting Medical Statistics from Proposal to Publication,* on presenting statistical data.[7]

- The table's title should explain what the table is about, and which subjects or observations are included;
- Give the number of subjects or observations overall and by the group where appropriate;
- Label rows and columns clearly;
- Give confidence intervals for comparison, not just p values;
- Give SD, SE, and Cis for means;
- Give percentages alongside frequencies, unless a group size is less than ten;
- Give range and interquartile range for medians;
- State the units used;
- Use consistent and appropriate decimal places;
- Refer to the table in the text; and
- Keep the table simple and check text size for legibility.

17.10. Statistical tests

17.10.1. t-test for two independent means

The independent samples t-test compares the means of two independent groups to determine whether statistical evidence shows that the associated population means are significantly different. Two samples should have some variance (spread between numbers in a data set). It is a parametric test (population data are normally distributed) and allows calculating a difference and confidence interval.

An online calculator is available at https://www.socscistatistics.com/tests/studentttest/.

17.10.2. Z test for two independent proportions.

The z test for two independent proportions is used to know whether two populations or groups differ significantly on some single (categorical) characteristic. It is a parametric test (population data are normally distributed) and allows calculating a difference and confidence interval.

An online calculator is available at https://www.socscistatistics.com/tests/ztest/.

17.10.3. Chi-squared test for two categorical variables (values >5)

The chi-squared test tests for an association between two categorical variables. The sample must be quite large, with 80 per cent of the values >5. The cell count must be 5 or above for each cell in a 2x2 contingency table (Table 2). The test gives a p-value but no direct estimate or confidence interval.

	Disease	No Disease	Total
Exposed	a	b	a+b
Unexposed	c	d	c+d
Total	a+c	b+d	a+b+c+d

Table 2. A 2x2 contingency table

An online calculator is available at https://www.socscistatistics.com/tests/chisquare/.

17.10.4. Fisher's exact test for two categorical variables (values <5)

Similar to the chi-squared test, where sample sizes are small. The test gives a p-value but no direct estimate or confidence interval. Use the two-sided p-value.

An online calculator is available at https://www.socscistatistics.com/tests/fisher.

17.10.5. Estimates for tests of proportions and effect sizes

Chi-squared and Fisher's exact tests do not measure effect sizes or the strength of the relationship. There are three main choices.

Risk difference (RD) ($p_1 - p_2$) presents the actual size of the difference of interest.

Relative risk (RR) (p_1 / p_2) presents the relative difference. A RR of 1.5 means that the risk of the outcome of interest is 50 per cent higher in the exposed group than in the unexposed group, and a RR of 0.8 means that the risk of the outcome of interest is 20 per cent lower. They are easier to interpret than odds ratios.

Odds ratio (OR) $\left(\frac{p_1}{1-p_1} / \frac{p_2}{1-p_2} \right)$ The odds ratio is similar to the relative risk if the outcome under investigation is rare but can be misinterpreted if the outcome is common. OR tend to give a larger effect size than RR, which has led to their overuse in many dental research papers. It is recommended to restrict their use to case-control studies only.[8]

17.10.6. Standardised mean difference (SMD) $\left(\frac{\text{treatment-comparator}}{\text{pooled standard deviation}} \right)$

The SMD measure of effect is used when studies report efficacy as a continuous measurement, such as a score on a pain-intensity rating scale. The SMD is also known as Cohen's d.[9]

17.10.7. One way analysis of variance (ANOVA)

This test is similar to the t-test but compares the means from three or more estimates.

Note: It is incorrect to do multiple t-tests instead of an ANOVA, increasing the risk of random error.

An online calculator is available at https://www.socscistatistics.com/tests/anova/.

17.10.8. Correlation and regression

Correlation and simple linear regression are used to investigate the relationship between two continuous variables.

17.10.8.1. Correlation quantifies the direction and strength of the relationship x and y, and the output gives a value r that lies between -1.0 and 1.0. A negative value of r indicates that as one variable increases, the other decreases; for a positive value, both variables increase. Pearson's correlation requires the distribution of data to be normal and gives a p-value and confidence interval. It is essential to plot the data before a Pearson's correlation analysis to check that the relationship is linear to avoid a false result (Figure 6).

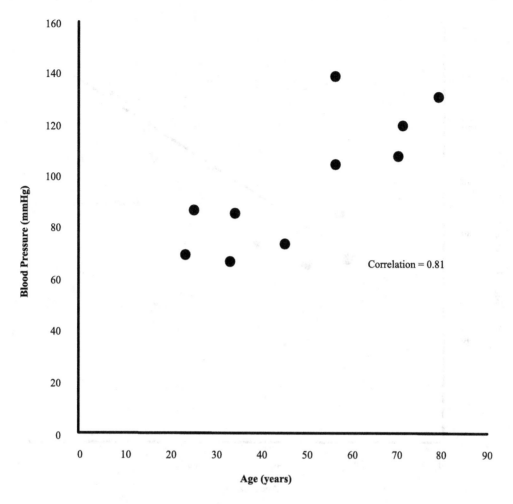

Figure 6. Correlation between blood pressure and age

17.10.9. Simple linear regression

The simple linear regression relates variable x to y through the equation y = a + bx. One variable is considered the outcome, and the other predicts the variable. Y represents the outcome, a the intercept where it crosses the y axis, b is the slope of the line (regression coefficient), and x is the predictor variable (Figure 7).

- The regression coefficient gives the change in the outcome (y) for the unit change in the predictor variable x.
- The intercept gives the value of y when x is 0.
- The line gives the mean or expected value of y for each value of x. Therefore, the mean blood pressure for a 60-year-old patient is 60 x 1.03+48= 109.8mmHg.

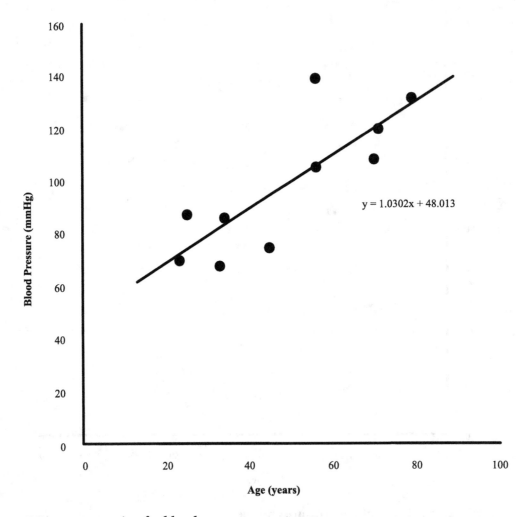

$$y = 1.0302x + 48.013$$

Figure 7. Linear regression for blood pressure versus age

17.10.10. Wilcoxon two-sample signed-rank test (Mann-Whitney U test)

The Wilcoxon two-sample signed-rank test is an analogue to the t-test but based on the rank or order of the data rather than the values themselves. The test is non-parametric, meaning it is based on the data either being distribution-free or having a specified distribution but with the distribution's parameters unspecified. The output gives a p-value but no estimate. A Mann-Whitney U test gives a similar p-value but is mathematically more complex.

An online calculator is available at https://www.socscistatistics.com/tests/signedranks.

17.11. Survival data (time-to-event analysis)

Survival analysis, or more generally, time-to-event analysis, refers to a set of methods for analysing the length of time until a well-defined endpoint of interest occurs. A good example would be a hip implant survival over ten years from the time of placement.

17.11.1. Censoring

Censoring is a way of handling incomplete survival data. For example, not all the test subjects may be entering the study simultaneously, and the survival data may only be known up to a certain point or lost-to-follow-up and is known as censored data. Survival methods such as a Kaplan-Meier curve can incorporate the censored data in its analysis.

17.11.2. Kaplan-Meier curves[10, 11, 12]

A Kaplan-Meier curve depicts the survival time on the x-axis and the cumulative survival probability on the y-axis. When an event such as restoration failure or death occurs, it is depicted as a step on the curve (the graph is not smooth). Censored data are indicated on the curve as a small vertical dash. A 95 per cent CI bands dashed lines can also be placed on the chart to signify uncertainty (Figure 8).

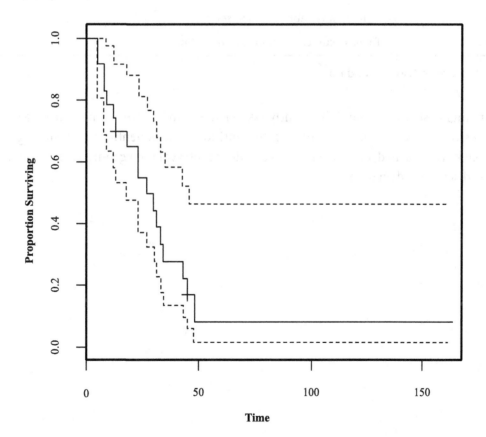

Figure 8. A Kaplan-Meier curve

The three dots in Figure 8 are level with the 0.5 proportion surviving value on the x-axis, represents that 50% of the events had occurred at time point 30 (95% CI: 18 to 45).

Online calculator is available at https://www.easymedstat.com/kaplan-meier-survival-analysis-online-calculator.

17.11.3. Log-rank test

The log-rank test allows the researcher to compare the survival distribution of two or multiple curves on one chart, such as a control group and an intervention group. It is a non-parametric test and appropriate to use when the data are right-skewed and censored. However, it is a significance test only and gives a p-value but no estimate of difference.

17.12. Transforming data

Data transformation is the process of changing the format, structure, or values of data. Common reasons are noted in Table 3:

Normal distribution	To make skewed data fit a more normal distribution
Variance	To make a variable more constant
Linearity	To make curved relationships more linear

Table 3. Reasons to transform data

If data are highly skewed to the right (positive skew), they can be transformed on a log scale, and then the estimates back-transformed using the anti-log or exponential function (Figure 9). If data are back-transformed, one can create a confidence interval for a geometric mean but *not* the p-value and standard deviation.

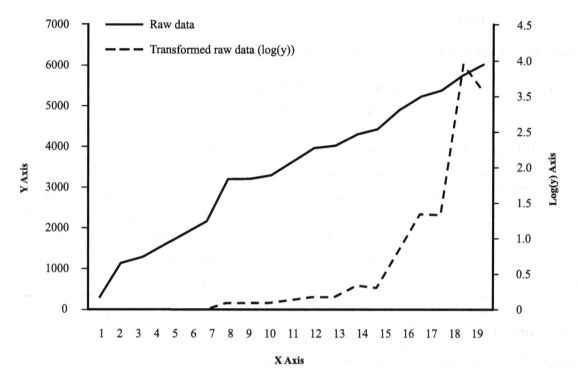

Figure 9. Log transformed skewed data

17.13. Kappa

Kappa is a statistic that measures the level of agreement between two raters. Kappa considers the possibility that a degree of interrater agreement could be by chance and corrects for this (Table 4). It is used in a variety of circumstances, including when training examiners for epidemiological surveys and during the survey(s) to ensure that they are assessing variables consistently, both between examiners (inter-examiner consistency) and for individuals (intra-examiner consistency).

Value of kappa	Strength of agreement
<0.00	Poor
0.00 – 0.20	Slight
0.21 – 0.40	Fair
0.41 – 0.60	Moderate
0.61 – 0.80	Good
0.81 – 1.00	Very good

Table 4. Interpretation of kappa

17.14. Diagnostic tests

Sensitivity and specificity are characteristics of a diagnostic accuracy test.

- **Sensitivity** (Sn) refers to the proportion of results that are true positives.
- **Specificity** (Sp) refers to the proportion of results that are true negatives.

To calculate Sp and Sn of a diagnostic/screening test, construct a 2x2 contingency table (Table 5).

Disease status				
		Positive	Negative	Total
Test	Positive	True positive (a)	False-positive (b)	a+b
	Negative	False-negative (c)	True negative (d)	c+d
	Total	a+c	b+d	n

Sensitivity = a/(a + c)

Specificity = d/(b + d)

Table 5. A 2x2 contingency table for sensitivity/specificity

Online calculators are available at http://araw.mede.uic.edu/cgi-bin/testcalc.pl and https://www.medcalc.org/calc/diagnostic_test.php.

17.14.1. Receiver operating characteristic (ROC) curves

An ROC graph plots sensitivity (true positive rate) against 1-specificity (false positive rate) or a diagnostic test. Perfect accuracy is represented by a point in the top left corner and the area under the curve= 1.0. A diagnostic test can be considered effective; if it produces a curve above the 45° line (line of no effect) (Figure 10).

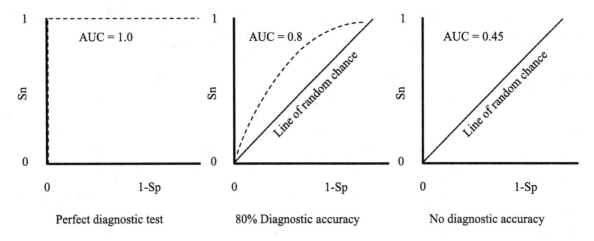

| Perfect diagnostic test | 80% Diagnostic accuracy | No diagnostic accuracy |

Figure 10. The area under the curve for ROCs

17.15. Missing data and intention-to-treat

Missing data occur when there is no data value stored for a variable in a series of observations. Studies missing more than 20 per cent follow-up data may be vulnerable to a higher risk of bias in their results, especially if the loss to follow-up is not 'at random,' i.e. loss is related to repeated treatment failure.[13] There are two broad categories for the cause of missing data.

17.15.1. Missing completely at random (MCAR)

MCAR means there is no systematic reason for missing data, such as a missing birth date.

17.15.2. Missing not at random (MNAR)

MNAR is due to a systematic problem in how the data are collected, such as a device not measuring particles beyond a specific size in an aerosol.

Several techniques manage missing data, but they are unreliable and reduce the validity of the study.

- When there is a small amount of missing data and the cause is random, it is possible to ignore the missing data and undertake a "complete case analysis" (an analysis restricted to individuals with complete data).
- A single value can be replaced with an average estimate to complete the data set, such as age.
- If the last value in a data series is missing, then a "last observation carried forward" technique can be used.
- Multiple imputation techniques [14]

17.16. Analysing multiple variables

17.16.1. Multiple regression

Multiple regression is an extension of simple linear regression and allows for the analysis of two or more continuous variables. Multiple regression generally explains the relationship between multiple independent or predictor variables and one dependent or criterion variable. The data needs to be normally distributed as for simple linear regression.[15]

$$y = b_0 + b_1x_1 + b_2x_2 + b_3x_3 + \cdots b_xx_x$$

- y = outcome
- x_1, x_2 are the predictor variables
- b_0 is the intercept, and b_1, b_2 are the regression coefficients for the variables x_1, x_2.

Consider which predictor variables may be important and analyse them separately before undertaking a multiple regression analysis.

Continuous variables do a scatter plot and simple linear regression.

Binary and categorical data calculate summary statistics for each group.

An online calculator is available at https://www.socscistatistics.com/tests/multipleregression.

17.16.2. Logistic regression

Logistic regression can be used to undertake simultaneous analyses for binary outcome variables such as survival yes/no. It uses a logarithmic transformation to allow a linear relationship to be created. The model is similar to that used in multiple regression.

$$\log_e [p / (1 - p)] = b_0 + b_1 x_1 + b_2 x_2 + b_3 x_3 + \cdots b_x x_x$$

The differences are that

- p is the proportion of the outcome;
- b_0 is the intercept and b_1, b_2 are the regression coefficients for the variables x_1, x_2 which when back-transformed from the log scale to the natural scale are odds ratios;
- $\log_e [p / (1 - p)]$ is known as the logit transformation.

To interpret odds ratios; if the OR=1 there is no relationship, if it is <1, that relationship is protective, and >1 it is harmful.

17.16.3. Additional regression models

17.16.4. Cox proportional hazards regression

Cox proportional hazards regression is used for time-to-event analysis.

17.16.5. Poisson regression

This is used for modelling rates.

An online calculator is available at https://www.statskingdom.com/420logistic_regression.hl.

17.17. Meta-analysis

Shorten and Shorten (2013)[16] have defined meta-analysis as a research process used to systematically synthesise or merge the findings of single, independent studies, using statistical methods to calculate an overall or absolute effect. Meta-analysis does not simply pool data from smaller studies to achieve a larger sample size. Instead, analysts use well recognised, systematic methods to account for differences in sample size, variability (heterogeneity) in study approach and findings (treatment effects) and test how sensitive their results are to their systematic review protocol (study selection and statistical analysis).

Meta-analysis is a highly complex statistical process; for more detail on the methodology, Chapter 10 of the *Cochrane Handbook* gives a detailed overview.[17] The classic endpoint of a meta-analysis is a Forest plot (Figure 11).

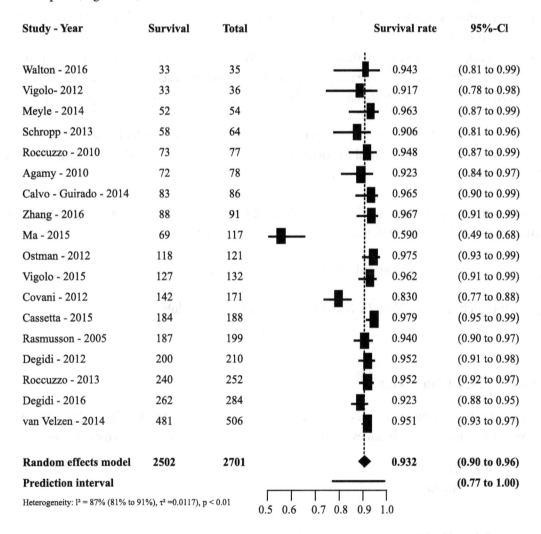

Study - Year	Survival	Total		Survival rate	95%-Cl
Walton - 2016	33	35		0.943	(0.81 to 0.99)
Vigolo- 2012	33	36		0.917	(0.78 to 0.98)
Meyle - 2014	52	54		0.963	(0.87 to 0.99)
Schropp - 2013	58	64		0.906	(0.81 to 0.96)
Roccuzzo - 2010	73	77		0.948	(0.87 to 0.99)
Agamy - 2010	72	78		0.923	(0.84 to 0.97)
Calvo - Guirado - 2014	83	86		0.965	(0.90 to 0.99)
Zhang - 2016	88	91		0.967	(0.91 to 0.99)
Ma - 2015	69	117		0.590	(0.49 to 0.68)
Ostman - 2012	118	121		0.975	(0.93 to 0.99)
Vigolo - 2015	127	132		0.962	(0.91 to 0.99)
Covani - 2012	142	171		0.830	(0.77 to 0.88)
Cassetta - 2015	184	188		0.979	(0.95 to 0.99)
Rasmusson - 2005	187	199		0.940	(0.90 to 0.97)
Degidi - 2012	200	210		0.952	(0.91 to 0.98)
Roccuzzo - 2013	240	252		0.952	(0.92 to 0.97)
Degidi - 2016	262	284		0.923	(0.88 to 0.95)
van Velzen - 2014	481	506		0.951	(0.93 to 0.97)
Random effects model	**2502**	**2701**		**0.932**	**(0.90 to 0.96)**
Prediction interval					**(0.77 to 1.00)**

Heterogeneity: I^2 = 87% (81% to 91%), τ^2 =0.0117), p < 0.01

0.5 0.6   0.7 0.8 0.9 1.0

Figure 11. Forest plot showing the proportion of dental implant survival at ten years[18]

Points to note concerning a forest plot are

- The y-axis is the line of no-effect;
- The x-axis displays the scale for the output statistic (OR, RR, AR, MD, proportion, or SMD);
- A black box represents each study's point estimate; the bigger the box, the more subjects in the sample;
- The horizontal line passing through the box represents the 95 per cent confidence intervals of the study result;
- The diamond represents the point estimate and confidence intervals when you combine and average all the individual studies;
- The prediction interval represents an estimate of the interval in which a future observation will fall;
- Random effects models allow for variation across individual studies, and fixed effects are constant; and
- Heterogeneity in meta-analysis refers to the variation in study outcomes between studies. The I^2 statistic describes the percentage of variation across studies that is due to heterogeneity rather than chance. In this meta-analysis, the heterogeneity is high (87 per cent).

Network meta-analysis goes one stage further in complexity and is a technique for comparing three or more interventions simultaneously in a single analysis by combining both direct and indirect evidence across a network of studies.[19]

Further information on meta-analysis is available at Students 4 Best Evidence blogs: https://s4be.cochrane.org/blog/2016/12/02/meta-analysis-what-why-and-how/.

https://s4be.cochrane.org/blog/2017/10/10/a-thorough-look-into-meta-analysis/.

https://s4be.cochrane.org/blog/2016/07/11/tutorial-read-forest-plot/.

17.18. Bayesian statistics

Bayesian statistics is a theory based on the Bayesian interpretation of probability where probability expresses a degree of belief in an event initially proposed by Rev Thomas Bayes in 1763.

$$Pr\ (A/B) = \frac{Pr\ (B/A)\ x\ Pr\ (A)}{Pr\ (B)}$$

- A and B are two events.
- Pr (A/B) is the probability that A will happen, given that B has happened already. This is also called the posterior probability.
- Prior probability is the probability of an event before new data are collected (Figure 12).

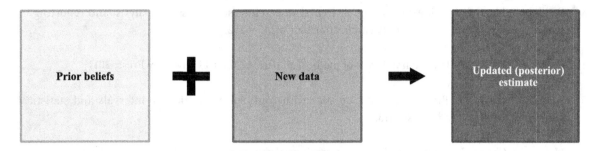

Figure 12. Bayesian inference

For more information, there is a good paper on Bayesian statistics in medicine.[20]

Useful free tools

- https://automeris.io/WebPlotDigitizer/ to convert images of charts into data for reanalysis.
- https://www.psychologie.hhu.de/arbeitsgruppen/allgemeine-psychologie-und-arbeitspsychologie/gpower.hl. G*Power calculates statistical power analyses for many different t-tests, F tests, χ2 tests, z tests and some exact tests.
- https://rstudio.com/ RStudio is an integrated development environment for R, a programming language for statistical computing and graphics.

Essential reading/reference

Peacock J., Peacock P. Oxford handbook of medical statistics: Oxford University Press; 2011.

D Alan, D Machin, T Bryant, et al. *Statistics with Confidence,* Hoboken, NJ: John Wiley & Sons, 2013.

JL Peacock, SM Kerry, and RR Balise. *Presenting Medical Statistics from Proposal to Publication*, Oxford University Press; 2017.

References

1   Koletsi D., Madahar A., Fleming PS., et al. Statistical testing against baseline was common in dental research. *Journal of Clinical Epidemiology.* 2015;68(7):776-781.

2   Gratsia S., Koletsi D., Fleming PS., et al. Statistical testing against baseline in orthodontic research: A meta-epidemiologic study. *European Journal of Orthodontics.* 2019;41(2):165-171.

3   Pandis N., Fleming PS., Katsaros C., et al. Dental research waste in design, analysis, and reporting: A scoping review. *Journal of Dental Research.* 2021;100(3):245—252.

4   Peacock J., Peacock P. Oxford handbook of medical statistics: Oxford University Press; 2011.

5   Alan D., Machin D., Bryant T., et al. Statistics with confidence: Confidence intervals and statistical guidelines: John Wiley & Sons; 2013.

6   University College London. Introduction research methods and statistics Great Ormond Street Institute of Child Health2010 (Available from: https://www.ucl.ac.uk/child-health/short-courses-events/about-statistical-courses/introduction-research-methods-and-statistics. (accessed on 17 March 2021)

7   Peacock JL., Kerry SM., Balise RR. *Presenting Medical Statistics from Proposal to Publication.* Oxford University Press; 2017. p. 48-63.

8   Bland JM. Statistics notes: The odds ratio. *British Medical Journal.* 2000;320(7247):1468-1468.

9   Faraone SV. Interpreting estimates of treatment effects: Implications for managed care. *Pharmacy and Theraputics*, 2008;33(12):700-711.

10   Pocock SJ., Clayton TC., Altman DG. Survival plots of time-to-event outcomes in clinical trials: Good practice and pitfalls. *The Lancet.* 2002;359(9318):1686-1689.

11   Layton DM. Understanding kaplan-meier and survival statistics. *International Journal of Prosthodontics,* 2013;26(3):218-226.

12   Rich JT., Neely JG., Paniello RC., et al. A practical guide to understanding kaplan-meier curves. *Otolaryngology-Head and Neck Surgery,* 2010;143(3):331-336.

13   Heneghan C., Goldacre B., Mahtani KR. Why clinical trial outcomes fail to translate into benefits for patients. *Trials.* 2017;18(1).

14   Hughes RA., Heron J., Sterne JAC, et al. Accounting for missing data in statistical analyses: Multiple imputations are not always the answer. *International Journal of Epidemiology.* 2019;48(4):1294-1304.

15   Peacock JL., Kerry SM., Balise RR. Multifactorial analysis. Presenting medical statistics from proposal to publication: Oxford University Press; 2017. p. 140-149.

16   Shorten A., Shorten B. What is a meta-analysis? *Evidence-Based Nursing.* 2013;16(1):3-4.

17   Deeks JJ., Alan DG. Chapter 10: Analysing data and undertaking meta-analyses. In: Higgins JPT TJ, Chandler J., Cumpston M., Li T., Page MJ., Welch VA. editors. Cochrane handbook for systematic reviews of interventions version 61 (updated september 2020): Cochrane; 2020.

18   Howe MS., Keys W., Richards D. Long-term (10-year) dental implant survival: A systematic review and sensitivity meta-analysis. *Journal of Dentistry.* 2019;84:9-21.

19 Chaimani A, Caldwell DM, Li T, Higgins JPT, Salanti G. Chapter 11: Undertaking network meta-analyses. In: Higgins JPT, Thomas J, Chandler J, Cumpston M, Li T, Page MJ, Welch VA (editors). *Cochrane Handbook for Systematic Reviews of Interventions* version 6.2 (updated February 2021). Cochrane, 2021. Available from www.training.cochrane.org/handbook.

20 Ashby D. Bayesian statistics in medicine: A 25-year review. *Statistics in Medicine*. 2006;25(21):3589-3631.

Chapter 18. Writing up and Disseminating the Results

Eaton K.A, Blum I.R., Wiles L.

18.1. Overview

This chapter will address the final stage of a research project. It outlines the steps that authors should take when seeking to publish research results in peer-reviewed journals and how to disseminate results through presentations at scientific conferences.

This chapter is divided into the following sections:

- Introduction;
- Steps to take before starting to write;
- Writing the paper or papers;
- Submitting the paper and the editorial process;
- Presenting results at meetings and conferences; and
- Further resources.

18.2. Introduction

Having performed research, it is the duty of the researcher(s) to disseminate the results and inform the scientific world and general population of the findings. Traditionally, this has been done via presentations at scientific conferences and by publishing in peer-reviewed journals. However, in the last twenty years, it has become possible to publish in e-journals (online) such as BioMed Central[1] as well as in traditional journals in printed form. Most journals now publish papers in both versions.

When disseminating research results, their potential to improve patient care and cost-effectiveness and change policy, both nationally and internationally, must be made clear and emphasised.

This chapter includes advice on how to structure a research paper and describes the stages in the publication process. Although the structure of such papers is different, many of the steps are identical for other types of scientific papers, such as reports of systematic reviews and case reports. In biomedicine, research methodology may be applied to research that seeks to identify answers to a new problem or to confirm the results of a previous study or studies, clinical audit, or service evaluation.

18.3. Steps to take before starting to write

18.3.1. Identify the target readership and journal

The study concerned has been completed, and the results analysed. It is now time to report them in a paper or papers. Before starting to write the paper(s), the following three questions should be asked:

- What message should the paper convey? Ideally, this should be summed up in one sentence.
- What impact will the research have? Apply the "so what?" test to the message.
- Who is likely to want to read the paper? Apply the "who cares?" test.

Each editor will have a very clear idea of their journal's readership and apply their versions of these tests to all the manuscripts that cross their desk. If a paper is to be considered, its topic will have to be within the journal's scope and will need to match the journal's audience. It is, therefore, very wise to review the contents of recent editions of the selected journal. An editor may be reluctant to publish yet another paper on a specific topic that has been covered comprehensively in recent issues.

Many editors welcome enquiries and the opportunity to give guidance to prospective authors.

When selecting a journal, authors should check that it is a bona fide journal and not a predatory journal (see Chapter 3 for details of predatory journals) before submitting the manuscript.

18.3.2. Information and guidance for authors

Authors should always read in detail the "information, instructions, or guidelines for authors" of any journal to which they wish to submit a paper and ensure that they follow the guidelines to the letter. They should ask themselves two questions:

1. Can they fulfil the requirements within the guidelines?
2. Will the selected journal do justice to their paper?

Some journals also provide checklists, as well as guidelines. The checklists are used by those who review papers submitted to the journal in question. An example of a checklist for papers reporting quantitative research[2] can be found at the end of this chapter (Figure 3). Such checklists detail the points that the reviewers will consider and which the authors should have covered in their paper. In addition, journals frequently require authors to follow specific guidelines for reporting results (for example, see the CONSORT guidelines for systematic reviews). Details of guidelines and checklists are shown in Appendix 1.

18.3.3. Preparing to write

Having read the guidelines for authors, refer to any checklists for reviewers or authors that the journal to which the paper is to be submitted may have produced, and read past editions to check its preferred style. The lead author is now ready to assemble all the material that should be on hand when writing. As far as style is concerned, it is usual to write in the third person and use the simple past tense as the report will detail what has happened rather than what is happening or will happen.

The materials may include all or some of the following: data generated by the study, questionnaires and letters to respondents used in the study, photographs, drawings, other images, letters from ethics committees, and so on. Make sure the data are complete and are organised into suitable tables and figures. Have copies of the papers that will be cited. Do not rely on memory or copy references from lists at the end of papers published in other journals, as they may not be in the style used by the journal to which the paper will be submitted.

Check any statistics before writing the first draft. If they are wrong, it will be necessary to carry out a major revision in a later draft. Before collecting any data, it will have been essential to obtain the advice of a biostatistician when designing a study and to refer to them any queries that may arise during the study and whilst writing a paper or an abstract for a conference presentation.

If the paper contains illustrations or any copyright-protected material, it is necessary to obtain permission from the copyright holders to reproduce the material in the paper. If a letter or an unpublished paper is cited in the paper, it is necessary to obtain permission from its author. It is also necessary to confirm with anyone acknowledged for their help that they are happy to be associated with the paper. It is possible that they may not wish to be associated publicly with the paper or wish the readers to infer that they have endorsed it.

18.4. Writing the paper or papers

18.4.1. The first draft

It is usual to produce several drafts of the paper, each of which is checked and commented on and corrected by co-authors (if there are any). Therefore, it is wise to add a date at the top of the first page of the first and all subsequent drafts and save the paper to a hard drive with the date in the file name (e.g. Draft 4, Paper 12 at 27 December 2020). This facilitates easy identification of the latest version of the paper when retrieving it for further work. As mentioned previously, as far as style is concerned, it is usual to write in the third person and use the simple past tense because the report will detail what has happened rather than what is happening or will happen.

As an alternative to using conventional word-processing software, a growing number of collaborative authoring tools allow multiple authors to work on a document—sometimes simultaneously—without the need to circulate it from person to person. These systems are usually cloud-based and synchronise changes online. Privacy features permit authors to decide who can read and edit documents, and there are tools for reviewing how the document has been changed. Such systems generally use plain-text format; thus, documents may easily be downloaded and edited offline with any basic text editor tool. Examples of authoring tools/systems include Authorea, HackMD, Manubot, and Overleaf.[3, 4]

The structure of the paper should follow the standard format for scientific papers and be written under the headings:

- Abstract (with keywords);
- Introduction;
- Aim(s);
- Methods;
- Results;
- Discussion;
- Conclusions;
- Acknowledgements; and
- References.

18.4.2. The title and the authors

Begin the first draft by devising a title, which should clearly state the paper's message. In effect, the title summarises the abstract, which in turn is a summary of the whole paper. It may be the case that the final version of the title is not agreed upon at the first draft stage, and it may be revised in subsequent drafts. Abbreviations should not be used in the title, and they should not imply more than the study shows. For example, a title such as "A study of dentists' use of washer-disinfectors" would be inappropriate if the study involved general dental practitioners in just one area. A better title would be "The use of washer-disinfectors in 2020 by general dental practitioners in Yorkshire."

The full names, qualifications, appointments, and addresses of all the authors should be listed under the title on the first page. In addition, the author to whom any correspondence relating to the paper should be sent should be identified and his or her e-mail address and contact telephone number provided.

18.4.3. The abstract

The abstract should summarise the paper. Abstracts reporting the results of research should be written under the sub-headings: aim(s), methods, results, and conclusion(s). The aims section may include a brief introduction as well as the aim(s). Each section should be one paragraph. References should not usually be cited in abstracts. Some journals have a word limit for the length of an abstract; it is usually 250-300 words. At the end of the abstract, keywords should be listed. These should be chosen carefully because they will be used by electronic databases, such as PubMed, to identify the paper when people perform online searches. For example, PubMed has lists of medical subject headings (MeSH) terms. Therefore, authors should check that their chosen keywords are listed as MeSH terms.

18.4.4. Referencing

Although they should not usually be cited in abstracts, references should be cited elsewhere throughout the paper and listed at the end of the paper. Many biomedical journals use the Vancouver style,[5] in which references are numbered in the order they are first cited in the text. The Vancouver style resulted from the International Committee of Medical Journal Editors in Vancouver in 1978. This committee has also produced Uniform Requirements for Manuscripts Submitted to Biomedical Journals (2019). More recently, the International Committee of Medical Journal Editors has also published recommendations for editors and authors,[6] and they form the basis for the guidelines or instructions to authors.

The other commonly used system is parenthetical referencing, generally referred to as the Harvard style.[5] In Harvard, the authors' names and the year of publication appear in the text instead of a number. Whichever system the journal uses, it is wise to follow the Harvard style until the final draft of the paper. This is because further references should be added or deleted during revisions to earlier drafts; it is easier to replace names and dates with numbers in the final draft rather than renumber references throughout all drafts.

18.4.5. Introduction (why was the research necessary?)

This is the most important part of the paper to the editor of a journal, along with the abstract. When a paper arrives in an editorial office, the editor is unlikely to read through its entirety in the first instance. Instead, many editors read the abstract to obtain an overall picture of the paper and then read the introduction to understand the author's skills as an investigator and writer. By the end of the abstract, the editor (and readers) should know why the research was started and what gap in the existing knowledge it has tried to fill. An introduction should set the scene for the rest of the paper, commencing with a paragraph on the broad area in which the research has been performed and describing previous work relevant to the topic before leading to the reason why the author was prompted to carry out the study. When planning and designing the study, it is essential to perform a literature search (using search engines such as PubMed, EMBASE, and CINAHL) to help find previous key papers relevant to the research topic. These key papers should be cited in the introduction. Too few citations in the introduction may lead to suspicion by the editor (and discerning readers) that the relevant literature was not thoroughly investigated before the project was started. On the other hand, too many citations may suggest that they have been copied from a dissertation or thesis, and there has been no attempt to cite only the key references. The null hypothesis of the study and the statistical level of significance used in the study, i.e., $p < 0.05$, should be clearly stated.

18.4.6. Aims

The introduction must lead to a clear statement of the aim(s) of the research. This can be linked to the introduction by using such phrases as, "Against this background," or "In the light of previous work, the aim of this study was …"

18.4.7. Methods (what was done?)

The quality of research can be determined by the quality of the methodology used. Good research design is crucial to the success of a study/project. Therefore, the methodology used needs to be fully described in the methods section, such that someone with little knowledge of the research topic could repeat the study. If the reader cannot understand precisely what was done, the methods section is inadequate. The author(s) must not assume that readers have the same knowledge of the topic as they do, and it is necessary to give a detailed explanation. The following points should be covered in the methods section:

- A full description of the subjects and materials used;
- How and why the sample was selected, including details of random sampling methods, or if applicable, why random sampling was not used;
- The numbers involved and details of a power calculation to justify the size of the sample;
- How and why those chosen were truly representative of the population that was studied;
- Inclusion and exclusion criteria;
- A full explanation of the methodology used;
- A description of how the methodology was piloted to test it before commencing the study;
- Details of ethical approval, or if this was not sought, the reason why;
- If relevant, details of patient consent and how it was obtained;
- A description of how data were collected;
- Copies of any questionnaire used, together with a copy of the explanatory letter to subjects/patients, if this was not included in the questionnaire;
- A full description of any drugs, chemicals, and other materials used, including their trade names and manufacturers' details; and
- Details of any statistical tests that were used and why they were selected.

The reasons for using the methods that have been described and a comparison with the methods used in previous similar studies should be given as part of a critique of the methodology at the beginning of the discussion section of the paper and not in the methods section.

Details of the response rate, the number of subjects who dropped out, and the reasons why this happened should also not be given in the methods but in the results section (see 18.4.8.).

Results (what was found?)

Although editors, reviewers, and discerning readers consider the scientific validity in terms of the methods section, they look to the results section for the factual findings. Some journals restrict the number of tables that can be published in a paper. However, this is less of a problem with the increasing use of online publishing because printed papers can have annexes including such items as long questionnaires and multiple tables published online. Key features of a results section are that it should

- Present data and any statistical tests used unambiguously, using tables, figures, graphs as appropriate;
- Account for any missing data which may be due to drop-outs or non-response to questions;
- Provide raw data (numbers) as well as percentages;
- Not present data (numbers) with several decimal points when the potential error in measurements is greater than 1 per cent; and
- Comment on any problems experienced during data collection which may have led to statistical errors or a deviation from the study design described in the methods section.

18.4.9. Discussion (what do the results mean?)

This section should start with a discussion and critique of the methodology that was used, including an explanation of why it was used and a comparison with the methodologies used previously in similar studies. The results should then be discussed and compared with previous studies, indicating where they confirmed or differed from those obtained in these studies and suggesting why this might have happened. Finally, the section should end with a brief summary outlining what the study has shown and a suggestion for any further research relating to the research topic presented in the paper that is necessary.

18.4.10. Conclusions

Conclusions may be listed in the summary at the end of the discussion. It is essential not to overstate the findings (results) or generalise them when only a small sample was involved. It is often wise to list the key findings as bullet points, making it easier for a reader to identify them. They should reflect the results accurately and not draw inferences over and above the results.

18.4.11. Acknowledgements

This section should

- Thank anyone who has helped in the production of the paper or the study that it reports;
- Identify any sources of funding for the study;
- Include a statement of conflicts of interest, should any of the authors have them;

- State precisely what each author contributed to the paper (the International Committee of Medical Journal Editors [ICMJE][6] has produced guidelines for who qualifies to be an author); and
- Give the authors ORCID identification codes (the Open Researcher and Contributor ID is a non-proprietary, alphanumeric code to identify scientific and other academic authors and contributors uniquely. Further information is available at https://info.orcid.org/what-is-orcid/).

18.4.12. References

All references, including electronic sources, cited in the paper should be numbered and listed in this section and numbered at the final draft stage. Personal communications are not generally included in the reference list. However, details of these should be included at the point within the text where they are cited. As mentioned previously, the style of the references will be either Vancouver or Harvard.

18.4.13. Revising drafts

If time permits, it is wise to leave drafts for some days before revising them. This helps authors take an objective view when looking for errors. These may be in the content and structure or style. Look for disparities between statements in the text and data presented in tables or figures. Ensure that there is continuity in the use of terms and that the full version of all abbreviations is given when they are first used (e.g. General Dental Council (GDC) should appear when first used in a paper, and then the abbreviation GDC throughout the rest of the paper). As mentioned previously, to ensure an objective style, check that the third person and simple past tense are used consistently throughout the paper. The use of the first person suggests a degree of subjectivity and the second person one of condescension, which should be avoided.

For simplicity reasons, the references should remain in the Harvard style, both in the text and in the list of references until the final stage. If the journal to which the paper is submitted requires, they should then be converted to the referencing style of the targeted journal.

If the journal to which the paper is submitted publishes a checklist for reviewers, the author(s) should go through the draft with the checklist to help identify any errors or omissions.

When the author(s) are happy with the final draft, it is wise to ask a colleague who is knowledgeable in the field of the paper to read the manuscript before it is submitted.

18.4.14. The final manuscript

Having completed any revisions, the last stage before submitting the paper is preparing the final manuscript. This involves

- Reviewing the manuscript requirements of the journal, as detailed in the information/guidelines for authors;
- Checking that the final version contains all the essential sections—such as title pages, abstract, keywords, and references—and that they conform to the journal's requirements;
- Ensuring that the width of the page margins conforms to the journal's requirements, the lines are double-spaced, each page is numbered, all tables and figures are numbered, and each appears on a separate page; and
- Obtaining permission from all the authors for the final version to be submitted.

18.5. Submitting the paper and the editorial process

18.5.1. Submitting the paper

Most journals require papers to be submitted electronically, either as e-mail attachments or via the journal's or publisher's online manuscript submission system, such as ScholarOne. Unfortunately, many online systems are very inflexible and do not allow manuscripts to be submitted unless every stage in the submission process has been performed in the manner required by the system. For example, the manuscript should be accompanied by a covering letter signed by the corresponding author. Photographs may be sent electronically with the manuscript, tables, figures and the covering letter. However, to obtain high-quality reproduction, some journals may also require photographs to be posted to the editor in hard copy.

18.5.2. The covering letter

Although the contents of the covering letter may vary from journal to journal, most require it to include a list of all the authors' names, the address and the contact details (e-mail, postal addresses, and telephone number) of the corresponding author, together with a statement that the paper is not being submitted to another journal, and has not been published or accepted by another journal as a whole or in part. An example of a covering letter is in Figure 1. In addition, some journals require all the contributing authors to sign the covering letter; others do not require this as long as the e-mail accompanying the manuscript and covering letter is copied to all the authors and has been signed by the corresponding author.

18.5.3. The editorial process (what happens next?)

When a paper arrives at an editorial office, it is given an identification number and subsequently forwarded to the journal's editor, who decides whether it is on a topic that falls within the scope of the journal concerned and should be sent out for peer review. If the paper does not fall within the journal's scope, an e-mail or a letter is sent to the author(s) to explain this.

18.5.4. Peer review

The editor nominates two or more colleagues who have particular knowledge of the paper's topic to peer review it. This process may be performed blind, in which case the author details are removed before the paper is sent to the reviewers. Most journals provide a checklist of points against which the reviewers assess the paper. Reviewers are given a deadline by which they should return their reviews to the editor. Apart from commenting on specific points, reviewers are also asked to recommend whether a paper should be accepted without revision, accepted following revisions, or rejected.

18.5.5. The editorial letter

The editor considers both reviews and then decides whether to accept or reject the paper. Very few papers are accepted without revision; some are rejected; many are accepted subject to minor or major revision. Finally, the editor writes to the author(s) with a decision on the paper. The authors are free to disagree with the comments made by the reviewers and can challenge any of them; if they do so, they must provide evidence to support their challenge. Generally, authors do not challenge comments made by reviewers and requests made by editors. A typical editorial letter is shown in Figure 2 and a typical review, using a checklist of a research paper is presented in Figure 3.

18.5.6. Revisions made by the author(s)

The authors are given a deadline by which to make revisions and resubmit the paper to the editor. A revised manuscript should be accompanied by a list of the revisions highlighted in the revised manuscript.

18.5.7. Editing

If it meets the editor's requirements, the manuscript is edited either by the editor or by an associate editor. This involves ensuring that the paper is written in the journal's house style, that it is consistent and unambiguous, that illustrative material meets the required standard, and that the references are accurate. Many journals will immediately return manuscripts to the authors where references either are incomplete or do not conform to the house style, and it is the responsibility of the author(s) to rectify these. Some journals may also revise the text to make it easier to read or emphasise important points. Depending on the extent of revisions, the edited version may then be returned to the authors for their approval.

18.5.8. Production of a proof and publication

Once approval has been given to the author(s), the paper is laid out in the graphic style of the journal, and a proof of all its pages is produced. The editorial team checks the proof, and a copy is also sent to the author(s) for proof-reading. Authors are provided with instructions on how to submit corrections (this varies from journal to journal) and a deadline for receipt of these. Substantial changes are not generally permitted at this stage, and the journal may levy a charge if the author deems such changes necessary. Any errors are reported and rectified. The corresponding author is generally sent a copyright form requiring the corresponding author to assign copyright to the publishing journal. Once this completed form has been returned to the editorial office, the paper's final copy can be printed. After publication, most journals send the corresponding author a PDF file of the paper in its published form. A PDF file is provided to ensure rapid dissemination of scholarly work, on the understanding that it should only be distributed in small numbers by the author(s) for educational purposes and at no cost to those receiving it. The publishers hold the copyright. It is understood that the PDF file will only be used in a manner consistent with the fair use provisions of the relevant copyright laws. Authors may not use it for any commercial enterprise.

18.6. Presenting results at meetings and conferences

Before publishing the research results, it is common to present them at a national or international scientific meeting that is relevant to the topic of the research. This is not compulsory but is another method for disseminating results. The convention is that only results that have not been published should be presented at such meetings or conferences. Authors must bear this in mind when seeking to publish their results. Such presentations at meetings or conferences usually present only the "highlights" of the research, either through a poster or a short (no more than fifteen minutes, including questions from the audience) oral presentation. Abstracts of such presentations are usually published in the meeting/conference programme book and often in the journal(s) of the organising society or association.

Further resources

Pears R, Shields G. Cite *Them Right*. The *Essential Referencing Guide*. 11th ed. London: Macmillan Education UK; 2019. Available from: www.citethemright.com. [Accessed 2020 Dec 29]

References

1   BioMed Central. Available from: www.biomedcentral.org. Accessed 29 Dec 29 2020.

2   Eaton KA. This is an example of the critical review of a paper submitted to *Oral Health and Dental Management in the Black Sea Countries*, 2009;8(4):53–60.

3   Perkel JM. Synchronised editing: the future of collaborative writing. Nature. 2020;580:154–155. Available from: https://doi.org/10.1038/d41586-020-00916-6.

4   Three ways to collaborate on writing. Document-sharing tools for scientists. 2020 Jan 10 (cited 2021 Jan 7). In: *Nature index. News Blog* (Internet). London: Springer Nature Limited c 2021. Available from: https://www.natureindex.com/news-blog/three-ways-to-collaborate-on-writing.

5   International Committee of Medical Journal Editors (ICMJE). Style—Citation Style Guide and Help, accessed 29 December 2020, www.researchguides.uic.edu/styleguides/icmje.

6   International Committee of Medical Journal Editors (ICMJE). Recommendations for the conduct, reporting, editing, and publication of scholarly work in medical journals. Updated Dec 2019. (cited 2020 Dec 29) Available from: www.icmje.org/recommendations/.

Figure 1. A fictional example of a covering letter from the author:

> Department of Children's Dentistry
> Someplace Dental Hospital & School
> Rose Tree Street
> Someplace
> SP1 4HR

Professor Smith, editor
Dental Journal
3 Whitehall Square
Manchester
M23 5RE   1 November 2022

Re GDPs' Views of Preformed Metal Crowns—Report of a Clinical Trial

Dear Professor Smith,

My co-authors and I would like the attached paper considered for publication in *Dental Journal*. My co-authors have all consented to the submission of the paper to your journal. It has not been submitted to another journal in full or in part.

I am the corresponding author. Details of my contact details and those of my co-authors and the contribution that each has made to the paper are set out below.

Dr Margaret Adams, BDS, MFDS, M Clin Dent, clinical lecturer in paediatric dentistry, Department of Children's Dentistry wrote the paper and planned the study. Reach her by e-mail: madams@someplace.ac.uk or telephone: 09862 753412.

Data collection and study coordination was managed by Shashi Patel, BDS, MFGDP (United Kingdom). General dental practitioner, 53, South Street, Some Place, SP6 7ED. e-mail whiteteeth@yahoo.co.uk or telephone 09862 754819.

Data collection and analysis were conducted by Norman Barnes, BDS, MSc, MGDS, General Dental Practitioner. 71 Orange Grove, Some Place, SP4 8TX e-mail npbarnes@btinternet.com or telephone 09862 836541.

Yours sincerely,
Margaret Adams
cc: Shashi Patel
        Norman Barnes

Figure 2. Fictional example of an editorial letter to the authors:

Margaret Adams

Clinical Lecturer in Paediatric Dentistry

Some Place Dental Hospital and School

Rose Tree Street

Someplace

SP1 4HR   14 December 2020

Re MS 421—GDPs' Views of Preformed Metal Crowns—Report of a Clinical Trial

Dear Margaret,

Thank you for submitting the above paper to *Dental Journal*. I have now received reports from its two reviewers. They are attached to this letter. As you will see, one review was extremely brief. However, you will be pleased to see that both reviewers liked the paper and have recommended that I accept it.

I am happy to do so subject to you and your co-authors agreeing to the following minor revisions or additions, as well as those suggested by the second reviewer:

- Add the words "A group of" at the beginning of the title.
- Revise the section currently headed "Objectives" such that it is headed "Aims."
- Add a brief explanation of why you did not seek ethics approval for the study.
- Add more detail to the methods section including: where the interviews took place, how many sessions there were, how many interviewers were used.
- If there was more than one interviewer, please explain how you ensured consistency.

I am sure that the second reviewer meant to write "Care Index" and not "Core Index" in the suggested amendments section of her report.

Could you please send me a revised manuscript by Jan 31 2022?

Best wishes,
Roger Smith
Editor, *Dental Journal*

Figure 3. Fictional example of a review using the checklist for papers reporting quantitative research[2]

Peer Reviewer's checklist and report form for papers reporting quantitative research

MS 421—GDPs' Views on the use of Preformed Metal Crowns—Report of a Clinical Trial

General

1. Is the topic of the paper appropriate for the journal? **yes**
2. Does the paper conform to the published guidelines for authors of the journal? **yes**
3. Is it an important or significant topic? **yes**
4. Does the study add to the existing knowledge base? **yes**

Presentation

5. Does the title accurately reflect the content of the paper? **yes**
6. Does the paper have a logical construction? **yes**
7. Does the length of the paper need adjusting (too long or short)? **no**
8. Is the paper written in a clear and easily understandable style? **yes**
9. Is the paper free of grammatical or typographical errors? **yes**

Abstract

10. Is there an abstract that conforms to the journal's published guidelines for authors? **yes**
11. Does the abstract present an accurate synopsis of the paper? **yes**
12. Are there keywords, and do they seem to be appropriate? **yes**

Introduction and Aims

13. Is the introduction appropriate to the paper's subject? **yes**
14. Is the literature that has been reviewed relevant, and is it comprehensive? **Not entirely; in the last six months, three relevant papers on the Hall technique have been published. However, they are not referred to in the introduction or the discussion**
15. From the introduction, does the study seem original in concept? **yes**
16. Do the aims of the study follow logically from the literature review, and are they clearly stated? **yes**
17. If appropriate, is a null hypothesis stated? **Not applicable**

Methods

18. Is the design of the study consistent with its aims? **yes**
19. If applicable, was a pilot study performed to test the methodology? **No, the authors should explain why this was not done**

20. Is the sample representative of the population in question? **yes**
21. Are controls needed and used in the study? **no**
22. If controls are used, are they appropriate? **no**
23. Is the method of selecting the sample/cases and controls clearly described? **yes**
24. Are other details such as numbers, periods, and statistical tests used clearly described and consistent? **yes**
25. If relevant, have examiners been trained and calibrated? **Calibration and training are not mentioned in the methods section; they should be**
26. Are details of such training and calibration given? **See 25 above**
27. If questionnaires and proforma have been used, have they been tested, are they relevant to the study, and are they presented either as figures in the paper or via a link to a website? **yes**
28. Could there be ethical objections to the study? **I do not think so**
29. Does the paper include a clear statement on whether ethical approval was sought, and if so, from whom? **Yes see page 12 of the paper**
30. If ethical approval was not sought, is there a clear explanation why? **yes**
31. If applicable, has patient/parental consent been sought? **yes**

Results

32. Are the results and any statistical tests presented clearly and unambiguously (tables, figures, and graphs)? **yes**
33. Are any missing data? If so, are they accounted for (e.g. dropouts, non-responders)? **missing data accounted for**
34. Are the numbers, percentages, statistical values accurate and precise? **As far as I can tell**
35. If statistical tests have been used, are they appropriate? **As far as I can tell**
36. If statistical tests have not been used, can this be justified? **yes**
37. Is the sample too small to justify the findings? **it is small, but this paper follows on from other studies when the sample must have been considered acceptable**
38. Although they may be statistically significant, are the findings clinically significant? **yes**
39. Are the results believable? **yes**

Discussion

40. Does the discussion critique and discuss the methodology used? **yes**
41. Does the discussion comprehensively discuss the results? **yes**
42. Are the results discussed concerning other important literature on the topic area of the study? **No, the three recent studies referred to in answer to question 14 were not mentioned**
43. Does the discussion extend beyond the methods and results of the study? **no**

Conclusions

44. Do the conclusions accurately reflect the results of the study? **yes**
45. Are the conclusions clearly set out? **yes**

Acknowledgements

46. Is any source of funding identified? **No, the authors should clarify this point**
47. Is there a statement of conflict of interest? **No, one should be added**
48. Is there a statement of exactly how each author contributed to the paper? **No, it should be added.**

References

49. Are the references accurate, up-to-date, and relevant? **No, the three recent papers mentioned in answer to questions 14 and 42 should be added.**

Rating:

1 excellent	4 poor
2 good	5 very poor
3 satisfactory	6 not applicable

Please phrase your suggested amendments on this page so that they may be passed directly to the author(s).

Page three

The Hall Technique is critical to the article and the understanding of this paper.

I should like to see the explanation of the Hall Technique on page 3 be given a bold sub-heading so that PDC readers can, at a glance, find its explanation. This may encourage them to read the article.

Page six (last paragraph)

A short sentence, possibly in parenthesis, of the core* index, could be of use to readers.

If the authors can address the points raised in this review, I recommend that the paper be accepted for publication.

*The reviewer meant "Care Index."

Appendix 1. Guidelines and Checklists

Santini A.

Introduction

This appendix provides further details of the guidelines and checklists cited in chapters 1 to 18. Most apply to the assessment of the reports of research. However, some are clinical guidelines, which aim to improve clinical effectiveness and efficiency. They are based on a combination of research evidence, experience and expert opinion. They provide advice on assessment, treatment modalities and management strategies for patients. Their recommendations are predicated on published high-quality research and can help clinicians keep abreast of the current literature.

Methodological assessment of studies selected as potential sources of evidence is based on several criteria that focus on those aspects of the study design that research has shown to significantly affect the risk of bias in the results reported and conclusions drawn. These criteria differ between study types, and a range of checklists is used to bring a degree of consistency to the assessment process.

Local, national, and international organisations produce clinical guidelines, though different guidelines can differ in their value. They need to be critically appraised in the same fashion as reports of research studies. There is a view that guidelines may be too prescriptive and hinder research. As far as clinical practice is concerned, they do not consider human variability and specific circumstances. Thus in some circumstances, it may be reasonable to ignore a clinical guideline for a specific patient. The knowledge, skills and clinical judgment of clinicians are not intended to be superseded by clinical guidelines. A sensible interpretation and application of all guidelines are required.[1, 2]

The legality of guidelines

It is questionable whether courts would consider standards of care promoted by clinical guidelines as legal "gold standards." However, if litigation ensues, when most medical professionals have recognised a guideline, a convincing rationale for not following the guidance would be required. The standard of care for professionals is a comparison with their professional peers. The case *Bolam v. Friern Hospital Management Committee* (1957) WLR 583[1] established that if a doctor acts following a responsible body of medical opinion, he or she will not be negligent. The test, known as the Bolam test, was arrived at following the case of Bolam (1957) and remains good law.[3] It is pertinent to mention that although the ruling of the Supreme Court on the Montgomery (2015) case did override the Bolam (1957) test for consent, it did not do so for clinical decision making.

The process of guideline development is summarised in Table 1:

• Confirm a need for the proposed clinical guideline.
• Identify individuals and stakeholders who will help develop the guideline.
• Identify the evidence for the guideline.
• Evaluate current practice against the evidence.
• Write the guideline.
• Agree on how the change will be introduced into practice.
• Engage in consultation and peer review and amend guidelines if necessary.
• Gain ratification.
• Implement and disseminate the guideline.
• Audit the effectiveness of the guideline

Table 1. The process of guideline development

The following guidelines and checklists are presented in this appendix:

1. AGREE II (Appraisal of Guidelines Research Evaluation Enterprise II)
2. CARE (Case Report guidelines)
3. CASP (Critical Appraisal Skills Programme)
4. CONSORT (Consolidated Standards of Reporting Trials)
5. GRADE (Grading of Recommendations Assessment, Development and Evaluation)
6. Qualitative studies (guidelines for reporting)
7. Quantitative research (checklist for peer reviewers)
8. PRISMA (Preferred Reporting Items for Systematic Reviews and Meta-Analyses)
9. STARD (Guidelines for reporting diagnostic accuracy studies)
10. SIGN (Scottish Intercollegiate Guidelines Network)
11. STROBE (Strengthening the Reporting of Observational studies in Epidemiology)

Because this manual is on the topic of research, clinical guidelines, such as those produced by the National Institute for Health and Clinical Excellence (NICE) and those found in many College of General Dentistry publications, such as *Standards in Dentistry,* are not included.

The reader should note that guidelines and checklists are updated from time to time. They should therefore check that they are using the most up to date version before appraising literature.

1. AGREE II (Appraisal of Guidelines Research Evaluation Enterprise II)

AGREE 11 is an international tool to assess the quality and reporting of practice guidelines. It is summarised in Table 2:

• **Scope and purpose** are concerned with the overall aim of the guideline, the specific clinical questions, and the target patient population.	
• **Stakeholder involvement** focuses on the extent to which the guideline represents the views of its intended users.	
• **Rigour of development** relates to the process used to gather and synthesise the evidence and the methods used to formulate and update the recommendations.	
• **Clarity and presentation** deal with the language and format of the guideline.	
• **Applicability** pertains to the likely organisational, behavioural and cost implications of applying the guideline.	
• **Editorial independence** is concerned with the independence of the recommendations and acknowledgement of possible conflicts of interest from the guideline development group.	

Table 2. Summary of AGREE II checklist

Each item is rated on the extent to which a criterion has been fulfilled and scored on a four-point scale where 4 = strongly agree, 3 = agree, 2 = disagree, and 1 = strongly disagree.

Further details for AGREE II are at www.agreetrust.org.

2. CARE (case report guidelines)

The CARE guidelines, including a reporting checklist, have been drawn up to aid in the robust reporting of case reports. The thirteen-item checklist includes the title, keywords, abstract, introduction, patient information, clinical findings, timeline, diagnostic assessment, therapeutic interventions, follow-up and outcomes, discussion, patient perspective, and informed consent. Well-written case reports provide feedback on clinical practice guidelines and offer a framework for early signals of effectiveness, adverse events, and cost. In addition, they can be shared for medical, scientific, or educational purposes (Table 3):

Section	Item	Checklist item description	Reported on page
Title	1	The words case report and the area of focus should appear in the title (such as diabetes, a therapeutic approach, an outcome)	
Keywords	2	Two to five keywords that identify areas covered in this case report	
Abstract	3a	Introduction—what is unique about this case? What does it add to the medical literature? Why is this important?	
	3b	The patient's primary concerns and important clinical findings	
	3c	The primary diagnoses, therapeutic interventions, and outcomes	
	3d	Conclusion—what are the takeaway lessons from this case?	
Introduction	4	One or two paragraphs summarising why this case is unique, regarding the relevant medical literature	

Patient information	5a	Anonymized demographic and other patient-specific information	
	5b	Main concerns and symptoms of the patient	
	5c	Medical, family, and psychosocial history, including relevant genetic information (this should also appear in the timeline)	
	5d	Relevant past interventions and their outcomes	
Clinical findings	6	Describe the relevant physical examination (PE) and other significant clinical findings	
Timeline	7	Relevant data from the patient's history is organised as a timeline.	
Diagnostic assessment	8a	Diagnostic methods (PE, laboratory testing, imaging, surveys)	
	8b	Diagnostic challenges (access, financial, cultural)	
	8c	Diagnostic reasoning, including other diagnoses, considered	
	8d	Prognostic characteristics when applicable (staging)	
Therapeutic intervention	9a	Types of intervention (pharmacological, surgical, preventive)	
	9b	Administration of intervention (dosage, strength, duration)	
	9c	Any changes in the interventions (with rationale)	
Follow-up and outcomes	10a	Clinician and patient-assessed outcomes (when appropriate)	
	10b	Important follow-up diagnostic and other test results	
	10c	Intervention adherence and tolerability (how was this assessed)	
	10d	Adverse and unanticipated events	
Discussion	11a	Strengths and limitations in your approach to this case	
	11b	Discussion of the relevant medical literature	
	11c	The rationale for your conclusions (causality assessment)	
	11d	The primary takeaway lessons from this case report	
Patient perspective	12	When appropriate, the patient should share his or her perspective on the treatments received	
Informed consent	13	Did the patient give informed consent? Provide if requested.	

Table 3. The thirteen-item CARE checklist

Further details are available at www.care-statement.org/.

3. CASP (Critical Appraisal Skills Programme)

The critical appraisal skills programme (CASP) is housed at the Oxford Centre for Triple Value Healthcare Ltd.

CASP appraisal checklists are a set of eight critical appraisal tools designed to be used when reading research reports. CASP has appraisal checklists for systematic reviews, randomised controlled trials, cohort studies, case-control studies, economic evaluations, diagnostic studies, qualitative studies, and clinical prediction rules.

The CASP randomised controlled trial standard checklist is one example. It includes eleven questions that help the reader make sense of a randomised controlled trial (RCT). These questions are designed to assist the reader think about these aspects systematically.

Aspects that need to be considered when appraising a randomised controlled trial are set out in Table 4:

• Is the basic study design valid for a randomised controlled trial? (Section A)
• Was the study methodologically sound? (Section B) What are the results? (Section C)
• Will the results help locally? (Section D)

Table 4. Aspects to consider when appraising a randomised controlled trial

The first three questions (section A) are screening questions about the validity of the primary study design and can be answered quickly. If, in light of responses to section A, it appears that the study design is valid, the reader continues to section B to assess whether the study was methodologically sound and if it is worth continuing with the appraisal by answering the remaining questions in sections C and D.

The CASP RCT checklist was initially based on the *Journal of the American Medical Association* users' guides to the medical literature in 1994 (adapted from Guyatt, Sackett, and Cook) and piloted with healthcare practitioners. The current version has been updated, taking into account the CONSORT 2010 guideline (http://www.consort-statement.org/consort-2010).

Further details are available at www.casp-uk.net

4. CONSORT (Consolidated Standards of Reporting Trials)

A complete and transparent description of clinical trials' results is vital to comprehensively assess the quality of healthcare interventions. To meet this requirement, a series of guidelines have been developed. The CONSORT (consolidated standards of reporting trials) statement in 1996 was the first to provide recommendations for the publication of randomised controlled clinical trials, the gold standard to assess healthcare interventions.

Subsequently, the CONSORT 2010 Statement was developed. It is an evidence-based set of recommendations for reporting RCTs. The checklist contains twenty-five items focusing on "individually randomised, two-group, parallel trials," which are the most common type of RCT (Table 5). It is recommended that the statement be read in conjunction with the CONSORT 2010 explanation and elaboration for necessary clarifications of all the items.[4]

Section/Topic	Item No.	Checklist item	Reported on page No.
Title and abstract			
	1a	Identification as a randomised trial in the title	
	1b	Structured summary of trial design, methods, results, and conclusions (for specific guidance, see CONSORT for abstracts)	
Introduction			
Background and objectives	2a	Scientific background and explanation of the rationale	
	2b	Specific objectives or hypotheses	
Methods			
Trial design	3a	Description of trial design (such as parallel, factorial), including allocation ratio	
	3b	Important changes to methods after trial commencement (such as eligibility criteria), with reasons	
Participants	4a	Eligibility criteria for participants	
	4b	Settings and locations where the data were collected	
Interventions	5	The interventions for each group with sufficient details to allow replication, including how and when they were administered	
Outcomes	6a	Completely defined pre-specified primary and secondary outcome measures, including how and when they were assessed	
	6b	Any changes to trial outcomes after the trial commenced, with reasons	
Sample size	7a	How sample size was determined	
	7b	When applicable, explanation of any interim analyses and stopping guidelines	
Randomisation			
Sequence generation	8a	The method used to generate the random allocation sequence	
	8b	Type of randomisation; details of any restriction (such as blocking and block size)	
Allocation concealment mechanism	9	The mechanism used to implement the random allocation sequence (such as sequentially numbered containers) describes any steps taken to conceal the sequence until interventions were assigned	
Implementation	10	Who generated the random allocation sequence, who enrolled participants, and who assigned participants to interventions?	

Blinding	11a	If done, who was blinded after assignment to interventions (for example, participants, care providers, those assessing outcomes) and how	
	11b	If relevant, a description of the similarity of interventions	
Statistical methods	12a	Statistical methods used to compare groups for primary and secondary outcomes	
	12b	Methods for additional analyses, such as subgroup analyses and adjusted analyses	

Results

Participant flow (a diagram is strongly recommended)	13a	For each group, the randomly assigned participants received intended treatment and were analysed for the primary outcome	
	13b	For each group, losses and exclusions after randomisation, together with reasons	
Recruitment	14a	Dates defining the periods of recruitment and follow-up	
	14b	Why the trial ended or was stopped	
Baseline data	15	A table showing baseline demographic and clinical characteristics for each group	
Numbers analysed	16	For each group, the number of participants (denominator) included in each analysis and whether the analysis was by original assigned groups	
Outcomes and estimation	17a	For each primary and secondary outcome, results for each group, and the estimated effect size and its precision (such as 95 percent confidence interval)	
	17b	For binary outcomes, presentation of both absolute and relative effect sizes is recommended.	
Ancillary analyses	18	Results of any other analyses performed, including subgroup analyses and adjusted analyses, distinguishing the pre-specified from the exploratory	
Harms	19	All important harms or unintended effects in each group (for specific guidance, see CONSORT for harms)	

Discussion

Limitations	20	Trial limitations, addressing sources of potential bias, imprecision, and, if relevant, the multiplicity of analyses	
Generalisability	21	Generalisability (external validity, applicability) of the trial findings	
Interpretation	22	Interpretation consistent with results, balancing benefits and harms, and considering other relevant evidence	

Other information			
Registration	23	Registration number and name of trial registry	
Protocol	24	Where the full trial protocol can be accessed, if available	
Funding	25	Sources of funding and other support (such as the supply of drugs), the role of funders	

Table 5. CONSORT 2010 checklist of information to include when reporting a randomised trial

Treatment studies compare the effects of a new treatment drug, intervention, or method with a previously used treatment drug, intervention, or method. The latter is usually the recognised best treatment drug, intervention, or method used at the study time. Any recorded improvement determined by the study can be quantified in absolute or relative terms or by the number needed to treat (NNT). The protocol of a treatment study should be clearly stated, with due attention paid to the points set out in Table 6:

Methodology protocol of a treatment study
• A clearly stated, focused clinical question and primary hypothesis;
• A randomisation process is clearly explained;
• Comparable groups allocated at the start of the study;
• Concealed allocation used in the apportionment of interventions;
• Groups should be treated equally except for the experimental intervention;
• Use effective blinding methods.

Results of a treatment study
• Control event rate;
• Experimental event rate;
• Absolute risk reduction/benefit increase;;
• Relative risk reduction/benefit increase;
• Numbers needed to treat;
• The precision of the estimate of treatment effect-confidence intervals.

Generalizability of a Treatment Study
• Does the target population relate to your patients?
• Will your patients benefit from the intervention?
• Are the benefits of the intervention worth the risks and costs?
• Have patients' values and preferences been considered?

Table 6. Points to include in the protocol for an RCT

Further information about CONSORT is available at www.consort-statement.org.

5. GRADE (Grading of Recommendations Assessment, Development and Evaluation)

The Grading of Recommendations Assessment, Development and Evaluation (GRADE) Working Group produced a grading system in which the quality of evidence is categorised as "high," "moderate," "low," or "very low." In addition, recommendations are graded as being "strong or weak."

More details can be obtained at http://www. gradeworkinggroup.org/.

6. Qualitative studies (guidelines for reporting)

Chapter 6 describes qualitative research processes, which concentrate on natural settings and are dependent on inductive reasoning processes. The results are less generalisable than those from quantitative studies. Data from qualitative research can be used to generate theories compared to the deductive inquiry processes used in quantitative research, where data are used to confirm or refute a hypothesis.

As with other forms of research, a checklist such as the one set out in Table 7 aids in the evaluation of a qualitative research study:

Methods
Was a significant clinical problem stated clearly? Was a qualitative approach appropriate?
Were the methods used to choose the participant clear?
Was the setting clearly described?
Were the data collection methods sufficiently described?
Were the data collection methods appropriate to the research question?
Data Results
Were appropriate the data analyses methods used?
Was the data analysis sufficiently precise and thorough?
Are the resulting data plausible?
Were any quantitative methods used appropriately?
Could the study be repeated to corroborate the results?
Are the findings and conclusion clearly stated?

Table 7. A checklist for evaluating a qualitative study

Qualitative research is grounded in specific theories, the discussion of which is beyond the remit of this appendix. The reader is referred to chapter 6 and to the CASP guideline for assessing reports of qualitative research.

7. Quantitative studies (checklist for peer reviewers)

The checklist (Eaton 2009),[5] which appears at the end of Chapter 18 was designed to guide peer reviewers of papers reporting quantitative research studies.

8. PRISMA (preferred reporting items for systematic reviews and meta-analyses)

The original PRISMA statement (Moher et al. 2009) was designed to help authors improve the reporting of systematic reviews and meta-analyses. Peer reviewers and journal editors widely use it: It can be helpful in the critical appraisal of published systematic reviews. However, according to a statement on the PRISMA website, "it is not a quality assessment instrument to gauge the quality of a systematic review."[6]

There have been several updates, including

- PRISMA-P for developing review protocols (Shamseer et al. 2015);[7]
- PRISMA-IPD (individual patient data) (Stewart et al. 2015);[8]
- PRISMA-NMA (Network Meta-Analyses) (Hutton et al. 2016). [9]

9. STARD (Guidelines for reporting diagnostic accuracy studies)

This section should be read in conjunction with Chapter 10. It presents tables 8 and 9, as well as Figure 1.

• Which patients could develop the disease? (Predisposition)
• Which patients have asymptomatic disease? (Screening)
• Which patients have symptomatic disease? (Diagnosis)
• How advanced is the disease?
• Will the disease progress over time? (Prognosis)
• Is a drug effective?
• Is the disease controlled? (Monitoring)
• Has the disease recurred? (Relapse)

Table 8. Checklist for diagnostic test accuracy

Methodology
• Did the patient sample have a suitable range of patients?
• Was the reference standard applied despite the consequences of the index test result?
• Was there was an independent and blind comparison between the reference standard and the index test?

Table 9. Checklists for methodology, generalisability, and accuracy

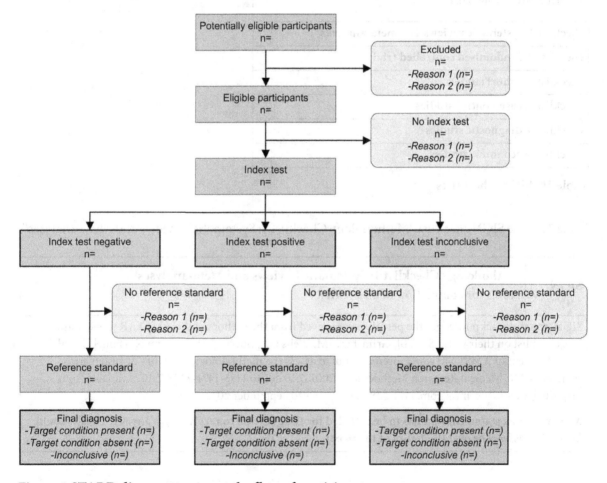

Figure 1 STARD diagram to report the flow of participants through a DIAGNOSTIC TEST accuracy study.

10. SIGN

The Scottish Intercollegiate Guidelines Network (SIGN) was launched in 1993 to sponsor and support the development of evidence-based national clinical guidelines for NHS Scotland. SIGN is part of the Evidence Directorate of Healthcare Improvement Scotland, and core funding supports the SIGN guideline programme.

A Guideline Developer's Handbook (SIGN 50), which describes their approach to levels of evidence and grades of recommendation, was printed in 2008. In 2012 an updated memorandum of the understanding between the Scottish Intercollegiate Guidelines Network and the National Institute for Health and Care excellence was produced.

The following SIGN checklists were subjected to evaluation and adaptation to meet SIGN's requirements for balancing methodological rigour and practicality of use. These are available at sign@sign.ac.uk. They include those shown in Table 10:

Available **SIGN Checklists**
checklist 1: **systematic reviews and meta-analyses**
checklist 2: **randomised controlled trials**
checklist 3: **cohort studies**
checklist 4: **case-control studies**
checklist 5: **diagnostic studies**
checklist 6: **economic studies**

Table 10. SIGN Checklists

Table 11 is the SIGN checklist "Methodology Checklist 1: Systematic Reviews and Meta-analyses":

SIGN	**Methodology Checklist 1: Systematic Reviews and Meta-analyses** **Notes for completion of a checklist**
SIGN gratefully acknowledges the permission received from the authors of the AMSTAR tool to base this checklist on their work: Shea BJ, Grimshaw JM, Wells GA, Boers M, Andersson N, Hamel C et al. "Development of AMSTAR: a measurement tool to assess the methodological quality of systematic reviews." BMC Medical Research Methodology 2007, 7:10 doi:10.1186/1471-2288-7-10. Available from http://www.biomedcentral.com/1471-2288/7/10 (cited 10 September 2012). **Must refer to a statement that has to be fulfilled for the question to receive a yes answer. These should be used to assess the overall quality of the paper.**	

Section 1: Internal validity		
In a well-conducted systematic review:		**Notes**
1.1	The research question is clearly defined, and the inclusion/exclusion criteria must be listed in the paper.	The PICO must be evident in the paper, even if not directly referred to. The research question and inclusion criteria should be established before the review is conducted.
1.2	A comprehensive literature search is carried out.	At least two relevant electronic sources must be searched. The report must list the databases used (e.g., Central, EMBASE, and MEDLINE). (Cochrane register/Central counts as two sources; a grey literature search counts as supplementary).
		(PubMed and MEDLINE count as one database.)
		Keywords or MESH terms must be stated, and the search strategy should be provided where feasible. In addition, dates for the search should be provided.
		The paragraph above is the minimum requirement.
		All searches should be supplemented by consulting current contents, reviews, textbooks, specialised registers, or experts in the particular field of study and reviewing the references in the studies found.
		The paragraph above is a quality criterion that affects the overall rating of the review.
		Notes
		This criterion will not apply in the case of prospective meta-analysis—this is where meta-analysis is based on pre-selected studies identified for inclusion before the results of those studies are known. However, such reports must state that they are prospective.
1.3	At least two people should have selected studies.	At least two people should select papers. Then, there should be a consensus process to resolve any differences.
1.4	At least two people should have extracted data.	At least two people should extract data and should report that a consensus was agreed upon. For example, one person checking the others data extraction is accurate is acceptable.
1.5	The status of publication was not used as an inclusion criterion.	The authors should state that they searched for reports regardless of their publication status. In addition, the authors should state whether or not they excluded any reports (from the systematic review) based on their publication status.
		If the review indicates that there was a search for "grey literature" or "unpublished literature," indicate "yes." For example, the SIGLE database, dissertations, conference proceedings, and trial registries are all considered grey for this purpose. If searching a source that contains both grey and non-grey, must specify that they were searching for grey/unpublished lit.

1.6	The excluded studies are listed.	Limiting the excluded studies to references is acceptable.
1.7	The relevant characteristics of the included studies are provided.	In an aggregated form such as a table, data from the original studies should be provided on the participants, interventions and outcomes. In addition, the ranges of characteristics in all the included studies, e.g., age, race, sex, relevant socioeconomic data, disease status, duration, severity, or other diseases, should be reported. (Note that a format other than a table is acceptable, as long as the information noted here is provided). The absence of this will make it impossible to form guideline recommendations. Mark as (-) original papers would need to be examined.
1.8	The scientific quality of the included studies was assessed and documented	It can include the use of a quality scoring tool or checklist, e.g. risk of bias assessment, or a description of quality items, with some result for EACH study ("low" or "high" is OK, as long as it is clear which studies scored "low" and which scored "high"; a summary score/range for all studies is not acceptable. The absence of this will make it impossible to form guideline recommendations. Mark as (-).
1.9	Was the scientific quality of the included studies used appropriately?	Examples include sensitivity analysis based on study quality, exclusion of poor-quality studies, and statements such as "the results should be interpreted with caution due to poor quality of included studies." The methodological rigour and scientific quality results should be considered in the analysis and the conclusions of the review and explicitly stated in formulating recommendations. Cannot score yes for this question if scored no for question 1.8.
1.10	Appropriate methods are used to combine the individual study findings.	Studies that are very clinically heterogeneous should not be combined in a meta-analysis. Look at the forest plot—do the results look similar across the studies? A test should be done to assess statistical heterogeneity for the pooled result, i.e. Chi-squared (c^2) test for homogeneity and/or I^2 test for inconsistency. The authors should have explored possible explanations using sensitivity analysis or meta-regression methods if significant heterogeneity is apparent. A random-effects analysis may be used to account for between-study variation but is not a "fix" for heterogeneity. Planned subgroup analyses should be pre-specified and limited because conducting many subgroup analyses increases the probability of obtaining a statistically significant result by chance. Therefore, conclusions based on post-hoc subgroup analyses must be interpreted with caution. Cannot score yes for this question if scored no for question 1.8.

1.11	The likelihood of publication bias was assessed appropriately.	The possibility of publication bias should be assessed where possible, commonly done by visual inspection of a funnel plot together with a statistical test for asymmetry (e.g., Egger regression test), although other statistical and modelling approaches may be reported. The absence of a funnel plot does not mean the likelihood of publication bias was not assessed appropriately (there are other methods); 10 studies are just a ball-park minimum number for a funnel plot, and a plot is of little use when there are few studies.
1.12	Conflicts of interest are declared.	Potential sources of support should be acknowledged in both the systematic review and the included studies.

SECTION 2: OVERALL ASSESSMENT OF THE STUDY

2.1	What is your overall assessment of the methodological quality of this review?	Rate the overall methodological quality of the study, using the following as a guide: **High quality** (++): The majority of criteria met. Little or no risk of bias. **Acceptable** (+): Most criteria met. Some flaws in the study with an associated risk of bias. **Low quality** (-): Either most criteria not met, or significant flaws relating to key aspects of study design. **Reject** (0): Poor quality study with significant flaws. Wrong study type. Not relevant to the guidelines.

Table 11. SIGN: "methodology checklist 1: systematic reviews and meta-analyses"

Full details of SIGN can be obtained at http://www.sign.ac.uk/.

11. STROBE (strengthening the reporting of observational studies in epidemiology)

The STROBE guidelines aim to provide a readily available checklist to present what was planned and carried out in an observational study.

Available Titles of the STROBE Guidelines
• STROBE checklist for **cohort, case-control, and cross-sectional studies** (combined)
• STROBE checklist for **cohort, case-control, and cross-sectional studies**
• Checklist for **cohort studies**
• Checklist for **case-control studies**
• Checklist for **cross-sectional studies**
• Draft STROBE checklist for **conference abstracts**

STROBE was an international, collaborative initiative of epidemiologists, methodologists, statisticians, researchers and journal editors involved in conducting and disseminating observational studies, with the common aim of strengthening the reporting of observational studies in epidemiology. The titles of the STROBE guidelines are set out in Table FF.

Table 12. Titles of the STROBE guidelines

The STROBE statement checklist (Table 13) is available for free on the websites of PLoS Medicine at http://www.plosmedicine.org/, Annals of Internal Medicine at http://www.annals.org/, and Epidemiology at http://www.epidem.com/). In addition, information on the STROBE Initiative is available at www.strobe-statement.org.

STROBE Statement—a checklist of items that should be addressed in reports of observational studies.		
	Item number	Recommendation
Title and Abstract	1	(a) Indicate the study's design with a commonly used term in the title or the abstract
		(b) Provide in the abstract an informative and balanced summary of what was done and what was found
Introduction		
Background/rationale	2	Explain the scientific background and rationale for the investigation being reported
Objectives	3	State-specific objectives, including any prespecified hypotheses
Methods		
Study design	4	Present key elements of study design early in the paper
Setting	5	Describe the setting, locations, and relevant dates, including periods of recruitment, exposure, follow-up, and data collection
Participants	6	(a) Cohort study—give the eligibility criteria and the sources and methods of selection of participants. Describe methods of follow-up Case-control study—give the eligibility criteria and the sources and methods of case ascertainment and control selection. Give the rationale for the choice of cases and controls.

		Cross-sectional study—give the eligibility criteria and the sources and methods of selection of participants.
		(b)
		Cohort study—For matched studies, give matching criteria and number of exposed and unexposed case-control studies—for matched studies, give matching criteria and the number of controls per case
Variables	7	Clearly define all outcomes, exposures, predictors, potential confounders, and effect modifiers. Give diagnostic criteria, if applicable
Data sources/measurement	8[a]	For each variable of interest, give sources of data and details of assessment methods (measurement).
		Describe comparability of assessment methods if there is more than one group
Bias	9	Describe any efforts to address potential sources of bias
Study size	10	Explain how the study size was arrived at
Quantitative variables	11	Explain how quantitative variables were handled in the analyses. If applicable, describe which groupings were chosen and why
Statistical methods	12	(a)
		Describe all statistical methods, including those used to control for confounding
		(b)
		Describe any methods used to examine subgroups and interactions
		(c)
		Explain how missing data were addressed
		(d)
		Cohort study—if applicable, explain how the loss to follow-up was addressed case-control study—if applicable, explain how matching of cases and controls was addressed cross-sectional study—if applicable, describe analytical methods taking account of sampling strategy
		(e)
		Describe any sensitivity analyses

Results			
Participants	13[a]	(a)	Report the numbers of individuals at each stage of the study—e.g., numbers potentially eligible, examined for eligibility, confirmed eligible, included in the study, completing follow-up, and analysed
		(b)	Give reasons for non-participation at each stage
		(c)	Consider the use of a flow diagram
Descriptive data	14[a]	(a)	Give characteristics of study participants (e.g., demographic, clinical, social) and information on exposures and potential confounders.
		(b)	Indicate the number of participants with missing data for each variable of interest
		(c)	Cohort study—summarise follow-up time (e.g., average and total amount)
Outcome data	15[a]		Cohort study—report numbers of outcome events or summary measures over time
			Case-control study—report numbers in each exposure category or summary measures of exposure
			Cross-sectional study—report numbers of outcome events or summary measures
Main results	16	(a)	Give unadjusted estimates and, if applicable, confounder-adjusted estimates and their precision (e.g., 95 per cent confidence interval). Make clear which confounders were adjusted for and why they were included.
		(b)	Report category boundaries when continuous variables were categorised
		(c)	If relevant, consider translating estimates of relative risk into absolute risk for a meaningful time.
Other analyses	17		Report other analyses undertaken —e.g., analyses of subgroups and interactions, and sensitivity analyses

Discussion		
Key results	18	Summarise key results regarding study objectives
Limitations	19	Discuss limitations of the study, taking into account sources of potential bias or imprecision. Discuss both direction and magnitude of any potential bias
Interpretation	20	Give a cautious overall interpretation of results considering objectives, limitations, the multiplicity of analyses, results from similar studies, and other relevant evidence
Generalisability	21	Discuss the generalisability (external validity) of the study results
Other information		
Funding	22	Give the source of funding and the role of the funders for the present study and, if applicable, for the original study on which the present article is based.

**Table 13. STROBE statement checklist of items that should be
addressed in reports of observational studies**

References

1   Röhrig B, du Prel J-B, and Blettner M. Study design in medical research. Part 2 of a series on the evaluation of scientific publications. *Deutsch Arzteblatt, Imternational* 2009;106(11):184–189.

2   Besen J, Gan SD. A critical evaluation of clinical research study designs. *Journal of Investigative Dermatology* 2014;134,e18.

3   Hurwitz B. Legal and political considerations of clinical practice guidelines. *British Medical Journal* 1999; 318:661- 664.

4   Alan DG, Schulz KF, Moher D, Egger M, Davidoff F, Elbourne D, Gøtzsche PC, Lang T; The revised CONSORT statement for reporting randomised trials: explanation and elaboration. CONSORT GROUP (Consolidated Standards of Reporting Trials). *Annals of Internal Medicine.* 2001 17 April;134(8):663-694.

5   Eaton KA. This is an example of the critical review of a paper submitted to *Oral Health and Dental Management in the Black Sea Countries. Oral Health Dent Management in Black Sea Countries.* 2009;8(4):53–60.

6   Moher D, Liberati A, Tetzlaff J, Alan DG. Prefered reporting items for systematic reviews and meta-analysis: The PRISMA Statement. The PRISMA Group. *Open Medicine.* 2009; 3(3): e123–e130. Published online 2009 21 July.

7   Shamsser L., Moher D, Clarke M., Ghersi D., Liberati A., Petticrew M., Shekelle P., Stewart L.A.,— PRISMA—P Group. Preferred reporting terms for systematic review and meta-analysis protocols (PRISMA P) 2015 elaboration and explanation. *British Medical Journal* 2015 2 January:350:G7647. Doi 10.1136/bmj. g7847.

8   Stewart L.A., Clarke M., Rovers M., Riley R.D., Simmonds M., Stewart G., Tierney F. PRISMA- PD Development Group. Preferred reporting items for systematic review and meta-analysis of participant data the PRISMA-IPD statement. *Journal of the American Medical Association* 2015 Apr 28; 313(16): 1657-1665. Doi 10.10001/jama 2015.3656.

9   Z. Hutton B., Catalá-Lopez F., Moher D. The PRISMA statement extension for systematic reviews incorporating network meta-analysis PRISMA NMA. *Medica Clinica* (Barcelona) 2016 Sep 16; 147(6) ; 262–266. Doi 10.1016/j.medcli. 2016.02.025. Epub 2016 31 March

10   Bossuyt PM, Reitsma JB, Bruns DE, et al. Stard 2015: An updated list of essential items for reporting diagnostic accuracy studies. *British Medical Journal* 2015:h5527.

11   Cohen J.F., Korevaar D.A., Alan D.G., Bruns De.Gatsois C.A., Hooft L., Irwig L., Levine D., Reitsma J.B., de Vet H,C,W., Bossuyt P.M.M. STARD 2015 guidelines for reporting diagnostic accuracy studies: explanation and elaboration. *BMJ Open* 2016 Nov 14; 6(11)e12799. Doi 101136/bmjpoen-2916-012799.

Additional reading

World Health Organisation. Recommended format for a research protocol. World Health Organization website. www.who.int/rpc/research_ethics/format_rp/en/ accessed on 10 March 2021.

NHS Health Research Authority. *Defining Research.* London: Health Research Authority; 2009 (rev. 2013). www.hra.nhs.uk/documents/2013/09/defining-research.pdf (Accessed Dec 2014).

SPIRIT (Standard Protocol Items: Recommendations for Interventional Trials): an international initiative that aims to improve the quality of clinical trial protocols by defining an evidence-based set of items to address in a protocol. www.spirit-statement.org accessed on 10 March 2021.

CONSORT (Consolidated Standards of Reporting Trials) encompasses various initiatives developed to alleviate the problems arising from inadequate reporting of randomised controlled trials. *www.consort-statement.org* accessed on 10 March 2021.

www.equator-network.org accessed on 10 March 2021.

Appendix 2. Glossary of Terms with Some Explanatory Notes

SANTINI A.

A

Absolute risk reduction (ARR) is the number of percentage points risk goes down if the individual concerned does something protective, such as stop drinking alcohol. The size of absolute risk reduction depends on what is initially decided as risk.

Accuracy: Accuracy and precision reflect how close a measurement is to an actual (true) value. Accuracy reflects how close a measurement is to a known or accepted value. (c.f. Precision). In terms of shooting at a target:

Accurately hitting (accuracy) the target means you are close to the target's centre, even if all the marks are on different sides of the centre.

Advanced clinical practice apprenticeships: This programme is for experienced health and social care practitioners who are currently working in an advanced clinical practice role or have obtained a trainee advanced clinical practitioner role before starting the programme. It is designed to support a person's development under the four pillars of advanced practice, which are

- clinical practice;
- leadership and management;
- education; and
- research.

Advanced clinical practice embodies the ability to manage clinical care in partnership with individuals, families and carers. It includes analysing and synthesising complex problems across various settings, enabling innovative solutions to enhance people's experience and improve outcomes. Students will be required to demonstrate core capabilities and area-specific clinical competence.

Algorithm is a procedure or formula for solving a problem. A computer programme is essentially an elaborate algorithm. In mathematics and computer science, it usually refers to a method that solves a recurrent problem. For example, treatment algorithms are used to systematise research study protocols, practice guidelines, and clinical decisions.

Alpha value (significance level): denoted as alpha or α, is the probability of rejecting the null hypothesis when it is true. For example, an $\alpha = 0.05$ indicates a 5 per cent risk of concluding that a difference exists when there is no actual difference.

Alternative hypothesis: The alternative or experimental hypothesis reflects that there will be an observed effect during an experiment. This hypothesis is denoted by either Ha or by H1. The alternative hypothesis is that an attempt is being made to demonstrate, in an indirect way, by the use of our hypothesis test that:

> If the null hypothesis is rejected, then the alternative hypothesis is accepted. For example, when studying a new treatment, the alternative hypothesis is that the new treatment does, in fact, affect patients in a meaningful and quantifiable manner.

> Alternative hypothesis versus null hypothesis: The null hypothesis and alternative hypothesis are frequently incorrectly stated. Both hypotheses should concern population means or proportions rather than sample means or proportions. The null hypothesis is an initial claim that is based on previous analyses or specialised knowledge. The alternative hypothesis states that a population parameter is smaller, greater, or different from the null hypothesis's hypothesised value.

Anonymity is the ethical practice designed to protect the privacy of human subjects while collecting, analysing, and reporting data. Confidentiality refers to separating or modifying any personal, identifying information provided by participants from the data.

Attributable risk (AR) or risk difference is the difference between the incidence rates in exposed and non-exposed groups. AR is calculated as the difference in cumulative incidences (*risk difference*) or incidence densities (rate difference) in a cohort study.

B

Background questions: Background questions ask for general knowledge about a condition or thing (cf. Foreground questions)

Bias is a systematic distortion of the real (true) effect that results from how the study in question was conducted. This can lead to invalid conclusions about whether an intervention works. Bias in research can make a treatment look better or worse than it is. Inferences about validity fall into two primary categories, which are internal or external. Types of bias include

> **Confirmation bias,** which occurs when researchers are predisposed to perceive, focus on, and give greater weight to data that fits their existing theories.

> **Neyman bias,** which is a selection bias where the very sick patients, very well patients, or both are excluded from a study.

> **Observation bias or Hawthorne Effect,** which is the alteration of behaviour by the study subjects due to their awareness of being observed.

Publishing bias, which is the failure to publish the results of a study "based on the direction or strength of the study findings." Non-publication introduces a bias that affects the ability to accurately synthesise and describe the evidence in a given area.

Recall bias: When survey respondents are asked to answer questions about things that happened to them in the past, the researchers must rely on the respondents' memories of the past.

Selection bias, which occurs when the selection of individuals, groups or data for analysis are not correctly randomised. This results in the obtained sample obtained not being representative of the population intended to be analysed.

Blinding refers to the concealment of group allocation from one or more individuals involved in a clinical research study, such as a randomised controlled trial.

R plot—also called a box plot or boxplot—displays the five-number summary of a data set. The five-number summary is the minimum, first quartile, median, third quartile, and maximum. In a box plot, a box is drawn from the first quartile to the third quartile. A vertical line goes through the box at the median. **Bracketing:** Bracketing in qualitative research refers to a researcher's identification of interests, personal experience, cultural factors, assumptions that could influence how the or study's data is interpreted.

C

Caldicott Principles are fundamentals that organisations should follow to protect information that could identify patients, such as their names and records. They also ensure that this information is only used and shared when it is appropriate to do so.

Case-control studies: A study that compares two groups of people: those with the disease or condition under investigation (cases) and a very similar (such as age or gender) group of people who do not have the disease or condition (controls).

Categorical variable: Variables can be classified as categorical (qualitative) or quantitative (numerical). Categorical variables take on values that are names or labels. The colour of a ball (e.g., red, green, blue) or the breed of a dog (e.g., collie, shepherd, terrier) are examples of categorical variables (cf. Quantitative variables).

Chain-referral sampling: see Snowball sampling.

Clinical practice guidelines: As defined by the Institute of Medicine, clinical guidelines are "systematically developed statements to assist practitioner and patient decisions about appropriate healthcare for specific clinical circumstances." They are statements that include recommendations intended to optimise patient care. They are informed by a systematic review of evidence and assessing the benefits and harms of alternative care options.

Cluster randomised control trials is a randomised controlled trial in which pre-existing groups, or clusters, of individuals, are randomly allocated to treatment arms. CRTs can be used when individual randomisation to treatment arms is not possible, or the intervention is applied to a whole cluster.

Cochrane Collaboration's primary purpose is to develop systematic reviews of the most robust evidence available about healthcare interventions. Consumers and health practitioners can then work together to make the best possible decisions about healthcare.

Coding in qualitative research is "how you define the data you are analysing" (Gibbs 2007). Applied codes enable data to be organised, examined and analysed in a structured way (e.g. by examining relationships between codes).

Cohort studies investigate disease causes and establish links between risk factors and health outcomes. The word cohort means a group of people. These types of studies look at groups of people.

Confidence intervals: Attached to every confidence interval is a level of confidence. This probability or per cent indicates how much certainty should be attributed to the confidence interval. If all other aspects of a situation are identical, the higher the confidence level, the wider the confidence interval. This level of confidence indicates the success of constructing a confidence interval. It is often expressed as a per cent whereby a population mean lies between an upper and lower *interval*. For example, confidence intervals with a confidence of 80 per cent will, in the long run, miss the true population parameter one out of every five times.

Confidence level refers to the percentage of all possible samples expected to include the true population parameter. For example, suppose all possible samples were selected from the same population. A confidence interval was computed for each sample. A 95 per cent confidence level implies that 95 per cent of the confidence intervals include the true population parameter.

Confidentiality is the ethical practice designed to protect the privacy of human subjects while collecting, analysing, and reporting data. Confidentiality refers to separating or modifying any personal, identifying information provided by participants from the data (cf. anonymity).

Confounding: A confounder is a variable that influences both the dependent variable and the independent variable, producing a false association.

CONSORT statement offers a standard way for authors to prepare reports of trial findings, facilitating their complete and transparent reporting and aiding their critical appraisal and interpretation. The CONSORT Statement comprises a twenty-five-item checklist and a flow diagram (see Appendix 1 for further details).

Contamination: Contamination is the process through which knowledge, expectations, or communication about the experimental treatment has an unintended influence on the non-experimental condition. Contamination occurs when those in the control condition are unintentionally exposed to aspects of the experimental situation.

Contingency table: Sometimes called a two-way frequency table, this is a tabular mechanism with at least two rows and two columns used in statistics to present categorical data in terms of frequency counts. r x c A contingency table shows the observed frequency of two variables, the observed frequencies of which are arranged into r rows and c columns. The intersection of a row and a column of a contingency table is called a cell.

Continuous variable: A continuous variable is a variable that can take on an infinite number of values; that is, a variable measured on a continuous scale, as opposed to a categorical variable.

Construct validity: The extent to which the study tests underlying constructs as intended.

Control condition: A control condition can refer to a group of participants in a study exposed to the experiment conditions that do not involve treatment or exposure to the independent variable.

Control event rate: See Magnitude of effect.

Correlation is a statistical measure that expresses the extent to which two variables are linearly related (they change together at a constant rate). It is a standard tool for describing simple relationships without making a statement about cause and effect.

Correlation coefficient: In statistics, a correlation coefficient is a quantitative assessment that measures this tendency's direction and strength to vary together.

Counterbalanced design: Where a comparison is made between two or more groups who receive the treatment and control conditions in different orders. There is no randomisation of participants.

Critically appraise: The issues to be accounted for in the critical appraisal of a scientific paper.

Does the study add anything new to the evidence in that practice?

What type of research question is being asked?

Was the study design appropriate for the research question?

Did the methodology address important potential sources of bias?

Critical appraisal: Critical appraisal is the course of action for watchfully and systematically examining research to assess its reliability, value, and relevance to clinical decision-making professionals.

D

Data: The plural of datum. There are different types which include:

> **Ordinal data:** Ordinal measurements report the ranking and ordering of the data without establishing the degree of variation between them. "Ordinal" indicates "order." They can be named, grouped, and also ranked. It reports the ranking and ordering of the data without actually establishing the degree of variation between them.

> **Continuous data:** Continuous data are numerical data that can theoretically be measured in infinitely small units. For example, blood pressure is usually measured to the nearest 2mm Hg but could be measured with a much higher resolution.

> **Dichotomous data:** A dichotomous variable takes on one of only two possible values when observed or measured. Dichotomous variables are most commonly measured using 1 and 0 as the two possible values. The use of 1 and 0 usually has no specific meaning relating to the variable itself.

Declaration of Helsinki: The World Medical Association (WMA) has developed the Declaration of Helsinki as a statement of ethical principles for medical research involving human subjects, including research on identifiable human material and data.

Dependent variable is the variable that is being measured or tested in an experiment. For example, in a study looking at how tutoring affects test scores, the dependent variable would be the participants' test scores since that is what is being measured.

Descriptors: Common descriptors are listed below. It is desirable to use the same descriptors as in the national census when possible.

Gender
Years of residence
Self-assigned ethnicity
Religion
Country of birth
Ethnic group
Parents' country of birth.

Diagnostic accuracy studies: The clinical performance of medical tests can be evaluated by diagnostic accuracy studies. Such studies assess a diagnostic test's ability to correctly distinguish between patients with and without a target condition by comparing the test results against the results of a reference standard.

Diagnostic study: A diagnostic procedure is an examination to identify an individual's specific areas of weakness and strength to determine a condition, disease or illness. Diagnostic tests are either invasive or non-invasive. Invasive diagnostic testing involves puncturing the skin or entering the body. Examples are taking a blood sample, biopsies, and colonoscopies. Non-invasive diagnostic testing does not involve making a break in the skin (cf. Prognostic study).

Diagnostic test is performed to confirm or determine the presence of disease in an individual suspected of having a disease, usually following the report of symptoms or based on other medical test results.

Diagnostic test accuracy: A diagnostic test's ability to distinguish between people with a health condition and people without one.

Dissertation is an extended piece of writing, usually between ten and twenty thousand words, on a topic set by a department or one chosen by the student. It is normally divided into chapters and may contain headings and sub-headings. These are sometimes (though not always) numbered as in a report. Dissertations answer a particular research question and either report on an empirical study or a literature-based study.

Doctoral fellowships: A fellowship provides financial support to graduate students to pursue graduate studies without associated teaching or research responsibilities. Fellowships are generally internal or external merit-based awards to support a student in a full-time course of study.

Double-blinding: In a double-blinding study, neither the participants nor the investigator knows the participants' treatment assignment.

E

Effect size refers to the magnitude of a treatment effect, independent of sample size. The effect size can be measured as either: a) the standardised difference between the treatment and control group means, or b) the correlation between the treatment group assignment (independent variable) and the outcome (dependent variable).

Effectiveness is defined as producing a result that is wanted, having an intended effect. Effectiveness studies attempt to examine interventions under conditions approximating to those in the real world. They tend to deal with heterogeneous patient populations, less-standardised treatment protocols, and delivery in routine clinical settings.

> Effectiveness trials without any apparent effect may be related to several factors, including an ineffective intervention, poor implementation, lack of provider acceptance, or lack of patient acceptance and adherence (cf. Efficiency). Assertions may not always be supported by the methods used and the results obtained. For example, claims of "difference" or "similarity" are often made not by thoughtful examination of the data but by statistical significance tests that are often misapplied or accompanied by inadequate sample sizes. These methodologic flaws can lead to false claims, inconsistencies, and harm to patients.

Efficacy: Efficacy studies use highly controlled conditions to research the benefits and harms of an intervention. This has the disadvantage of requiring significant deviations from accepted or everyday clinical practice with the advantage of creating high internal validity. Essentially it measures the capacity of an intervention to produce an effect under optimal conditions.

> Efficacy trials are often conducted in an academic environment by well-trained researchers as interventionists and exclude participants with comorbid conditions other than the target problem. A placebo-controlled randomised controlled trial (RCT) design is ideal for efficacy evaluation because it minimises bias through multiple mechanisms, such as standardisation of the intervention and double-blinding.

Efficiency is the ability to do something or produce something without wasting materials, time, or energy (cf. Effectiveness).

Endpoint: A clinical endpoint refers to the occurrence of a disease, symptom, sign, or laboratory abnormality that is one of the target outcomes of the trial in question.

Epistemological assumption in qualitative research is defined as "reality can be described in terms of meanings that people attach to communication experiences". cf. Ontological assumption.

Equipoise: Clinical equipoise means genuine uncertainty over whether or not the treatment will be beneficial. Even if the researcher truly believes in a hypothesis, there is no proof that the benefit exists. Equipoise provides an ethical basis for research that assigns patients to different treatment arms of a clinical trial.

Equivalence: Equivalence occurs when parallel versions of the same measure show consistent responses. Note: Most clinical studies show comparative superiority, but many reports claim equivalence between the investigated entities. These assertions may not always be supported by the methods used and the results obtained. Claims of "difference" or "similarity" are often made not by thoughtful examination of the data but by statistical significance tests that are often misapplied or accompanied by inadequate sample sizes. These methodologic flaws can lead to false claims, inconsistencies, and harm to patients.

Error, types 1 and 2: In statistical hypothesis testing, a type I error is the rejection of a true null hypothesis (also known as a "false positive" finding or conclusion; for example: "an innocent person is convicted"), while a type II error is the non-rejection of a false null hypothesis (also known as a "false negative" finding or conclusion).

Ethnography: Ethnography in qualitative research gathers observations, interviews and documentary data to produce detailed and comprehensive accounts of different social phenomena

Evidence-based: The term is derived from contextualised decision-making that integrates the best available research evidence considering patient characteristics (including preferences) and resources.

Evidence-based practice is the conscientious, explicit, and judicious use of current best evidence in making decisions about the care of individual patients.

Evidence hierarchy: The hierarchical system of classifying evidence is the cornerstone of evidence-based medicine. This hierarchy is known as the levels of evidence. Researchers and physicians are urged to find the highest level of evidence to answer clinical questions.

Exclusion criteria: Exclusion criteria are those characteristics that disqualify prospective subjects from inclusion in a study.

Experiment: A study where a series of observations are performed under controlled conditions to study a relationship between two or more circumstances and derive inferences about this relationship. Experiments involve manipulating an independent variable, the exposure of different groups of participants to one or more conditions being studied, and the measurement of a dependent variable.

External validity: External validity refers to how results from a study can be applied (generalised) to other situations, groups or events. It is a measure of the validity of an experiment's dependence on the experimental design (cf. Internal validity).

F

Factorial study design: Factorial design is a research methodology that allows for investigating the main and interaction effects between two or more independent variables and one or more outcome variables.

False-positive is an error resulting from the incorrect indication of a disease's presence (i.e. the result is positive when, in reality, the patient is disease-free).

False-negative is an error resulting from the incorrect indication that the patient does not have the disease (i.e. the result is negative when, in reality, the patient has the disease).

Field research: Field research in qualitative research is a qualitative method of data collection that aims to observe, interact and understand people in a natural environment. Although field research is generally characterised as qualitative research, it often involves multiple aspects of quantitative research.

FINER: fixed allocation randomisation: Each participant has an equal probability of being assigned to either treatment or control. The probability remains constant throughout the study. Tables of random digits or randomisation software can be used to achieve this.

Fixed block size: In a randomised block design, participants are first classified into groups (blocks) of a fixed length (usually four, six, or eight) based on a variable that the experimenter wishes to control. Individuals within each block are then randomly assigned to one of several treatment groups.

Focus groups: A focus group is a form of qualitative research in which a group of people are asked about their perceptions, opinions, beliefs, and attitudes towards a concept, interests, personal experiences, and other issues relative to the researcher's quest.

Foreground questions: Ask for specific knowledge to inform clinical decisions or actions (cf. Background questions).

G

Gaussian distribution: A sample of data forms a distribution. The most well-known distribution is the Gaussian distribution or Normal distribution. This bell-shaped distribution provides a parameterised mathematical function that can be used to calculate the probability for any individual observation from the sample space.

Generalisability: Generalisability refers to which results or findings can be transferred to situations or people other than those studied initially or, in other words, the accuracy of extending research findings and conclusions from a study conducted on a sample population to the population at large. While the dependability of this extension is not absolute, it is statistically probable. Quantitative research on large sample size populations provides the best basis for generalizability. The larger the sample population, the more one can generalise the results.

Gold standard test is usually the diagnostic test or benchmark that is the best available under reasonable conditions.

Grounded theory refers to systematic inductive methods for conducting qualitative research aimed toward theory development. These analyses provide focused, abstract, conceptual theories that explain the studied empirical phenomena.

H

Harmonic mean is a type of numerical average. It is calculated by dividing the number of observations by the reciprocal of each number in the series. Thus, the harmonic mean is the reciprocal of the arithmetic mean.

Harvard style: Harvard is a referencing style primarily used by university students to cite information sources. In-text citations are used when directly quoting or paraphrasing a source. They are located in the body of the work and contain a fragment of the complete reference in brackets. For example (Smith and Jones 2011).

Reference lists are located at the end of the work and list full references, in alphabetical order, for sources used in the assignment. For example: Santini A., Eaton K.A. "An introduction to research for primary dental care clinicians part 4: Stage 6a, obtaining ethical approval." *Primary Dental Care,* Vol os18, Issue 3, 2011, 127–32, https://doi.org/10.1177/205016841os1800312.

Hawthorne Effect (observation bias): The alteration of behaviour by the study subjects due to their awareness of being observed.

Heterogeneity: In statistics, heterogeneity arises in describing the properties of a dataset or several datasets. It relates to the validity of the often convenient assumption that any part of an overall dataset's statistical properties is the same as any other part; it is the opposite of homogeneity. Thus, for example, clinical heterogeneity is defined as differences in participant, treatment, outcome characteristics or research setting.

Histogram: A histogram is a graphical display of data using bars of different heights. It is similar to a bar chart; a histogram groups numbers into ranges. The height of each bar shows how many fall into each range. A histogram is used to summarise discrete or continuous data. In other words, it provides a visual interpretation. This requires focusing on the main points and numerical data by showing the number of data points that fall within a specified range of values (called "bins"). It is similar to a vertical bar graph.

Homogeneity: In statistics, homogeneity arises in describing the properties of a dataset or several datasets. It relates to the validity of the often convenient assumption that any part of an overall dataset's statistical properties is the same as any other part. Thus, it is the opposite of homogeneity.

Hypothesis: A hypothesis is a supposition or proposed explanation based on limited evidence as a starting point for further investigation. a proposition made as a basis for reasoning, without any assumption of its truth. "The hypothesis that every event has a cause."

Hypothesis testing: In statistics, the topic of statistical significance tests or hypothesis testing can be complex for a newcomer to the topic. There are type 1 and type 11 tests (vide infra). In addition, there are one-sided and two-sided tests and the concepts of a null or alternative hypothesis.

> The essential question is whether events in a study are caused by chance or caused by certain factors. Thus, it is necessary to differentiate between events that occur by random or chance and those that are highly unlikely to occur randomly. Therefore, hypothesis testing involves carefully constructing two statements: the null hypothesis and the alternative hypothesis.

> The **Null Hypothesis** reflects that there will be no observed effect arising from the experiment. In a mathematical formulation of the null hypothesis, there will typically be an equal sign. H0 denotes this hypothesis. The null hypothesis is that an attempt is being made to overturn the hypothesis test. A *p*-value less than the stated (a priori) alpha value justifies the null hypothesis's rejection.

Care must be given to the meaning of *not* rejecting the null hypothesis. Just because a null hypothesis is not rejected does not mean that the statement is true. For example, when a study investigates a new treatment or drug, the null hypothesis is that a new treatment or medication will not affect the subjects in any meaningful way.

The **Alternative Hypothesis**: The alternative or experimental hypothesis reflects that there will be an observed effect for the experiment. This hypothesis is denoted by either Ha or by H1. The rejection of the null hypothesis is an acceptance of the alternative hypothesis. For example, when the study investigates a new treatment or drug, the alternative hypothesis is that the treatment does affect the subjects in a meaningful and measurable way.

The **p-Value**: The null hypothesis is rejected if the *p*-value is less than or equal to the alpha value. The null hypothesis is not rejected if the *p*-value is greater than the alpha value. Thus, either the null hypothesis is rejected, or the null hypothesis is not rejected. If the null hypothesis is rejected, the consequence is the acceptance of the alternative hypothesis. This does not mean that that null hypothesis is accepted, but only that there is insufficient evidence to reject it. Moreover, "Not rejecting" is not the same as "accepting."

The essential question is whether events in a study are caused by chance or caused by certain factors. Therefore, it is important to differentiate between events that occur randomly or by chance and those that are highly unlikely to occur randomly. The standard method is the p-value method.

The null hypothesis is rejected if the *p*-value is less than or equal to the (a priori) alpha value. The null hypothesis is not rejected if the *p*-value is greater than the alpha value.

I

IMRAD stands for introduction, methods, results, and discussion. In this format, research is presented and discussed logically.

Impact factor (IF) or journal impact factor (JIF) of an academic journal is an index that reflects the yearly average number of citations of articles published in the last two years in a given journal. It is frequently used as a proxy for the relative importance of a journal within its field; journals with higher impact factor values are often deemed more important, or carry more intrinsic prestige in their respective fields, than those with lower values.

Independent and dependent variables: An independent variable is a variable that stands alone and is not changed by the other variables that are being measured. In contrast, a dependent variable is the effect. In an experiment, the independent variable is manipulated, and the outcome in the dependent variable is measured.

Index test: A diagnostic test is evaluated against a reference standard test in test accuracy studies. Evaluations of diagnostic test accuracy require a comparison between the diagnostic test being assessed, referred to as the index test and a reference standard to categorise participants as having or not having a target condition.

Inductive reasoning: Understanding gained when information is collected and conclusions are drawn from what is observed.

Informed consent is the permission granted in full knowledge of the possible consequences; typically the permission a patient gives to a doctor with an understanding of the potential risks and benefits: "written informed consent was obtained from each patient." For consent to be valid, it must be voluntary and informed. In addition, the person consenting must have the capacity to make the decision.

Integrative diagrams: These are used to pull study detail together to help make sense of the emerging theory's data. The diagrams can be any form of graphic that is useful at that point in theory development.

Internal validity: Internal validity is the extent to which one can be confident that other factors cannot explain a cause-and-effect relationship established in a study. Internal validity is the degree of confidence that the causal relationship being tested is not influenced by other factors or variables (cf. External validity).

Intent to treat (ITT): Randomized controlled trials often suffer from two major complications, i.e., noncompliance and missing outcomes. A statistical concept called intention-to-treat (ITT) analysis helps overcome this inconvenience. Every subject who is randomised according to the randomised treatment assignment is included in the analysis. All noncompliance subjects, protocol deviations, withdrawals, and anything that happens after randomisation are ignored. In ITT analysis, an estimate of the treatment effect is generally conservative. The per-protocol population is defined as a subset of the ITT population who completed the study without any major protocol violations.

Intention to treat analysis is performed to avoid crossover and dropout effects, which may break the random assignment to the treatment groups. ITT analysis provides information about the potential impact of treatment policy rather than on the possible effects of specific treatment (see *p*er-protocol analysis).

Internal consistency: Responses to questionnaire items that measure the same construct and are highly intercorrelated.

Internal validity is the extent to which the results of a study are true. That is, the intervention did cause a behaviour change. The change was not the result of other extraneous factors, such as differences in assessment procedures between intervention and control participants.

Interquartile range measures where the "middle fifty" is in a data set. The interquartile range is a measure of where the bulk of the values lie.

K

Kaplan Meyer: The Kaplan-Meier estimator is used to assess the survival function. The visual representation of this function is termed the Kaplan-Meier curve. The curve shows the probability of an event (e.g. survival) at a specific time interval. If the sample size is large enough, the curve should approach the true survival function for the population under investigation. Usually, two groups are compared, e.g. a Group A, receiving treatment A versus a G B, not receiving treatment B.

Keyword is a word or concept of great significance. In medical publications, keywords are words that capture the essence of the paper. Keywords make the document searchable from literature databases. Therefore, it is essential to include the most relevant keywords to help other authors find the concerned paper (cf. MEsh terms).

L

Level of evidence chart has been adapted from OCEBM Levels of Evidence Working Group, "The Oxford 2011 Levels of Evidence," Oxford Centre for Evidence-Based Medicine, http://www.cebm.net/ocebm-levels-of-evidence/. A glossary of terms can be found here: http://www.cebm.net/glossary/.

> Level-I through IV studies may be graded downward based on study quality, imprecision, indirectness, or inconsistency between studies or because the effect size is very small; these studies may be graded upward if there is a dramatic effect size. For example, a high-quality randomised controlled trial (RCT) should have ≥80 per cent follow-up, blinding, and proper randomisation. The level of evidence assigned to systematic reviews reflects the ranking of studies included in the review (i.e., a systematic review of Level-II studies is Level II). A complete assessment of individual studies' quality requires a critical appraisal of all aspects of study design.
>
> Features were assessed when deciding the level of evidence arising from a study:
>
> - Investigators formulated the study question before the first patient was enrolled;
> - In these studies, cohort refers to a nonrandomised comparative study. For therapeutic studies, patients treated one way (e.g., cemented hip prosthesis) are compared with those treated differently (e.g., cement-less hip prosthesis);
> - Investigators formulated the study question after the first patient was enrolled;

- Patients identified for the study based on their outcome (e.g., failed total hip arthroplasty), called "cases," are compared with those who did not have the outcome (e.g., successful total hip arthroplasty), called "controls"; and
- Sufficient numbers are required to rule out a common harm (affects >20 per cent of participants). In addition, for long-term harms, follow-up duration must be adequate.

Level of significance: In conducting a test of significance or hypothesis, two numbers can be confused. One number is the level of significance or alpha value; the other is called the p-value of the test statistic. These numbers are easily confused because they are both numbers between zero and one, and both are probabilities. The alpha number is the threshold value against which the p values are measured. It indicates how extreme observed results must be to reject the null hypothesis of a significance test. The value of alpha is associated with the confidence level of the test. The alpha value gives us the probability of a type 1 error, which occurs when a null hypothesis that is actually true is rejected. In the long run, for a test with a significance level of $0.05 = 1/20$, a true null hypothesis will be rejected one out of every twenty times.

The following lists some confidence levels with their corresponding alpha values: For results with a 90 per cent confidence level, the alpha value is $1 - 0.90 = 0.10$. For results with a 95 per cent level of confidence, the value of alpha is $1 - 0.95 = 0.05$. For results with a 99 per cent level of confidence, the value of alpha is $1 - 0.99 = 0.01$.

For results with a C per cent level of confidence, the value of alpha is $1 - C/100$. The most commonly used is 0.05 because the general accord is that this level is appropriate. Historically, it has been accepted as the standard.

(Cf. Levels of Significance, p-values, Type 1 & 11 errors.)

Likelihood ratio for a positive test result (LR+) is how much more likely is a positive found in a person with, as opposed to without, the disease. The likelihood ratio for a negative test result (LR-) is how much more likely a negative test is found in a person with the disease than not having the disease.

Linear regression: Linear regression is used to predict the value of a variable based on the value of another variable. The variable to be predicted is called the dependent variable, or sometimes, the outcome variable. It is the next step up after correlation (cf. Correlation with multiple regression).

Logistic regression: Logistic regression is a statistical model that, in its basic form, uses a logistic function to model a binary dependent variable, although many more complex extensions exist. In regression analysis, logistic regression (or logit regression) estimates the parameters of a logistic model (a form of binary regression). Logistic regression is used to obtain an odds ratio in the presence of more than one explanatory variable. The procedure is quite similar to multiple linear regression, except that the response variable is binomial. The result is the effect of each variable on the odds ratio of the observed event of interest.

M

Magnitude of effect: Effect size is a quantitative measure of the magnitude of the experimental effect. The larger the effect size, the stronger the relationship between two variables. The effect size is assessed when comparing any two groups to see how substantially different they are. In statistical analysis, the effect size is usually measured in three ways: (1) standardised mean difference, (2) odds ratio, (3) and correlation coefficient. For example, the effect size of the population can be found by dividing the two population mean differences by their standard deviation.

Margin of Error is a statistic expressing the amount of random sampling error in survey results. The larger the margin of error, the less confidence one should have that a poll result would reflect the result of a survey of the entire population

Maximum likelihood: This technique models all the obtained data, adds some error variance and estimates the parameter values that make the observed data maximally likely.

Mean is the average of a data set (cf. Mode, Median).

Measures: measures ascertain the size, amount, or degree of something, using an instrument or device marked in standard units. They can be continuous, dichotomous, or ordinal (cf. Continuous data; Dichotomous data; Ordinal data).

Median: In statistics, the median separates the higher half from the lower half of a data sample, a population, or a probability distribution. The "middle" of a sorted list of numbers. To find the median, place the numbers in value order and find the middle number.

Mediator: In statistics, it is a variable that helps account for the association between an independent and a dependent variable. A mediation model seeks to explain the mechanism that underlies an observed relationship between an independent variable and a dependent variable via the inclusion of a third explanatory variable, the mediator variable. Rather than hypothesising a direct causal relationship between the independent and dependent variables, a mediational model hypothesises that the independent variable causes the mediator variable, which causes the dependent variable.

Memoing is the act of recording reflective notes about what the researcher, fieldworker, data coder, and analyst are acquiring from the data: memos accrue as written ideas or records about concepts and their relationships

Member checking: Asking participants in one-on-one interviews or focus groups to check the transcript of these events, confirm that they are accurate, point out any inaccuracies, and ask for them to be corrected.

MeSH terms: MeSH (medical subject headings) is the United States of America's National Library of Medicine's controlled vocabulary or subject heading list. It is used by indexers, who are subject analysts and maintain the PubMed database, to reflect journal papers' subject content as they are published. When labelling an article, indexers select terms only from the official MeSH list; never use other spellings or variations.

Meta-analysis: A meta-analysis is a statistical analysis that combines the results of multiple scientific studies. Meta-analysis can be performed when numerous scientific studies address the same question, with each study reporting measurements that are expected to have some degree of error.

Missing at random (MAR) is the alternative of MCAR, suggesting that what caused the data to be missing does not depend upon the missing data itself.

Missing completely at random (MCAR) describes the assumption that data are missing completely at random. MCAR assumes that, at any time point, a missing subject or missing data point occurs for entirely random reasons.

Mode is the most common number in a data set (cf. Mean, Median).

Moderator: In statistics, a variable alters the direction or strength of the association between other variables. For example, if gender moderates their relationship, two variables may be positively associated among women but negatively correlated among men.

Monograph is a specialist-written work on a single subject or an aspect of a topic, often by a single author and usually on an academic subject. It may not be peer-reviewed before publication.

Multiple regression generally explains the relationship between numerous independent or predictor variables and one dependent or criterion variable. A dependent variable is modelled as a function of several independent variables with corresponding coefficients and the constant term. Multiple regression requires two or more predictor variables, which is why it is called multiple regression (cf. Linear regression).

N

Narrative research is a literary form of qualitative research; it concerns collecting and detailing a story or stories. Researchers write narratives about an individuals' experiences, describe a life experience, and discuss the meaning of the experience with the individual.

Negative predictive value: The proportion of people with a negative test result who do not have the disease or characteristic. It is different from specificity. (Specificity: if a patient does NOT have the disease, what are the chance of getting a negative result in the new test? If a patient has a negative result on the new test, what are the chances of not having the disease?

Nonprobability sampling is defined as a sampling technique in which the researcher selects samples based on the researcher's subjective judgment rather than random selection. It is a less stringent method and depends heavily on the expertise of the researcher.

Null hypothesis refers to a default position that there is no relationship between two measured phenomena (or that a potential medical treatment has no effect).The null hypothesis reflects that there will be no observed effect from the experiment in question. In a mathematical formulation of the null hypothesis, there will typically be an equal sign. H0 denotes this hypothesis. The null hypothesis attempts to overturn the stated hypothesis test. The hope is to obtain a small enough *p*-value that justifies the rejection of the null hypothesis. If the null hypothesis is not rejected, then care must be taken to say what this means. It is generally assumed true until evidence indicates otherwise. For example, given the test scores of two random samples, does one group differ from the other? A possible null hypothesis is that: The mean male score is not the same as the mean female score (cf. Alternative hypothesis).

Number needed to treat (NNT): The NNT is the average number of patients who need to be treated to prevent one additional bad outcome. In other words, the number of patients who need to be treated for one of them to benefit is weighed against a clinical trial control.

Number needed to treat (NNT) = 1/ARR. A specific risk reduction may appear impressive, but how many patients must be treated before seeing a benefit? This concept is called "number need to treat" and is one of the most intuitive clinical-practice statistics.

For example, if

	Yes	No
Exposed	8	992
Not Exposed	10	990

The RR = (8/1000) / (10/1000) = 0.8 making the RRR = (1-0.8/1)=0.2 or 20%. Although this sounds impressive, the absolute risk reduction is only 0.01-0.008=.002 or 0.2%. Thus the NNT is 1/0.002=500 patients. The pre-intervention risk or probability is a major determinant of the degree of possible post-intervention benefit, yield, or risk reduction on an individual patient basis.

Observational studies are ones where researchers observe the effect of a risk factor, diagnostic test, treatment or other intervention without trying to change who is or is not exposed to it. Cohort studies and case-control studies are two types of observational studies.

Odds ratio (OR) is a statistic that quantifies the strength of the association between two events, A and B. Odds of an event happening is defined as the likelihood that an event will occur, expressed as a proportion of the possibility that the event will not occur. Therefore, if A is the probability of subjects affected and B is the probability of subjects not affected, then odds = A/B.

Ontological assumption in qualitative research is that reality is subjective.

Open-ended questions do not provide participants with a predetermined set of answer choices but allow them to respond in their own words.

P

***p*-Values:** Like the alpha value, the *p*-value is a "measure" of probability. Every statistical test generates a probability or *p*-value. This value is the probability that the observed statistic occurred by chance alone. There are several different ways to find a *p*-value which depends on the different test statistics. The *p*-value of the test statistic is a way of saying how extreme that statistic is for the sample data, and it gives a measurement of evidence against the null hypothesis.

> Tests of statistical significance all begin with a null hypothesis and an alternative hypothesis. The null hypothesis is the statement of no effect or a statement of the commonly accepted state of affairs. The alternative hypothesis is what is being attempted to prove. The working assumption in a hypothesis test is that the null hypothesis is true.

> To calculate a *p*-value, the appropriate software or statistical table that corresponds with the test statistic is used.

> The *p*-value is a probability. This means that it is a real number from 0 and 1. In general, the smaller the p-value, the more evidence there is against the null hypothesis. How small is a *p*-value needed to reject the null hypothesis? The answer to this is, "It depends." A common rule of thumb in clinical studies is that the *p*-value must be less than or equal to 0.05, but there is nothing universal about this value. Typically a threshold value is chosen a priory. If the *p*-value is less than or equal to this threshold, then the null hypothesis is rejected. This threshold is called the level of significance of the hypothesis test and is denoted α. There is no value of α that always defines statistical significance. It should be set a priori and is usually 0.05 but can be lower.

Parallel study design ("between patient"; "non-crossover"): A parallel study is a type of clinical study where two groups of treatments, A and B, are given so that one group receives only treatment or intervention A while another group receives only treatment or intervention B.

Patients' rights outlines how patients are to be treated with dignity and respect, may accept or refuse treatment, and may only be physically examined with consent. Patients must be given information about any available tests and treatment options, what they involve, their risks and benefits, and to have access to your records.

Peer review evaluates scientific, academic, or professional work by others working in the same field. It is a process of subjecting an author's scholarly work, research or ideas to the scrutiny of experts in the same field. It functions to encourage authors to meet the accepted high standards of their discipline and control the dissemination of research data to ensure that unwarranted claims, unacceptable interpretations or personal views are not published without prior expert review.

Per protocol analysis is a comparison of treatment groups that include only those patients who completed the treatment initially allocated. If done alone, this *analysis* leads to bias (cf. Intention to treat analyses).

Phenomenology is qualitative research that focuses on studying an individual's lived experiences within the world. Understanding the ontological and epistemological assumptions underpinning these approaches is essential for successfully conducting phenomenological research.

Phenomena is a fact or situation observed to exist or happen, especially one whose cause or explanation is in question.

Placebo is a substance made to resemble drugs but not containing an active drug but an inert substance. In a placebo-controlled trial, the group randomised to a placebo arm receives an inert substance indistinguishable in appearance from the active drug under investigation. The inclusion of a placebo arm holds expectations about treatment benefit and adherence constant across the control and intervention groups while testing the active drug's actual pharmacological effects.

Plagiarism is to steal and pass off the ideas or words of another as one's own. Also, to use another's work without crediting the source. Finally, it is to commit literary theft and to present, as new and original, an idea or product derived from an existing source.

PICO: PICO stands for patient/population, intervention, comparison, and outcomes.

Positive predictive value (PPV) is the proportion of subjects who give a positive test result and have the disease.

Power: In terms of statistics, power is the probability that a test of significance will identify an effect in the population studied. Power is the probability that a test of significance will detect a deviation from the null hypothesis, should such a deviation exist. Power is the probability of avoiding a type II error.

Precision reflects how reproducible measurements are, even if they are far from the accepted value (cf. Accuracy). Think of precision and accuracy in terms of hitting a bullseye. Precisely hitting (Precision) a target means all the hits are closely spaced, even if they are very far from the target's centre. Accurately hitting (Accuracy) the target means they are close to the target's centre, even if all of the hits are on different sides of the centre.

Poisson regression is used to model count variables. Poisson regression is similar to regular multiple regression except that the dependent (Y) variable is an observed count that follows the Poisson distribution. Thus, Y's possible values are the non-negative integers: 0, 1, 2, 3, and so on. Furthermore, it is assumed that large counts are rare. Hence, Poisson regression is similar to logistic regression, which also has a discrete response variable. However, the response is not limited to specific values as it is in logistic regression (cf. Logistic regression; Multiple regression).

Predatory journals are scam publishers that charge authors fees upfront but do not provide the service they promise. The majority of these predatory journals will take payments without ever publishing the work. Other predatory journals publish articles without any form of an editorial or peer review process.

Probability is how likely something will happen. The probability is a number that reflects the chance or likelihood that a particular event will occur. For example, a probability of 0 indicates that there is no chance that a specific event will occur. In contrast, a probability of 1 indicates that an event is certain to occur.

Prognostic studies: The standard prognostic study is a cohort study in which a group of people with a particular condition or set of characteristics is followed over a period of time. At the start of the period, a range of factors that may influence outcomes are measured, and outcomes are measured over the period. The best design for a prognostic study is a cohort study. It would usually be impossible or unethical to randomise patients to different prognostic factors (cf. Diagnostic studies).

Prospective Study investigates outcomes, such as developing a disease, during the study period and relates this to other factors such as suspected risk or protection factor(s). The study usually involves taking a cohort of subjects and watching them over a long period.

Protocol is a system of rules that explain the correct conduct and procedures to be followed in formal situations. It is a detailed plan for a scientific experiment or medical treatment (cf. Research protocol).

Pseudo-anonymity is the appearance but not the reality of online anonymity. Most commonly, pseudo-anonymity enables anonymous posting of patient data and commenting on it.

Publishing bias occurs when there is a failure to publish the results of a study "based on the direction or strength of the study findings." This non-publication introduces a bias that impacts the ability to accurately synthesise and describe the evidence of the study in question in a given area.

Purposeful sampling in qualitative research is used to identify and select information-rich cases related to the phenomenon of interest. The researcher relies on his judgment when choosing members of a population to participate in the study. It is also known as judgment, selective, or subjective sampling.

Q

Qualitative study seeks to answer why or how questions. When designing a research question for a qualitative study, the researcher will need to ask a why or how question about that research topic. Numerical data are not usually collected, and consequently, statistical analysis is rare in qualitative research.

Quantitative study consists of a mathematical analysis of the research topic. The research outcomes will result from an assessment that measures variables numerically to produce data that can then be analysed statistically.

Quantitative variables are numerical. They represent a measurable quantity. For example, when one speaks of a city's population, the number of people in the town is considered; this is a measurable attribute of the town. Therefore, the population would be a quantitative variable (cf. Qualitative variables).

Questionnaire is a research instrument that consists of a set of questions or other prompts that aim to collect information from a respondent. A questionnaire may or may not be delivered in the form of a survey, but a survey always consists of a questionnaire.

Quota sampling is a nonprobability sampling method in which the researcher creates a sample involving individuals representing a population. The researcher then decides and creates quotas so that the research samples can help collect data. These samples can be generalised to the entire population.

R

Random assignment: In this case, participants or other sampling units are assigned to an experiment's conditions at random so that each participant or sampling unit has an equal chance of being assigned to any particular intervention or treatment.

Randomisation: Clinical trial randomisation is assigning patients by chance to groups that receive different treatments. In the most straightforward trial design, the test group receives the new treatment, and the control group receives standard therapy.

Randomly permuted blocks: Blocks of patients are created such that balance is enforced within each block. For example, let E stand for the experimental group and C for the control group, then a block of 4 patients may be assigned to one of EECC, ECEC, ECCE, CEEC, CECE, and CCEE, with equal probabilities of 1/6 each. In each block, there are equal numbers of patients assigned to the experimental and the control group. (CER) = c/c+d.

Randomised controlled trials: A study in which people are allocated by chance alone (at random) to receive one of several clinical interventions. The subjects are randomly assigned to one of two groups: one (the experimental or test group) receiving the intervention that is being tested, and the other (the comparison group or control) group receiving an alternative (conventional) treatment.

Recall bias: When survey respondents are asked to answer questions about things that happened to them in the past, the researchers have to rely on the respondents' memories of the past. As a result, they may or may not be accurate.

Reference standard test: The best available method of determining whether people have a condition. The reference standard is the test, considered the best available way of categorising participants as having a target condition in a diagnostic test accuracy study (cf. Gold standard; Reference test).

Regression: Regression is a statistical method that attempts to determine the strength and character of the relationship between one dependent variable and a series of other variables, known as independent variables.

Relative risk (RR): Relative risk is a ratio of the probability of an event occurring in the exposed group versus the likelihood of the event occurring in the non-exposed group.

Relative risk reduction (RRR): Cf. Magnitude of effect.

Reliability is the extent to which a measurement gives consistent results (cf. Validity).

Reliability, inter-rater refers to the reproducibility or consistency of decisions between two reviewers and is a necessary component of validity c.f. inter-consensus reliability

> **Inter-consensus reliability** refers to the comparison of consensus assessments across pairs of reviewers in the participating centres.

Research ethics are the moral principles that govern how researchers should carry out their work. These principles are used to shape research regulations agreed by groups such as university governing bodies, communities or governments. The application of moral rules and professional codes of conduct to collect, analyse, report, and publish information about research subjects, particularly active acceptance of subjects' right to privacy, confidentiality, and informed consent. All researchers should follow any regulations that apply to their work.

Research protocol is a document that describes the background, rationale, objectives, design, methodology, statistical considerations, and organisation of a clinical research project. It is the guidebook for a research study. It describes what the researchers intend to do and how they will do it. Writing a protocol ensures that all the major issues are considered in designing and developing a particular research project.

Response bias is a general term that refers to conditions or factors that occur while responding to surveys, affecting how responses are provided. Such circumstances lead to a non-random deviation of the answers from their actual value.

Risk difference (attributable risk) is the difference in the risk of a condition such as a disease between an exposed group and an unexposed group.

ROC (receiver operating characteristic curve): An ROC curve is a graph showing a classification model's performance at all classification thresholds. This curve plots two parameters, the true positive rate and the false positive rate. A ROC curve plots the true positive rate and the false positive rate at different classification thresholds. For example, lowering the classification threshold classifies more items as positive, thus increasing both false positives and true positives.

> **Area under ROC curve:** The area under ROC curve (AUC) measures the entire two-dimensional area underneath the whole ROC curve from (0,0) to (1,1). In general, an AUC of 0.5 suggests no discrimination (i.e., ability to diagnose patients with and without the disease or condition based on the test), 0.7 to 0.8 is considered acceptable, 0.8 to 0.9 is deemed to be excellent, and more than 0.9 is deemed to be outstanding.

Rosenthal effect is a psychological phenomenon in which high expectations lead to improved performance.

S

Sample size refers to the number of participants or observations included in a study. This number is usually represented by n. Two statistical properties are influenced by the size of a sample: the precision of the estimates and the power of the study to draw conclusions.

Sample size calculation: The sample size is the number of participants in a sample. A fundamental statistical principle is that the sample size is calculated before starting a clinical study to avoid bias in interpreting results.

Sampling methods: Standard sampling techniques are defined in Chapter 5.

Sensitivity analysis determines how different values of an independent variable affect a particular dependent variable under a given set of assumptions. In other words, sensitivity analyses study how various sources of uncertainty in a mathematical model contribute to the model's overall uncertainty.

Screening test detects potential health disorders or diseases in people with no disease symptoms. Screening tests are not considered diagnostic but are used to identify a subset of the population who should have additional testing to determine the presence or absence of disease.

Selection bias is a systematic distortion of evidence that arises because people with specific important characteristics were disproportionately more likely to wind up in one condition. This results in the obtained sample obtained not being representative of the population intended to be analysed. Although random assignment theoretically eliminates selection biases, a bias can still occur.

Sensitivity measures the proportion of people with the condition that the measure correctly identifies. Sensitivity also indicates how often the test will be positive (true positive rate) if a person has a disease? If the test is highly sensitive and the test result is negative, one can be nearly confident that the patients do not have the disease. Thus, sensitivity relates to the test's ability to identify a condition correctly.

Clinical significance measures how significant the differences in treatment effects are in clinical practice. Clinical significance implies that the difference between treatments' ineffectiveness is clinically significant, and clinical practice may change if such a difference is seen (cf. Statistical significance).

Significance level, also denoted as alpha or α, is the probability of rejecting the null hypothesis when it is true. For example, a significance level of 0.05 indicates a 5 per cent risk of concluding that a difference exists when there is no actual difference.

Snowball sampling or chain-referral sampling: Snowball sampling techniques are used to identify study participants. The researcher first identifies one or two people he would like to include in the study and then relies on those initial participants to identify additional study participants.

Specificity measures the proportion of people without a condition that the measure correctly classifies. If a person does not have a disease, how often will the test be negative (true negative rate)? In other words, if the test result for a highly specific test is positive, there is reasonable certainty that the subjects have the disease. Specificity relates to the test's ability to exclude a condition correctly.

Standard deviation is a statistic that measures the dispersion of a dataset relative to its mean and is calculated as the square root of the variance. If the data points are further from the mean, there is a higher deviation within the data set; thus, the more spread out the data, the higher the standard deviation.

Stratified randomisation is a technique in which a population is divided into subgroups (strata), and individuals or cases from each stratum are randomly assigned to conditions.

Statistical conclusion validity is the validity of inferences about covariation between two variables.

Statistical power is the power of any test of statistical significance and is defined as the probability of rejecting a false null hypothesis. Statistical power is inversely related to beta or the likelihood of making a type II error.

Power = 1 – β.

Statistical significance measures how likely any apparent differences in outcome between treatment and control groups are real and not due to chance. *p* Values and confidence intervals (CI) are the most commonly used measures of statistical significance. The p values give the probability that any particular outcome would have arisen by chance assuming that the new and the control treatments are equally effective as the null hypothesis. CI estimate the range within which the real results would fall if the trial is conducted many times. Hence, 95 per cent CI of the difference in treatment outcomes between the two groups would indicate the range in which the differences between the two treatments would fall on 95 per cent of the occasions if the trial is carried out many times.

Statistical stability is how well the results of a study or experiment hold up. More specifically, it is a measure of how well random errors are controlled in a study.

Survival analysis involves modelling time to event data, such as time to death or recovery.

Systematic review examines a formulated question that uses systematic and reproducible methods to identify, select, and critically appraise all relevant research and collect and analyse data from the studies included in the review.

T

Temporal stability occurs when a person scores consistently across assessments at two different time points.

Thesis is a long piece of writing on a particular subject involving personal research, written mainly by a candidate for a higher college or university degree, e.g. a doctoral thesis for a PhD. It is also a work embodying results of original research and especially substantiating a specific view (cf. Dissertation).

Time-series design: Measurements are taken before and after an intervention with no control group involved in a time series design.

Treatment condition is the specific intervention condition to which a group or individual is exposed in a research study.

Treatment fidelity is how accurately or faithfully a program (or intervention) is reproduced from a manual, protocol or model. Fidelity is usually measured using a checklist, which trained assessors complete.

Treatment integrity, or construct validity of an intervention, is the degree to which the treatment protocol operationalises the influences that the theory posits cause change. Pragmatically, treatment fidelity describes whether the interventionist delivered the treatment as planned.

Treatment manual provides specific operational guidelines to deliver an intervention. Dissemination and use of a manual maximise the probability of treatment being conducted consistently across settings, therapists, and clients.

Triangulation in qualitative research refers to using multiple methods or data sources to develop a comprehensive understanding of phenomena. Triangulation also has been viewed as a qualitative research strategy to test validity through the convergence of information from different sources.

Type I and II errors and hypothesis testing: Hypothesis testing requires both the statement of a null hypothesis and the selection of a level of significance. The null hypothesis is either true or false and denotes the default claim for a treatment or procedure (e.g. when testing the usefulness of a new procedure, the null hypothesis would be that the new procedure does not affect the operation outcome). Ideally, the null hypothesis should be rejected when it is false and not rejected when it is true. This may not always be the case, and two situations are possible, each of which will result in an error.

> **Type I error** involves the rejection of a null hypothesis that is true. This is called a type I error or an error of the first kind. Type I errors are equivalent to false positives. For example, if the null hypothesis is rejected in testing a "new drug," the claim is that the drug affects the outcome. If the null hypothesis is true, then the new drug is falsely claimed to positively impact the outcome when the actuality is that the new drug does not moderate the disease at all. Type I errors can be controlled. The alpha (α) value, which is related to the selected level of significance, directly affects type I errors. Alpha (α) is the maximum probability that a type I error can occur. For a 95 per cent confidence level, the value of alpha is 0.05. This means that there is a 5 per cent probability that a true null hypothesis is rejected. One out of every twenty hypothesis tests performed at this level of α will result in a type I error in the long run.

> **Type II error:** When a false null hypothesis is not rejected, this results in a type II error or the second kind error. Type II errors are equivalent to false negatives. For example, considering the new drug mentioned above. A type II error would occur if it was accepted that the new drug did not affect the outcome, but in reality, it did. The Greek letter beta gives the probability of a type II error. This number is related to the hypothesis test's power or sensitivity, denoted by 1 -beta.

V

Validity is the extent to which the results obtained meet the scientific research method's requirements. It describes how well a test measures what it is intended to measure. Internal validity questions the research design structure—has the scientific method been adhered to? External validity examines the results and seeks to determine if there are there any causal relationships? (cf. Reliability). Reliability is necessary for determining the overall validity of a scientific experiment and improving the robustness of the results. Significant results must be innately repeatable. The same experiment under the same conditions should generate the same results. The validity of an assessment is the degree to which it measures what it is supposed to measure.

Vancouver style is a numbered referencing style commonly used in medicine and science and consists of citations to someone else's work in the text, indicated by the use of a number and a sequentially numbered reference list at the end of the document providing complete details of the corresponding in-text reference.

Variance is a measure of the spread, or dispersion, of scores within a sample. A small variance indicates highly similar scores, close to the sample mean. A significant variance indicates more scores at a distance from the mean and possibly spread over a more extensive range.

Vertical bar chart is sometimes called a column chart. A bar graph shows comparisons among discrete categories. One axis of the chart shows the specific categories being compared, and the other axis represents a measured value (cf. Histogram).

W

Wilcoxon test is a non-parametric statistical hypothesis test used either to test the location of a set of samples or to compare the locations of two populations using a set of matched samples.

Appendix 3. Apprenticeship Scheme Further Details

REED D.

Since April 2017, in England, an apprenticeship levy has been paid automatically by employers whose wage bill is over £3million per year. The levy is collected via Paye As You Earn (PAYE) Real Time Information (RTI) system employer submission at a rate (in 2021) of 0.5 per cent of the employer's wage bill. Once collected, employers can access their available funding through the Digital Apprenticeship Service (DAS), and use the levy to fund the training of apprentices within their organisation. Any part of the funding within the DAS not used within the allotted twenty-four-month period is forfeited to the government.[1, 2] The government uses the expired funds to support existing apprenticeships and fund apprenticeships for smaller, non-levy paying employers.

Those employers with a wage bill of less than £3 million do not contribute to the apprenticeship levy but may draw down on apprenticeship funding. Non-contributing employers may enter their employees into apprenticeships (available from level 2 to level 7 MSc) for 5 per cent of the maximum funding for the apprenticeship. The maximum funding is different for each apprenticeship, and the current rate is stated on each of the apprenticeship standards sites[3]. For example, for a Senior Leader apprenticeship, a level 7 masters level, the typical apprenticeship maximum funding is £14k (as of 29 March 2021), a non-contributing employer would be liable for the 5 per cent of the cost, which would be £700 in total.

Regarding research, the senior leader apprenticeship standards, knowledge requirement (KR) K5, specifically include the acquisition "Systems thinking, knowledge/data management, research methodologies and programme management." Elsewhere, the senior leader apprenticeship standard requires the acquisition of skills to permit the apprentices to "undertake research, and critically analyse and integrate complex information."[3]

Meanwhile, the apprenticeship standard for those who wish to become an advanced clinical practitioner (pathways currently are being developed for dental professionals) can expect the opportunity to develop research knowledge (4.1- 4.6)[3] which permits the apprentice to "Engage in research activity; develop and apply evidence-based strategies that are evaluated to enhance the quality, safety, productivity and value for money of health and care," and this reinforced with the skills requirements (4.1- 4.6), which ensure the apprentices gains:

"The range of quantitative and qualitative research methodologies relevant for use in health and social care; the roles and responsibilities of those involved in research; the range of legal, ethical, professional, financial and organisational policies and procedures that will apply to your research activities; the importance and impact of research on advancing clinical practices."[3]

Those employees on an apprenticeship are required to spend 20 per cent of the time in "off-job" learning, although the form this 20 per cent takes will depend on the training provider; typically, it may be one day a week or in blocks.[4]

The government have been quick to dispel myths and misinformation related to apprenticeship via a myth buster leaflet.[1] This includes the myth that apprenticeships cannot be used for existing staff. The reality is that apprenticeships are available to employees of all ages and offer opportunities to existing staff as a means by which to upskill and or retrain.

There are currently several apprenticeship standards, many of which might be of interest to dental professionals wishing to extend their research skills and conduct a small research project as part of an apprenticeship. Examples include senior leader for those who may be interested in developing skills and research related to business and administration; or advanced clinical practice (for those wishing to focus on training and research related to clinical practice); or clinical scientist for dental professionals who might wish to perform practice-based research within their workplace.

Some higher education institutions offer premium rate programmes, such as master's in business administration (MBA), which can be partly funded by the apprenticeship levy and topped up with an additional payment to meet the commercial rate required by the training provider.

Thus apprenticeships can offer an excellent route for developing research skills and an opportunity to conduct a practice-based study funded through the apprenticeship levy.

Details on how to take advantage of apprenticeship opportunities can be obtained from local apprenticeship-training providers, who will advise the application process to those interested and their employer. In addition the government regularly provide an updated list of apprenticeship-training providers by postcode area for each apprenticeship standard.[4]

References

1   UK Government. Key Facts about the Apprenticeship Levy 2019. https://www.gov.uk/government/news/key-facts-you-should-know-about-the-apprenticeship-levy. Accessed 14 November 2021.

2   UK Government. Myths about the Apprenticeship programme 2019 https://assets.publishing.service.gov.uk/government/uploads/system/uploads/attachment_data/file/819164/Top_7_myths_about_the_apprenticeships_programme.pdf. Accessed 28 January 2021.

3   Institute for Apprenticeships The Apprenticeship Standards

    Institute for Apprenticeship Standards 2021 https://www.instituteforapprenticeships.org/apprenticeship-standards/. Accessed 14 November 2021.

4   UK Government. Apprenticeship Training Courses 2021. https://findapprenticeshiptraining.apprenticeships.education.gov.uk/Courses. Accessed 14 November 2021.

Index

A

absolute risk reduction 268, 281, 298

accuracy 5, 10, 11, 16, 94, 101, 118, 120, 121, 122, 123, 124, 125, 126, 127, 133, 134, 137, 193, 212, 220, 236, 262, 270, 271, 280, 281, 286, 287, 290, 293, 300, 303

allocation bias 64

alpha level 96

alpha value 281, 291, 292, 295, 299

alternative hypothesis 20, 282, 291, 292, 298, 299

anonymity 95, 107, 154, 172, 214, 282, 284, 301

ANOVA 230

applicability 11, 12, 77, 124, 263, 267

B

basic research designs 35

Berkson (admission rate) bias 99

bias 6, 9, 12, 13, 39, 42, 44, 45, 46, 47, 48, 49, 50, 53, 54, 55, 56, 57, 58, 60, 64, 66, 67, 77, 83, 87, 88, 90, 92, 93, 94, 98, 99, 100, 101, 107, 108, 110, 113, 114, 120, 124, 138, 140, 141, 142, 144, 149, 167, 177, 192, 193, 196, 198, 201, 213, 237, 261, 267, 274, 275, 277, 279, 282, 283, 285, 288, 291, 299, 301, 302, 303, 304

bias, allocation 64

bias, confirmation 282

bias, diagnostic purity 99

bias, historical control 99

bias, information 57, 100, 101

bias, interviewer 107

bias, membership 99

bias, Neyman 45, 99, 282

bias, observation 100, 282, 291

bias, publishing 283, 301

bias, recall 46, 48, 49, 50, 283, 302

bias, response 99, 303

bias, sampling 98

bias, selection 12, 42, 46, 49, 50, 53, 54, 55, 57, 58, 64, 98, 100, 101, 198, 213, 282, 283, 304

blinding 13, 56, 58, 60, 64, 67, 68, 70, 93, 100, 101, 154, 267, 268, 283, 287, 288, 294

blinding, double 67, 68

blinding, single 67

Box and whisker plot 227

bracketing 77, 283

C

Caldicott Guardian 172, 182, 214

Caldicott Principles 214, 215, 283

calibration 108, 193, 194, 195, 202, 216, 259

CARE checklist for case reports 264

case-control studies 34, 42, 44, 45, 46, 47, 48, 49, 50, 51, 54, 55, 230, 265, 272, 275, 277, 283, 298

case reports 6, 20, 22, 34, 36, 39, 40, 41, 42, 43, 74, 244, 262, 263, 264

case series 34, 36, 39, 40, 42, 43, 74

CASP checklists 264

categorical variable 205, 206, 226, 229, 283, 285

causality 39, 42, 44, 50, 51, 60, 264

Chi-square test 229

Classic Hierarchy of Evidence 6

clinical expertise 4, 6, 7, 8, 16

clinical practice apprenticeships 281

clinical research v, 5, 7, 22, 34, 37, 38, 65, 66, 67, 101, 149, 159, 161, 164, 165, 167, 172, 178, 179, 180, 181, 182, 192, 193, 198, 201, 202, 207, 279, 283, 303

clinical significance 13, 97, 305

closed-ended questions 103, 110, 112, 113, 114

cluster randomised 284

Cochrane, Archie 4, 16

Cochrane Collaboration 90, 284

coding 81, 82, 86, 107, 113, 211, 218, 284

Cohort studies 15, 34, 45, 50, 51, 52, 53, 54, 140, 145, 265, 272, 275, 284, 298

concealed allocation 93, 100, 101, 268

confidence interval 89, 91, 96, 97, 128, 145, 146, 148, 154, 220, 224, 225, 228, 229, 230, 234, 240, 242, 267, 268, 278, 284, 305

confidence intervals 89, 91, 96, 97, 128, 145, 146, 148, 154, 220, 224, 225, 228, 229, 230, 234, 240, 242, 267, 268, 278, 284, 305

confidence level 96, 97, 154, 284, 295, 307

confidentiality 78, 116, 154, 157, 165, 168, 169, 172, 173, 179, 182, 203, 213, 214, 215, 219, 282, 284, 303

confounding 11, 53, 56, 57, 58, 61, 64, 100, 141, 277, 284

congruence 77

consent 41, 60, 95, 116, 123, 140, 153, 154, 155, 159, 161, 162, 164, 165, 167, 169, 170, 171, 172, 175,

retrospective studies 35, 50, 53, 137, 139

reviews 2, 8, 9, 10, 11, 12, 15, 16, 17, 21, 22, 23, 24, 26, 33, 34, 37, 40, 60, 72, 78, 79, 82, 84, 87, 88, 89, 90, 92, 117, 149, 159, 162, 164, 165, 166, 167, 168, 174, 175, 176, 177, 190, 202, 204, 212, 216, 218, 220, 239, 242, 243, 244, 245, 252, 253, 254, 257, 258, 260, 262, 264, 270, 272, 273, 274, 275, 279, 280, 283, 284, 294, 299, 300, 306

ROC 121, 127, 128, 129, 130, 131, 132, 133, 220, 236, 303, 304

ROC curve, area under 304

Rosenthal effect 13, 42, 304

S

sample size 12, 13, 44, 52, 57, 60, 61, 65, 66, 70, 93, 94, 96, 97, 100, 101, 116, 124, 137, 138, 141, 142, 145, 154, 163, 191, 198, 204, 205, 224, 226, 229, 239, 266, 287, 288, 290, 294, 304

sample size calculation 93, 96, 97, 116, 304

sampling 12, 33, 40, 42, 43, 56, 58, 59, 63, 79, 80, 92, 93, 94, 95, 96, 98, 100, 103, 143, 153, 177, 204, 223, 224, 249, 277, 283, 296, 297, 301, 302, 304, 305

sampling bias 98

sampling methods 12, 56, 58, 63, 93, 94, 95, 249, 302, 304

sampling, types of random 93, 94, 95

scaling questions or ranking questions 110

schedules 150, 151, 152, 155, 189, 193, 194, 209

screening 10, 31, 33, 118, 119, 120, 122, 123, 124, 129, 204, 236, 265, 270, 304

screening test 118, 119, 129, 236, 304

selection bias 12, 42, 46, 49, 50, 53, 54, 55, 57, 58, 64, 98, 100, 101, 198, 213, 282, 283, 304

sensitivity 40, 41, 75, 91, 92, 96, 118, 119, 121, 125, 126, 127, 128, 129, 130, 134, 147, 236, 242, 271, 274, 277, 278, 304, 307

sensitivity analysis 91, 92, 274, 304

significance, clinical 13, 97, 305

significance, statistical 12, 73, 96, 226, 287, 288, 291, 299, 305

specificity 118, 119, 121, 122, 125, 126, 127, 128, 129, 130, 134, 236, 271, 297, 305

standard deviation 89, 91, 96, 97, 208, 222, 223, 224, 225, 230, 234, 296, 305

statistical significance 12, 73, 96, 226, 287, 288, 291, 299, 305

study closure 201

study duration 148, 200, 201

study initiation 197, 198, 200, 201

study plan 34

support requirements 196

survival analysis 145, 146, 147, 149, 233, 306

survival probability 146, 233

survival time 145, 146, 233

systematic review 10, 11, 15, 16, 33, 34, 60, 87, 88, 89, 90, 92, 117, 204, 218, 239, 242, 243, 244, 245, 262, 264, 270, 272, 273, 275, 280, 283, 284, 294, 306

T

thematic analysis 80, 81

time effects 42

training, data collector 216

transferability 72, 77

triangulation 83, 306

t-test 229, 230, 232, 241

type I error 97, 288, 307

type II error 97, 288, 300, 305, 307

types of bias 57, 98, 282

types of preclinical research 37

types of questionnaires 106

types of study 12, 33, 34, 35, 203, 204, 284

V

validity 8, 9, 11, 12, 13, 17, 19, 42, 56, 57, 60, 72, 93, 95, 96, 102, 111, 114, 115, 123, 142, 177, 185, 194, 217, 237, 250, 265, 267, 273, 279, 282, 285, 288, 289, 291, 293, 303, 305, 306, 307

validity, construct 115, 285, 306

validity, external 9, 11, 12, 13, 17, 60, 95, 96, 267, 279, 289, 293, 307

validity, internal 13, 42, 93, 95, 96, 194, 273, 288, 289, 293, 307

Vancouver style 248, 307

variance 77, 97, 208, 209, 229, 230, 234, 296, 305, 308

vertical bar chart 308

visual analogue scales 112

W

Wilcoxon test 308

Printed in the United States
by Baker & Taylor Publisher Services